Sports Supplement Review

W9-BNA-992

4th Issue

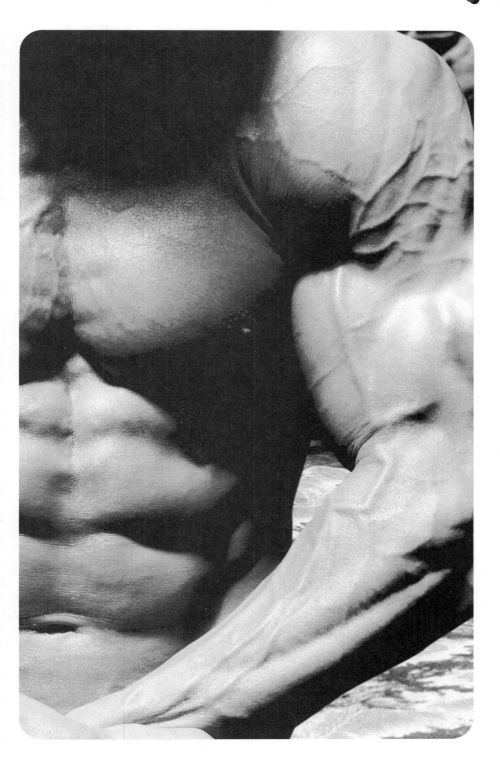

by Vince Andrich

ABOUT THE AUTHOR Vincent Andrich

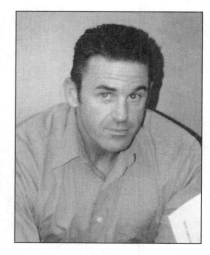

Vincent Andrich, the author of this book, is a self-taught nutrition and exercise fanatic. For over 15 years, Vince, once a successful amateur bodybuilder, has been both an executive and has consulted with the most highly regarded sports supplement companies in the world. In fact, when asked, Vince will tell you that his greatest asset is his network of colleagues that read like a "who's who" of supplement manufacturers, high-level athletes, exercise physiologists, and performance nutrition researchers. This unique vantagepoint lets Vince bridge the communication gap that exists between the individual needs of serious athletes and the latest nutritional concepts discovered by the world's leading researchers and scientists. These life experiences also allow Vince to quickly evaluate the scientific rationale and basis behind various supplements and most important, tell you, the consumer, if the supplement actually stands up to the acid test of cost versus performance.

Vince is highly respected by the sports supplement industry's "inner circle" for his insightful views on sports nutrition and athletic performance, and many regard him as one of the most intuitive sports supplement designers and writers in the field today. Vince joined Muscle Media and EAS, Inc. in 2000 to report on and lead the development of new scientifically viable performance-enhancing supplements. He pens the popular column in Muscle Media, fittingly called Sports Supplement Review, which is read by the thousands of fitness enthusiasts around the world who demand the latest forward-thinking, scientifically sound, yet practical, information on sports supplements. This latest installment of the Sports Supplement Review contains even more intense subject matter and breakthrough information on every aspect of performance nutrition.

Contributors to Sports Supplement Review, 4th Issue

I would like to thank all of the people who made this issue of the Sports Supplement Review a reality. It was only through their collaborative efforts that we were able to sift through the enormous amount of information that was available to us while putting this book together. This team utilized many diverse sources of information from athletes, textbooks, medical journals, scientific conference abstract presentations, and reports from supplement manufacturers and distributors. To give individual credit to each and every text consulted or each person interviewed would be impossible. Here is a list of the main contributors for this book and their respective backgrounds:

Ryan HornBuckle (The Franchise)

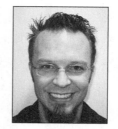

If you asked me to put together the sports supplement "dream team," Ryan HornBuckle would be my number one draft choice—giving him the nickname "The Franchise." Ryan has over nine years of health and fitness business experience, and has been intimately involved with product development from both research and marketing perspectives. Ryan and I have worked together for the last several years. His commitment to the health and fitness industry has taken his career through General Nutrition Centers, Weider Nutrition, and MET-Rx to his current post as an industry consultant. Ryan also has an expansive educational background ranging from consumer behavior to chemistry to business administration. This combination of academic training and on-the-job business skills, along with familiarity of the history and behaviors that mold the health and fitness business has made Ryan an immeasurable asset to many popular sports nutrition brands and, of course, this book. In addition to these "all star" industry qualities, Ryan has the type of personality and wit that can make any project we work on together both thought provoking and entertaining.

Peter Miller (Rainman)

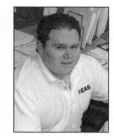

When I first joined EAS, it became apparent to me that Peter Miller was anything but "average." In fact, Peter has such a high intellect and comprehension level that it prompted me to nickname him "Rainman" very early on. A native of Colorado, Peter received his degree in kinesiology from the University of Colorado at Boulder, and has continued to amass an enormous amount of knowledge in nutrition and exercise science. Peter is an ISSA Certified Trainer, and has worked in many aspects of the health and fitness industry such as, Vitamin Logic Store Manager, EAS Tech Support (answering the questions no one else can answer), and his current position as Product Manager for EAS High Performance products. Peter has an incredible knack for building state-of-the-art product formulations because he understands both chemistry and biology, which can ultimately determine product efficacy. Of course, Peter can also articulate his thoughts very well, which has made him a key contributor to this project. Peter definitely has a very bright future in this industry.

Kevin Whetsell (The Freight Train)

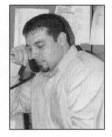

Kevin came to EAS several months ago as an intern right after he finished his master's degree in Sports Management from West Virginia University. Kevin has developed extensive experience in health- and fitness-related fields working at a hardcore bodybuilding gym for two years, teaching college weight training courses (WVU), and as a bone-crushing former college athlete. Kevin has been a frequent subscriber to health and fitness publications for the last eight years, which has given him a good overall understanding of the sports nutrition market. The day we met, Kevin displayed such intense drive and work ethic to back up his credentials that I immediately asked him to take on the responsibility as Managing Editor for this project. After the first few weeks in his new position, I realized I couldn't have made a better choice. Indeed a project of this scope and magnitude will ultimately "stall" somewhere in its tracks if there isn't someone with the personality of a Freight Train to keep it rolling. Kevin has been the Freight Train that this project needed to keep it on track. From editing to content planning, Kevin has made a long-lasting mark on this book. We'll all be hearing a lot from Kevin in the future.

Pavel Tsatsouline (The Evil One)

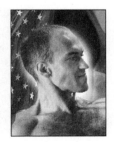

Finding new and effective training methods is never an easy task. However, when you do run across an author with a fresh perspective, they are always easy to spot. Pavel Tsatsouline, our resident training expert for this issue of the Sports Supplement Review, has such an immense understanding of training variables that his work stands out like a sore thumb. From the first time I read materials from Pavel, I knew he was easily one of the most brilliant trainers I had ever come across. We call Pavel the "Evil One" because his training methods are usually diverse and full of "PAIN"—the pain of a great exercise done correctly of course. Once you get acquainted with our training section in Chapter 16, called "Altered States," I am sure you will agree Pavel is the real deal when it comes to designing goal-specific training programs. With his contributions to this book, Pavel adds a new and much needed advanced training dimension to this fourth issue of the Sports Supplement Review.

Lorenzo Nicastro (Pudding to Protein)

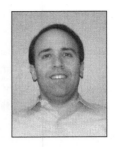

Another contributor to this book is Lorenzo Nicastro, the resident Director of Product Development for EAS' ready-to-drink beverages and functional foods. Lorenzo is unique in that he has a vast amount of experience developing products, but he also is a perfect example of the power of positive change through nutrition and exercise. For 10+ years, Lorenzo has worked in Research and Development for three Fortune 500 food companies. His career started with Campbell Soup Company, followed by Nabisco and then Kraft Foods. He worked from soup to nuts (literally). But during the course of his work formulating products, he constantly had to taste test the prototypes. In other words, he was always eating. (Remember, most great chefs are overweight.) This is not bad if you are formulating nutritionally balanced products—like the ones we talk about in this book. Unfortunately, prior to joining EAS, Lorenzo was formulating pudding and gelatin products, which either contained low amounts of high-quality protein or large amounts of sugar. Formulating these products (with the addition of minimal exercise) helped Lorenzo increase his body fat to 28%, causing him to become motivated by the idea of playing a role in making a difference in the health of other people, including himself. Lorenzo now "sports" a much leaner physique, and he attributes much of his success to simply changing the types of products he works on, plus weight training. Essentially Lorenzo went from formulating "pudding to protein," thus the nickname. Make no mistake; Lorenzo's life experience and vast formulation expertise allows him to be very picky when it comes creating products that help build and maintain a better body.

Andrea Silberman (Voice of Reason)

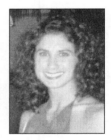

We have one female writer for this issue of the Sports Supplement Review who has turned out to be a real asset to the entire project. We found out by accident that when a group of Type-A males get together to write a book on sports supplements, having someone on the team who can present different points of view—and in our case keep you "grounded" by offering a voice of reason—is crucial for success. For all of us who contributed to this book, that "Voice of Reason" has been Andrea Silberman, who has quite the background in fitness, nutrition, and supplementation. Andrea has a degree in Biology from the University of Colorado, six years of personal training experience, five years in the supplement industry (including four years with EAS in sales, tech support, and product development), and she co-produced the popular EAS Fitness Guide. Andrea's unique point of view on several topics make this issue of the Sports Supplement Review one of the best ever.

I would also like to specifically thank:
• Gianni D'Ottavio and Ben Hall, our "buff" models who stayed late several nights to be photographed for the exercise sections in this book
• Brian Harvat, our awesome Graphic Designer who created the look and feel of this entire book
• Gretchen Ferraro, our number one Copy Editor who made all the words make sense
• Michael Sitzman, our Production Coordinator whose experience in producing the highest quality publications around made us all look good.

These professionals have all contributed immensely and without them this book would never have become a reality.
In case you were wondering, our front cover model is lifetime drug-free bodybuilder Roger Applewhite, and the photo is the work of Dennis Lane.

Important Information:

As with past issues of the Sport Supplement Review, this current issue evaluates and recommends a variety of supplements. It is the intent that all information pertaining to all supplement reviews are to be viewed and understood as the expression of the author's opinion and are in no-way meant to be interpreted as absolute scientific conclusions. None of the evaluations and recommendations contained herein; are intended to diagnose, treat, cure, or prevent any disease.

The information contained in this book is Copyright 2001 by Experimental and Applied Sciences, Inc. (EAS). Neither EAS nor the authors of this book assume any liability for the information contained in this publication. Be advised that this book does not provide medical advice. All medical advice should be sought out and obtained from licensed health-care practitioners. Please consult a physician before adhering to any of the nutrition, training or supplement programs contained in this publication.

Throughout this book you will find quotes from famous athletes and coaches that have used hard work and dedication to make the most of their talents. Whether it is building the ultimate physique, competing at the highest level possible or coaching a championship team these sports personalities know what it takes to be the best. By referring to these when you need a boost of confidence or pure motivation you will attain what each of these legends all have in common-DESIRE.

The quotes listed throughout this text are used for inspirational purposes only. The sources of these quotes do not in anyway endorse the information contained throughout this publication.

This book is dedicated to my dear mother Angela Andrich,
*my strong willed father Robert Andrich Sr., my mentor Angela
Andrich MD, my inspirational brother Robert Andrich Jr. my tough
sister Susan Andrich Cocchi, my perpetual driving force and wife
Jamie Hagan Andrich, my beautiful daughter Morgan Rose, and my
"other" family Catherine and Allan Farlow, Ed and Adele Hagan.
Not to mention my training partners over the last twenty years.*

Thanks for believing.

table of contents

Chapter 10 - SUPPLEMENT DELIVERY SYSTEMS:

"Double and triple the effectiveness of numerous supplements on the market right now."

Chapter 11 - THE BUILDING BLOCKS – AMINO ACIDS:

"Amino acids are the building blocks from which proteins can be manufactured in your body."

Chapter 12 - THE BASICS - VITAMINS AND MINERALS:

"They all contribute to the normal function, growth and maintenance of your body."

Chapter 13 - THE HERBAL TRUTH:

"Basically it is difficult to keep track of all the folklore and anecdotal support for the thousands of herbs."

Chapter 14 - BUYER BEWARE - BRAND AWARENESS AND REVIEWS:

"Supplement consumers should be now – more than ever – aware of those companies that are committed to great products and those committed to strictly great profits."

Chapter 15 - RATING THE INDUSTRY'S HOTTEST SUPPLEMENTS:

"Don't go bargain hunting before you're armed with the facts."

Chapter 16 - ALTERED STATES:

"The Information Age has spawned the misinformation age making it tougher for athletes to get the real inside scoop on maximum training methods."

Chapter 17 - MISCELLANEOUS SUPPLEMENTS:

"Rounding out products that you may have heard of, or think might be of interest to you."

Chapter 18 - ADDITIONAL HELP:

"Helping you to attain some of the best, most credible information out there."

"The mind is the limit.
As long as the mind can envision the
fact that you can do something,
you can do it, as long as you really
believe 100 percent."

-Arnold Schwarzenegger

Chapter

1

Introduction

I have to be honest; I am literally living a life-long dream. That is to say I was given the opportunity to take over 20 years of training, and 15 years of professional experience in this industry to lead the development of the *Sports Supplement Review, 4th Issue*. When the senior management at EAS first approached me to put this book together, I was flattered to say the least (really I said "who me?" to myself many times). To say that I was "chomping at the bit" so to speak to immediately start collaborating with my key contacts to outline the plan wouldn't be all that far from the truth. Actually, I literally slept no more than four hours per night from all the excitement, after all this book is arguably the most anticipated book sequels for fitness enthusiasts ever. The fact that there were hundreds of topics swirling around in my head that I felt must be covered in this project didn't help my sleeping situation much. All of this "stress" got me even more "fired up" with more energy than ever before to meet this tremendous challenge head-on.

As reality sunk in, though, I was reminded of an old saying that asserts "be careful what you wish for, you just might get it." This statement could have never been more timely to me as I pondered the months of hard work ahead. To say that I had my "work cut out" for me is an understatement. Then again, I knew that from the start. You see, I know I have a very tough act to follow: Bill Phillips. After all, this man had become an icon in the world of fitness on all levels. What is more, luck had very little to do with it. Over the last sixteen years Bill Phillips had touched virtually every aspect of the industry and re-shaped it. He created *Muscle Media*®, one of the most widely acclaimed and fastest growing fitness publications on the market today. His latest book Body-*for*-LIFE™ is still a runaway best seller and is living proof that his evangelistic style of inspiring everyday people to achieve what they never thought they could with their life and body is second to none. It is common knowledge to those who have been around the supplement industry since the late

'80s that Bill Phillips was the first writer with the guts to use a straightforward "no-holds-barred" style of reporting on the forbidden topics related to performance enhancement, nutrition, and exercise. Let's not forget he invented the concept of a comprehensive sports supplement review in the first place. Make no mistake Bill Phillips is THE MAN. A hard act to follow? You bet! In the end, Bill has cut a clear path for me to assemble the most comprehensive edition of the *Sports Supplement Review* ever.

What's Inside the *Sports Supplement Review, 4th Issue*

The first thing you will see in this updated edition of the *Sport Supplement Review* is that many of the sections are more concise. For example, we have added consistent formatting to many of the chapters so that you can get a quick snapshot of an herb or vitamin and mineral without sifting through a lot of explanatory text. Next, you'll get more individual and branded product reviews, which include some of the most advertised and popular supplements on the market. This issue also has two exciting new sections that thoroughly explain Periodized Nutrition and Training that I am sure you will quickly put to good use.

Let's get one thing right out in the open—**I am not a scientist**. However, I do have a considerable amount of "in-the-trenches" bodybuilding experience that has given me the knowledge to ask researchers and athletes the tough questions regarding the sports supplement marketplace. This means a full investigation of the most popular products, the latest science, the most recent advertising claims, and even the relevant "background" on nearly all the companies that are fighting for your supplement dollars.

In turn I'll work with experts in each specialty and provide concrete answers on topics such as:

- What's inside the industry's most popular supplements.

- What is the best overall diet for bodybuilders and athletes year around.

- How to simultaneously gain lean body mass while putting on minimum amounts of bodyfat.

- How to "amplify" the effects of even the best fat-burning supplements on the market today.

- How to maximize the anabolic effects of your training with a simple dietary modification used for post-exercise.

- How to "drive" more muscle-building nutrients into your muscle cells without ingesting boatloads of carbohydrates.

- What is the best way to structure a program that incorporates supplements for individual goals?

Plus I'll include the latest information on new cutting-edge compounds and supplement strategies that will take your physique to a new level such as:

- Manipulating insulin for Precise Carbohydrate Management and anabolic gains.

- The straightforward supplement combination that can turn your body into a nitrogen-retention machine.

- Unsurpassed supplement delivery systems that take sport nutritionals into the realm of pharmaceuticals.

OK Now that you can see I am dead serious about the exciting information contained in this edition, it should become clear to you this edition of the *Sports Supplement Review* will absolutely modernize the way you train, eat, and, of course, supplement your diet. My personal opinion (although I am a bit biased) is that this book will give you all of the answers to practically every question you could possibly ask about bodybuilding supplements. I say this because I am one of you and these are the same questions I would want answered if I had read this book when I first began bodybuilding. In my early bodybuilding days, I was just like many of you who are reading this: I was looking for ANSWERS. Early on, it wasn't uncommon for me to sift through two and three books at a time, hoping to find the answers to my questions. Unfortunately, to this day, I have yet to find one single publication that addresses all the questions an aspiring bodybuilder or weight trainer encounters on the quest to attain a bigger, stronger, and leaner physique. With the opportunity to write this book, I can take the 20 years of frustration of sifting through book after book to end up with no answers at all or worse yet more questions than before. I now extend the invitation to you to read through all of the information in this book and see whether I have done a good job in my quest to create a

publication that addresses virtually all questions bodybuilders and fitness enthusiasts share. In the end, we both get what we want: the truth regarding the sport we love. So enough with all of this. Let's get right into this all new, completely modernized *Sports Supplement Review, 4th Issue*. I've got a STACK of exciting, new information to share with you (some of which has never before appeared in print!), so let's get to it…

"The will to win is important,
but the will to prepare is vital."

-Joe Paterno

Chapter

2

The Sports Supplement Explosion

The sports nutrition industry is fast becoming a major component of the bigger, more commonly referred to dietary supplement industry. According to the *Nutrition Business Journal*, the entire dietary supplement market has quadrupled in the last 10 years, going from $3.3 billion to $13 billion, and the market is projected to continue in this upward trend. The sports nutrition segment is growing at an even greater rate now that industry researchers have realized sport supplements are actually part of the fastest growing industry segment: diet aids. This combined sub-group of sports nutrition and diet aids now totals of over $5 billion in annual sales. So, why is the sport supplement market exploding to such an exceptional degree?

I think there are several reasons why we are seeing this phenomenon. First, scientific research on the associations between supplements, weight loss, and performance is accumulating rapidly. New research studies in the area of nutrition are being published in dozens of journals like the *Journal of Applied Physiology*, *Journal of Strength and Conditioning Research*, *Medicine & Science in Sports and Exercise*, and many more. It seems that just to stay in business in the dietary supplement industry, corporations need to interpret new information that seemingly evolves every day. The very best companies are really taking advantage of all this new information and applying it into a wide array of different products used for a number of purposes. All of that said, we now have performance and diet products for "immediate gratification," as well as many other items that can be deemed as preventative measures or alternatives to mainstream medicine.

The second reason for this growth is due to the aging baby boomer generation, which accounts for a large percentage of the population in the United States. Because they are getting older, many baby boomers are starting to become more aware of the status of their health. In an effort to take better care of their bodies and extend their life expectancy as long as possible, this segment of the population is seeking a variety of advantages available to assist them in their pursuit for improved health and fitness. Not to mention, most of them have children who have taken a serious interest in following a healthy lifestyle. In essence, this nutrition kick is catching on.

The final reason for the big boom in supplement sales is that many of these products provide young athletes with a legal, safe alternative to enhance performance. Athletes from high school swimmers to Olympians to professional football players are all enjoying the benefits that sports supplements can provide. Never before have so many safe and effective options been available to help athletes become bigger, faster, and stronger. There is already an impressive body of clinical research to support the benefits of many of these dietary supplements, and with new science being conducted and published every day, the newfound benefits and applications will likely expand the market rapidly as we move forward through the 21st century.

Now, I could probably continue to list the reasons behind the supplement boom, but I think you get the general idea. The bottom line is that health- and fitness-related topics in this country are gaining popularity. Even though hardcore bodybuilders or elite athletes are often the first group to understand the benefits of a new supplement, performance nutrition products aren't just for them any more. They are for the college track ath-

lete trying to improve his or her time to make the finals. They are for the busy mom trying to increase her calcium and protein intake. They are for the aging weekend warrior trying to strengthen and heal worn joints. Supplements are fast becoming a household word and commodity, and as they grow in popularity, questions regarding their efficacy, safety, and regulation are growing too.

Industry Regulation

I believe that the consensus among the population is still that dietary supplements are unsafe and unregulated. Some people even associate supplements with drugs. But dietary supplements are not drugs! (A drug is a synthetic or plant-derived substance that is intended to diagnose, treat, cure, or prevent disease.) Furthermore, the dietary supplement industry does have very rigorous laws and standards in place (albeit less than the pharmaceutical industry) that are enforced by the Federal Trade Commission (FTC) and the Food and Drug Administration (FDA). These two government agencies split the "police work" for the industry, which is no easy task, especially when the market for self-help products is growing at such a fast pace.

The FTC and FDA Supplement Regulators

The two government agencies listed above (FDA and FTC) have two different roles in policing the dietary supplement industry. Although their roles are unique, they fit together to cover every aspect related from consumer health and safety to truth in advertising. The FTC regulates the advertising aspects, including topics such as identifying claims, interpreting ad meaning, and substantiating claims. Items that the FTC is likely to review are advertisements and other product literature. The FDA oversees safety, manufacturing, product labeling, package inserts, and approval of any ingredients before they can be marketed. In many instances this simply means that an ingredient must pass the guidelines set up by the Dietary Supplement Health and Education Act (DSHEA) of 1994.

The DSHEA guidelines were put in place in 1994 when Congress realized that millions of consumers were using dietary supplements to improve their nutrition and obtain health benefits. DSHEA was created to ensure that safe and appropriately labeled products remain available to those who want to use them. The framework of DSHEA includes the following items: [1]

- Define dietary supplements and dietary ingredients which includes;

- If an ingredient is found in nature and can be consumed naturally in the diet, then it is normally considered DSHEA compliant.

- If an ingredient was marketed as a dietary supplement before 1994, it is considered "grandfathered" into DSHEA compliance.

- If an ingredient was not marketed as a dietary supplement before 1994 or cannot be found in nature, a manufacturer must submit a "new dietary ingredient" pre-market notification letter for approval to the FDA. It is then up to the FDA to allow or reject this notification based on their knowledge of the safety of the ingredient in question.

Using DSHEA's guidelines, both the FTC and FDA work together to monitor the dietary supplement industry with an emphasis on the following. The first is safety, which will include everything from health hazards and adverse events to Internet surveillance. The second is labeling, and this category will include substantiation of claims and related

"I believe that the consensus among the population *is still that* dietary supplements are unsafe and unregulated."

publications. Third are boundaries, which covers structure/function claims and explores how dietary supplements compare to other drug and food categories. The fourth category is enforcement activities, which allows the FDA and FTC to take appropriate action against incompliant companies that may include fines and/or recalls.

As you can see, there are many steps taken by the FTC and FDA to govern these products. In addition, the supplement industry for the most part does a good job of policing itself. The majority of companies and products are responsible, but as with any product, you, as a consumer, need to be scrutinizing and taking some of that responsibility upon yourself. Along with this responsibility comes many questions. To help answer those questions, let me give you a quick course in "Supplements 101."

How Do Supplements Work?

Without re-inventing the wheel, let's look at some of the information provided in the third issue of the *Sports Supplement Review*. For starters, the effects of supplements are described by identifying three categories. The first category describes how a supplement may help to make up for a deficiency in your diet. For example, USDA studies show that 68% of self-selected diets contain less than two thirds of the RDA for zinc[2] and 39% contain less than two thirds of the RDA for magnesium.[3] Between the increase in consumption of processed and fast foods, and the increasingly fast pace of life in the 21st century, meeting your daily requirements for nutrients is becoming more and more difficult. Supplements may be the answer to protecting you against deficiencies.

The second category relates to how supplements may provide a nutrient that is "under-supplied" to cells or not normally available in "optimal" levels in your diet. The *Sport Supplement Review, 3rd Issue* fluently described creatine as a good example of this type of supplement. Another good example are essential fatty acids (EFAs). Although we do ingest enough EFAs through our diet to support certain vital body functions, we do not necessarily take in enough to enjoy benefits such as fat loss or reducing LDL (bad cholesterol). Included in this category are many other substances that we ingest on a daily basis in sub-optimal amounts. Providing extra quantities of

these substances may allow your body to "up-regulate" its natural function.

The third category identified was supplements that may produce a pharmacological or "drug-like" effect on cellular processes. This is where I have to add a bit more detail to clarify the previous point. Specifically, I do not believe that supplements are in the same ballpark as pharmaceuticals such as real growth hormone or insulin. However, the parallel may be made that many sports performance supplements or health products that we do not ingest on a regular basis like ephedrine or St. John's wort can elicit **similar** effects to their pharmaceutical cousins when taken as directed. These substances are not necessary for normal cellular function, but may alter the normal function of cells when administered. This category includes many phytochemicals and herbs, which, next to vitamins and minerals, are one of the most widely used groups of supplements available.

Who Should Use Supplements and Why?

Based on these three categories used to describe how supplements work, anyone can use them. The trick is to figure out which ones suit your particular goals. I hope that after reading the rest of this book, you will have a much better sense of what is out there, and what the best choices are for you.

When Should You Use Supplements?

Supplements can be used on a daily basis. One critical factor to remember, however, is that supplements should not take the place of a healthy, whole-food diet. It is extremely important that you continue to consume a variety of healthy foods including fruits, vegetables, whole grains, lean meats, dairy, and unsaturated fats. Many of these foods contain ingredients that supplements don't, like phytochemicals and fiber. Another reminder that I would like to mention is that supplements are not the "magic" answer to your weight-loss or muscle-gain challenges or goals. Supplements must be combined not only with a healthy diet, but also a regular, effective exercise program in order to be successful. Supplements can help you get better gains faster by making meal planning easier and by offsetting the trauma associated with advanced exercise regimens, but only if used properly.

Okay, now that you have had a quick review of the sports supplement explosion, with a refresher course in Supplements 101, let me start answering that somewhat rhetorical question: "What supplements should I take?"

References Cited

1 fda.gov

2 Holden, M. J., et al., "Zinc and Copper in Self-Selected Diets," *J. Am. Diet. Assoc.* 75.1 (1999) : 23-28.

3 Morgan, J. K. et al., "Magnesium and Calcium Dietary Intakes of the U.S. Population," *J Am. Coll. Nutr.* 4.2 (1985) :195-206.

"You have to expect things of yourself before you can do them."

-Michael Jordan

Chapter 3

Rock Solid Nutritional Strategies

I get questions almost every day about so-called "breakthrough" bodybuilding nutrition, supplementation, and exercise routines. Rather than helping people build a better body, this seemingly endless proliferation of advice oftentimes confuses individuals to the point of despair and disinterest in pursuing their fitness goals.

The reason for all the questions is that bodybuilders and athletes are always on a quest to find the magic supplement, training, or diet program. This desire to find a better way makes them vulnerable to advice that is either not fully explained or is out of place for their current level of fitness or ultimate goals. I know that for you to actually gain valuable insights from this edition of the *Sports Supplement Review*, you need something more than the one magic idea or concept. I recognize this because in my own pursuit to figure out the magic formula, which has taken the better part of 20 years, I now know that an "integrated approach" with a broad understanding of how the body responds to supplements, nutrition, and training is what really works. I call this approach the Periodized Bodybuilding Nutrition System, which simply means that you do a specific program for a specific **period** of time to reach a specific goal. I believe you will see the difference between this book and others simply because this book covers **Real Bodybuilding Nutrition Strategies,** which in my opinion is the most critical area that an athlete must master. Let me explain.

Several years ago I decided to take control of my life and start bodybuilding. Early on, I believed that a militant approach to nutrition would be the key to my success. During the first five years of this pursuit, I literally tried every supplement and diet combination in print or overheard in the gym. Before long, I started making up my own diet programs, and I started to see trends that afford me the vantagepoint I have today. In retrospect, many of my gym acquaintances held very different viewpoints than I did on nutrition. In fact, most of these people thought I was miserably naïve to think nutrition was "all that important." Today, I feel as though my initial thoughts and hypotheses have been validated. Over the last several years, the science of performance nutrition has made such great strides that even "weekend warriors" are succumbing to a new way of life—nutrition.

Make no mistake; the nutritional strategies in the next three chapters will change your outlook on the entire subject of bodybuilding, because I've seen it firsthand through my own experiences. Case in point: It's been over 15 years since I first competed in a bodybuilding show, and I can still invariably control the way I look with simple dietary modifications. In contrast, many (but not all) of my old gym "friends" either don't train anymore or can't ever seem to get in shape. You see, back in the day, my detractors spent more time trying to find the ultimate pharmaceutical array to enhance their physiques than they did studying the art of bodybuilding nutrition. This is unfortunate for them, but if you read and use the information I'm going to share, you will avoid years of frustration and be able to take total control of your physique. Whether your goals are to increase lean mass, decrease bodyfat, or a combination of both, the following nutrition strategies will help you attain them.

The Periodized Bodybuilding Nutrition System—The Power is in the Strategy.

I assume that you, just like other athletes from all walks of life, want to know how real bodybuilders use nutrition and supplements to create their impressive physiques. As I said before, there is no magic program that works for everyone all the time. The solution to mastering the way your body looks can be achieved only by understanding basic principles and how to incorporate them into effective strategies for specific goals and time periods. The next three chapters allow you to understand several nutrition strategies that are all integrated parts of the Periodized Bodybuilding Nutrition System.

> "...if you read and use the information I'm going to share, you will avoid years of frustration."

Getting on Solid Ground

Chapter 4 begins with a discussion on building what I call "The Bodybuilding Foundation Diet," which I am sure will become the cornerstone of your nutrition planning. This is vitally important because I have found, more often than not, that when beginners or even very advanced trainees want direction on how to use supplements to speed up their progress, they somehow forget to cover the basics. This chapter also covers a simple, yet effective, technique that allows athletes to maximize their performance, recovery, and hormonal environment by manipulating how to plan out daily nutrition—**with real food.**

You'll learn how to do this without resorting to "old school" methods that just add additional calories that could otherwise turn into unsightly bodyfat. The Bodybuilding Foundation Diet sounds basic, but it is really an advanced bodybuilding eating plan that will allow you to make great gains and get your physique ready to go to the next level.

How to Systematically Get Lean and Muscular

Chapter 5 explores authoritative guidelines for achieving extreme leanness and muscularity. In this chapter, you'll learn how your body uses stored fat for energy. You'll also learn state-of-the-art tricks of the trade that will "turn on" your fat-burning machinery without drugs or chemicals. Additionally, we will cover the "practical" applications for the ever-popular low-carbohydrate or ketogenic diets, and expose the "best" supplements to maximize their effectiveness.

Overcoming Hardgainer Neurosis

Finally, Chapter 6 examines the age-old problem of gaining lean mass for the "hardgainer." This topic is of great interest to young athletes or those who seem to have a metabolism that just does not respond to mere mortal mass-gaining programs. In this chapter, you will learn how to take a traditional high-carbohydrate diet and turn it into an "anabolic primer" without gaining excess bodyfat. This information is absolutely essential for the hardgainer, and can put slabs of fat-free mass on your physique in as little as six weeks.

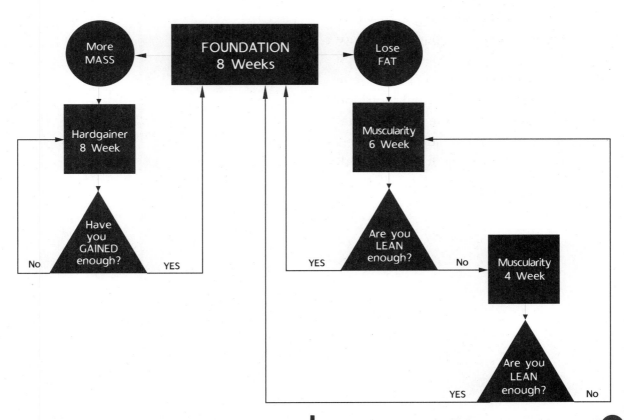

Real Bodybuilding Nutrition Strategies

The Periodized Bodybuilding Nutrition System covers supplement strategies based on the latest science and thousands of actual athlete testimonials. I cannot state this more forcefully—the next three chapters exploit the power of the Periodized Bodybuilding Nutrition System by continually manipulating your macronutrient ratios (proteins, carbs, and fats) to trigger different metabolic responses. By studying these chapters in depth, you will have the tools to forge ahead of the "pack" and get in your best physical condition ever. What you will learn will be invaluable in your quest to maximize your time in the gym. Even if you are an advanced trainee or personal trainer, you will take away some valuable nuggets of information. Remember that the following three chapters cover advanced and sometimes radically new concepts that will enhance your performance and build your ideal body in less time, so you should only use them after you have several months of exercise and sound nutrition under your belt. Please note that the concepts contained in the following chapters may seem difficult to grasp at first, but with a little time and persistence it will become almost second nature.

Chapter 4

Establishing a Nutritional Foundation

You've likely heard this before, but you must first lay the foundation when constructing a proper nutrition plan to get lean and gain muscle. For weight-training athletes, this means concentrating on eating five to six small meals per day that contain optimal amounts of proteins, carb, and fats. OK, now before you say "Duh, I already have my diet in order," remember how long it took you to grasp this concept when you were first learning about weight training (if in fact you already have). Remember, this diet is not in any way a maintenance plan. We will cover *variations* of the Foundation Diet later, so be patient, and try to grasp the basis of this critical base diet.

High Tech Made Simple

You don't have to be a rocket scientist or weigh out your food portions obsessively to understand this program. And although it has been proven to work in thousands of cases from everyday folks to very advanced athletes, I think you'll agree it is pretty easy to understand. To ensure optimal progress, all you need to do is learn how to meet certain nutrient requirements at each meal.

Protein—The Cornerstone of the Bodybuilding Foundation Diet

The first requirement is protein, protein, and more protein. I have yet to witness anyone with an impressive physique that has not taken protein intake serious. Protein is essential to providing the necessary materials for size, strength, and every other major metabolic process that our bodies go through in a 24-hour period. I am constantly amazed at the sheer number of avid weight trainers, who, while looking for that magic supplement, can't even tell you how many grams of protein they consume each day. This is a critical mistake, especially if your needs aren't met. I don't want to preach to you about all the studies that clearly show that successful weight trainers need more protein than sedentary individuals. But, I will tell you that after talking to some of the best physique athletes around, and from my own personal experience, protein consumption should equate to roughly 1.2 to 1.8 grams of protein per pound of bodyweight. This information has been verified in a study that examined the diets of nationally ranked bodybuilders.[1] This figure is a bit higher than the old body-building "standard" of one gram of protein per pound of bodyweight. However, there are quite a few health benefits beyond building muscle that leads me to urge you to get your protein intake in the range of about 1.35 grams of protein per pound of bodyweight.

"...protein consumption should equate to roughly 1.2 to 1.8 grams of protein per pound of bodyweight."

First of all, many high-level athletes have learned that by cutting back on their carbo-hydrate intake and ingesting additional lean protein, they can stay in better shape year around (and who doesn't want that). In addition, a recent study demonstrated that a high-protein diet may be beneficial for blood lipid profiles (cholesterol and triglyc-eride concentrations) even in individuals that don't exercise as frequently or inten-sively as bodybuilders.[2] Armed with these facts, you can see that getting a handle on protein consumption should be the basis of your program. And, with the plethora of protein and meal supplements in the form of powders, bars, or ready-to-drink shakes available today, there should be no excuse not to meet these needs.

The Protein Numbers Game

To figure out your individual protein needs, aim for an intake of about 1.35 grams of protein per pound of bodyweight based on your desired lean bodyweight (DLB). You must have realistic goals, though. If you weigh 150 lbs, you cannot jump directly to a lean mass goal of 250 lbs to cal-culate your protein needs. I suggest you cal-culate your protein needs based on a lean-mass number that is about 10 lbs over your lean bodyweight today. To get an accurate assessment of your current lean body mass, you need to start by having your bodyfat percentage taken. The best methods are skin calipers; underwater weighing, also called bio-electrical impedance; or the Bod Pod. If you are not familiar with these meth-ods, consulting with a personal trainer at most commercial gyms can provide you with an accurate testing procedure. I have put together a bodyfat testing fact sheet below to help get you started:

BODYFAT COMPOSITION WORKSHEET

SKINFOLD MEASUREMENTS
(All measurements are taken on the right side of body):

TRICEPS ___ ___ ___

(Vertical fold; on the posterior midline of the upper arm, halfway between the elbow and shoulder joint, with the arm held freely to the side of the body)

SUPRAILIAC ___ ___ ___
(Love Handle)

(Diagonal fold; in line with the natural angle of the iliac crest or hip bone, taken in the anterior axillary line immediately superior to the iliac crest)

UMBILICUS ___ ___ ___
(Belly)

(Vertical fold; 2 cm to the right side of the umbilicus or belly button)

THIGH ___ ___ ___

(Vertical fold; on the anterior midline of the thigh, midway between the proximal border of the knee cap and hip bone)

= SUM OF *SKINFOLDS* _____

(Add the averages of each site location as a sum)

MEN = [0.29288 x (Sum of 4 *Skinfolds*)] - [0.0005 x (Sum of 4 *Skinfolds*)2] + [0.15845 x (Age)] - 5.76377

WOMEN = [0.29669 x (Sum of 4 *Skinfolds*)] - [0.00043 x (Sum of 4 *Skinfolds*)2] + [0.02963 x (Age)] + 1.4072

PERCENT BODYFAT = _____%

Fat weight = (BF% x bodyweight)

Lean Body Mass = (Bodyweight - Fat weight)

For example, if you have a lean body mass of 190 lbs, then your goal should be set at a lean body mass of 200 lbs. With 200 lbs as a goal, your daily protein intake should be 270 grams. (200 lbs x 1.35 grams of protein per day = 270 grams)

Now, please forget about the notion, or rather myth, of not consuming more than 30 grams of protein per meal. Take a look around the gym or at photos of large natural bodybuilders like Bill Davey, and tell me a 210-lb man has the same protein digestion limitations as a 100-lb woman. I myself weigh about 200 lbs, and my protein intake borders 300 grams, sometimes 350 grams every day. But don't take my word for it. Just look at the 30-grams-per-meal notion from a human development perspective. Our ancestors at times went days without a meat kill or some type of sizeable protein meal. But when they were fortunate enough to feast on an animal, they ate it all—at times ingesting hundreds of grams in one sitting. Therefore, it is illogical that we would evolve from this feeding scheme to be able to process only 30 grams of protein at one time. Make sense? It does to me. Now, if protein consumption for a 200-lb athlete is roughly 270 grams and we strive for 5 to 6 meals, then protein intake should be 45 to 54 grams per meal. As a standard rule, this number should be kept at these levels whether you are trying to gain mass or get leaner. To achieve these goals, we will adjust carbohydrate and fat intake. An example of this plan is seen in Figure 1 on the next page.

The only time you should deviate from this protein intake is on workout days, which will be discussed later.

Figure 1

Desired Lean Bodyweight Multiplier 200 lbs.			
Standard Bodybuilding Foundation Diet	Protein	Carbs	Fat
Meal A	45	45	10
Meal B	45	45	10
Meal C	45	45	10
Meal D	45	45	10
Meal E	45	45	10
Meal F (Post-exercise example)	45	45	10
Total Grams per Macronutrient	270	270	60
Calories per Macronutrient	1080	1080	540
% Calories per Macronutrient + or - 1%	40%	40%	20%
Total Calories	2700		
Post-Exercise Meal Percentages (Example is Meal F)	17%	17%	17%

When deciding how to meet your protein needs, as I stated above, protein powders, meal replacements, bars, and ready-to-drink shakes are all excellent sources. When looking at whole foods, shoot for what nutritionists call "complete" proteins. Examples of lean complete proteins would be chicken, fish, lean cuts of red meat, cottage cheese, and so forth. Unfortunately, most grain and vegetable proteins (except soy) are incomplete, meaning they do not contain all of the necessary amino acids. For more information on protein types and quality, please refer to Chapter 8.

Protein Intake Calculations:

The 200-lb DLB multiplied by 1.35 grams of protein per day equals 270 grams. And 270 grams of protein per day divided into 6 meals equals 45 grams per meal.

Carbohydrate Intake for the Bodybuilding Foundation Diet

Your basic carbohydrate intake should be equal to your daily protein intake established above. Do not deviate from this figure. The Bodybuilding Foundation Diet is just that— The Foundation. Many athletes have "tuned out" the importance of carbs in favor of higher protein and/or higher fat regimens. For now, though, lets stick with the basics. We'll cover more creative programs later. What I will say is that, in over 20 years of studying or speaking to the best bodybuilders from coast to coast, rarely, if ever, have I seen anyone eat a truly low-carb diet (less than 15% of total calories) for more than 6 to 8 weeks at a time. The reason for this is that to perform the type of intense training bodybuilding requires, you need stored energy. And carbs are, for the most part, the energy currency your muscles need to train hard and recover. This energy comes from stored glycogen in muscle, and the amount of carbohydrates taken in is the primary factor in determining glycogen stores. If we use protein intake as our starting point, carb consumption for an athlete looking for a DLB of 200 lbs is 270 grams. (200 lbs x 1.35 grams of carbohydrate per day = 270 grams) As with protein, your goal should be to strive for 5 to 6 meals, with the carbohydrate content per meal between 45 to 54 grams of per meal. However, as with any good program, there will be a few exceptions, which we will discuss later.

Understanding Carbohydrate Selection

Carbohydrate selection can be a fairly tricky topic when it comes to performance nutrition. You may have heard the term "glycemic index." Simply put, various carbs elicit a different metabolic response in your body. The rate at which your body can process carbs is generally dubbed the glycemic index. I'm not going to bore you with all of the detail of this, but here is a brief explanation: Depending on the type and amount of carbs consumed, along with various other factors, insulin is released into circulation as a nutrient shuttle. Insulin is a protein peptide hormone (around 50 odd amino acids linked in an exact sequence) secreted by the pancreas. The job of insulin is to transport or drive nutrients into the cells of all organs in the body, including muscle tissue. So, it basically carries nutrients into various cells, such as those of skeletal muscle, fat tissue, and the liver. In particular, insulin dictates energy storage, that is, where the calories you consume go and to what degree. Sometimes, this results in the storage of energy in undesirable places and with undesirable consequences—bodyfat. Of course, this is the opposite of what we want to happen.

However, one time in which insulin is showing to be beneficial is immediately following a workout. This makes sense because your body has become depleted of glycogen, and energy stores need to be replenished quickly. Therefore, on the Foundation Diet, we recommend consuming foods that elicit a small response in insulin levels during normal meals, and foods that elicit an amplified insulin response after your workout. We will further cover this concept later in the chapter when I discuss post-workout recovery meals. Anyway, this seems to be the optimal way to add pounds of lean mass and not suffer the consequences around your "love handles." Examples of low-glycemic foods are brown rice, pastas, sweet potatoes, most fruits and vegetables, and oatmeal. One other way you can lower the glycemic response and subsequent rise in insulin is to add fiber to every carb-containing meal. To do this, for every 10 grams of carbs you ingest, consume an additional 1 gram of fiber to slow the absorption of nutrients and decrease insulin and fat storage. On the flip side, high-glycemic foods would include most "white" foods like potatoes, rice, flour, bananas, and other highly refined foods like breads. Remember, eat these only after a workout. For a comprehensive list of foods and their glycemic index, as well as additional information, go to www.glycemic.com. Understanding how to amplify insulin and manage the glycemic response to ingested carbs is truly one of the hottest areas in sports supplements today. You'll find more detailed explanations in Chapter 9, called "The Next Wave of Bodybuilding Supplementation."

How Much Fat Can I Eat on the Bodybuilding Foundation Diet?

I believe that the great debate between nutritionists over the last several years regarding optimal fat intake is really one borne out of marketing. You see, it is always easier to tell the public to stick to a plan that gives up one food at a time. Remember the nutritional pundits that swore that you have to avoid fats at all costs, yet eat all the carbs you want, and you'll be energetic and lose fat? And how about the current dogma that has us pursue a zero-carbohydrate diet while eating burgers, bacon, and eggs? While it seems that the fat-free school of thought is clearly losing the battle, a newer problem is that of proposing super high fat intake regardless of health status. I realize that many low-carb dieters are out in an attempt to lose bodyfat, and they are doing this diet to minimize insulin production (as we discussed above, excess insulin and carbs can lead to fat accumulation). This regimen will be discussed in a practical sense when we cover the Muscularity Diets in the next chapter. For the Foundation Diet, my guidelines for fat intake take into consideration that in other diet modules, dietary fat will be altered to meet specific nutritional needs. So in the Foundation Phase, which is likely to be adhered to more often throughout the year, I have set fat intake at 30% of your lean bodyweight goal. For example, using the same 200-lb DLB goal, this would mean a fat intake of 60 grams divided into 6 meals (200 lbs multiplied by the 30% multiplier for grams of fat per day equals 60 grams). When choosing fats, look for foods high in unsaturated fats and low in saturated fats. Most animal sources like ground beef, pork chops, and sausages contain saturated fats and should be avoided. Look for sources like flax, sunflower and olive oils, salmon, black olives, avocados, and others.

As you can see, the Foundation Diet is simple to understand, and like great German engineering, this diet eliminates the need for frills that take an athlete off course. This nutritional planning model can be used year round, and can be slightly altered depending on your goals and how your body responds in the mirror (not just the scale). Remember to keep protein, carbs, and fat in line with these recommendations until you start seeing your physique change according to your goals. At that time, you can evaluate which module is best to take you to the next level. However, since all muscular progress can be halted without proper recovery, the next strategy we will explore is the Maximum Recovery Foundation Diet for use on training days.

Post-Workout Dietary Manipulation on the Bodybuilding Foundation Diet

Now that you have an understanding of the basic tenets regarding the Bodybuilding Foundation Diet, we can work on maximizing this program into what I call the "Maximum Recovery Foundation Diet." This is often a great next step to maximize the Bodybuilding

Foundation Diet, or, as you will see later, any diet module you are in. Here's why: If you calculated the nutrient ratios in meal 6 in Figure 1, the Bodybuilding Foundation Diet allows you to get about 17% out of total daily intake of protein, carbs, and fat in your post-exercise meal. This is fine for overall meal planning, especially on non-training days. However, more and more evidence analyzing metabolic variables for muscle growth and even fat loss is pointing toward gearing an athlete's daily diet toward higher levels of carbs and protein to maximize post-exercise recovery. Therefore, the first step will be to maximize circulating levels of insulin for increased anabolic (muscle-building) support, followed by increased protein to maximize recovery and growth. When adjusting these macronutrient values for maximum post-exercise recovery, you will do so without resorting to adding additional calories to your overall diet. Let me explain how this strategy works.

Insulin and the Post-Workout Anabolic Sequence

In the carbohydrate section, we briefly touched on insulin, and if you remember, I said one exception where the body can utilize high insulin levels is after a workout. Why? Like I said before, your body is depleted of essential nutrients, and working out can leave you in a catabolic (muscle-wasting) state. Therefore, it is the goal of this portion of the diet to maximize as many anabolic pathways as possible. With insulin, it is difficult to determine precisely the effects on muscle-protein synthesis. However, it has been well known

for a long time that insulin plays a major role. The Maximum Recovery Foundation Diet should "amplify" the level of insulin we produce post exercise and "extend" its time in your blood to help drive more muscle-building nutrients into your targeted muscle cells. It is at this time that we specifically want to "up regulate" the amount of protein, creatine, and glycogen-stimulating glucose that can be loaded into our muscle tissue.

> "I believe that the great debate… regarding optimal fat intake is really one born out of marketing."

Triggering an Anabolic Cascade

If you happen to review the muscle magazines every month like I do, you may have read the current rhetoric about post-exercise recovery that preaches you should eat all the junk you want or just consume boatloads of sugar mixed with creatine, and you'll gain 10 pounds in 5 days. Let me tell you firsthand that this "old-school" approach is fine for the other guys, but if you want to be the best you can be, this tactic just doesn't cut it. Currently, the state of the art is to maximize post-workout hormonal environment by first setting the stage with a small amount of carbs stacked with insulinogenic (insulin-producing) amino

Figure 2

Desired Lean Bodyweight Multiplier 200 lbs.			
High-Performance Recovery Diet	Protein	Carbs	Fat
Meal A	40	30	14
Meal B	40	30	14
Meal C	40	30	14
Pre-Exercise Meal	20	2	0
Post-Exercise Meal A (1 hour after training)	65	90	4
Post-Exercise Meal B (3 hours after training)	65	90	14
Total Grams per Macronutrient	270	272	60
Calories per Macronutrient	1080	1088	540
	40%	40%	20%
Total Calories	2708		
Post-Exercise Meal Percentages	48%	66%	30%

acids and glucose-disposal agents. One of the best amino acid combinations to maximize insulin secretion is L-arginine and glutamine peptide from hydrolyzed wheat gluten. These two amino acids have recently been shown to amplify the insulin secretion set in motion by a meal that contains some simple sugar. Combining these compounds with alpha-lipoic acid, taurine, and d-Pinitol, which are often used as glucose-disposal agents, is truly a "can't-miss" synergistic one-two punch. We'll discuss this further in Chapter 10. Next, our strategy will be to "borrow" some proteins and carbs from other meals to maximize the anabolic processes that are available right after training. In essence, we are striving to post load almost 50% of our daily proteins and carbs into the critical post-workout window of opportunity.

In the example, (Figure 2) we see that we can effectively "push" over 130 grams of protein and 180 grams of carbs (using a 200-lb DLB) into the 4 hours immediately after training. This in contrast to the same 200-lb athlete whose Foundation Diet allows him to normally eat 45 grams of protein, 45 grams of carbs, and about 10 grams of fat every 3 hours (Figure1).

In this portion of the diet, we also recommend you add a pre-workout meal consisting of a small protein drink with low carbs or low-calorie energy compounds such as D-ribose and creatine. Excellent products for this are economical whey or casein protein powders and/or D-ribose, which helps your body restore energy. Therefore it makes sense to use something like this before your workout to support your body's energy stores during training. Many athletes who supplement with D-ribose immediately before or during exercise often report a greater ability to perform more reps per set. This could be big news to bodybuilders, because originally the ribose-performance connection was deemed to be best suited for recovery, when the body is laboring to make more energy for the next training session. Remember to adjust the values in your diet if you choose a pre-workout drink like EAS' RiboForce HP, which does contain some carbs.

Follow the standard format of the Foundation Diet on non-training days and the Maximum Recovery Foundation Diet on training days religiously for about two weeks, and I am confident you will see measurable results. Many athletes who follow it experience decreased recovery times, fuller muscles, and even less bodyfat due to the "cycling" effect of the program.

Advantages of Using the Maximum Recovery Foundation Diet

By taking a closer look at Figure 2, we can see that by increasing post-workout carbs and proteins as a percentage of calories from our original 17% to 48% and 66%, respectively, we can improve post-exercise glycogen storage and create an anabolic environment for new muscle growth. In addition, for the other meals, carb and protein intake is reduced, while fat is slightly increased, which will allow for superaphysiological levels of protein and carbs to be consumed post-exercise. This technique allows you to stay within your caloric boundaries while maximizing recovery. Here is how we get the adjusted figures:

Protein Intake Calculations:

The 200-lb DLB goal multiplied by 1.35 grams of protein per day equals about 270 grams. And 270 grams of protein per day divided into 6 meals equals about 40 grams per meal for three meals, 20 grams for one meal, and about 65 grams for two post-exercise meals.

Carbohydrate Intake Calculations:

The 200-lb DLB goal multiplied by 1.35 grams of carbohydrate per day equals 270 grams. And 270 grams of carbohydrate per day divided into 6 meals equals about 25 grams per meal for three meals, one low-carb meal, and about 90 grams for two post-exercise meals.

Fat Intake Calculations:

The 200-lb DLB goal multiplied by .30 grams of fat per day equals 60 grams. And 60 grams of fat per day divided into 6 meals equals about 10 grams per meal. However, if you can take in less fat in the first post-exercise meal, do so as it will increase the rate of gastric emptying and thus magnify insulin production.

How Long Do I Stay On the Bodybuilding Foundation Diet?

Each module in the Periodized Body-building Nutrition System runs in four-to-eight week intervals. However, if the Bodybuilding Foundation Diet is allowing you to reach your current goals, just continue on it for another eight weeks. Once you complete another eight weeks on the program, re-evaluate your progress, and repeat the cycle again or continue on to the muscularity or hardgainer programs in the next chapters.

SUPPLEMENTATION
FOR THE FOUNDATION DIET:

As I have said many times in the previous text, the Foundation Diet is your core nutrition program. And if you take a look at the Periodized Bodybuilding Nutrition Phases diagramed at the end of Chapter 3, it is easy to see that this is the program that must be mastered completely. In business we often say that the best companies master their core competencies, and to build a great physique you must also look at the Foundation Diet the same way.

I have taken a very close look at the dietary interventions and have also had the joy of going through some very grueling training that is designed for the Foundation phase. Let me tell you from experience that the exercise guidelines in this program will literally force your body to adapt with larger and stronger muscles—granted they have proper nutrition. The Foundation meal planner is nearly bulletproof but with additional support from supplements you may be able to recover quicker and get more training sessions in per week. I have compiled a list of recommended supplements, when to use them, and in what quantities. There are three programs to choose from—economy, mid-range, and high-end, depending on your supplement budget. To better evaluate your own personal supplement needs, my suggestion is to review the Foundation Diet based on your desired lean bodyweight goal and begin planning out your meals. Then armed with the information regarding how much protein you will be consuming each meal, you can go shopping for the rest of your supplies.

Economy $ Foundation Phase Supplementation

Meal Supplements—meal-replacement powders (MRPs), bars, ready-to-drink shakes (RTDs) and protein powders

- Usage: Use MRPs and protein powders to create two to four supplemental meals. Use RTDs and bars for convenience.
- Benefits: Increases protein and meal frequency, enhances recovery, and repairs damaged muscles.
- Examples: MRPs from reputable manufacturers: Myoplex (Regular and Deluxe), RTDs and bars, Precision Protein, and Simply Whey
- Notes: You can use similar products from reputable manufacturers. Remember, many meals may require additional carbohydrates and fiber.

Creatine

- Usage: Three to ten grams post-exercise. Be sure to drink eight to ten 12-ounce glasses of water per day.
- Benefits: Enhances recovery and ATP replenishment
- Examples: Phosphagen HP, Synthevol HP, or RiboForce HP
- Notes: Products with d-Ribose should be used right before or during exercise. You can use similar products from reputable manufacturers, but remember to ingest ample carbohydrates according to meal plan.

Glutamine

- Usage: One to two grams post-exercise

- Benefits: Enhances recovery and glycogen and glutamine replenishment
- Examples: CytoVol, glutamine powder
- Notes: Check to see if ample glutamine is included in your creatine product. If so, you're covered. You can use similar products from reputable manufacturers.

Mid-Range $$ Foundation Phase Supplementation

Meal Supplements—meal-replacement powders (MRPs), bars, ready-to-drink shakes (RTDs) and protein powders

- Usage: Use MRPs and protein powders to create two to four supplemental meals. Use RTDs and bars for convenience.
- Benefits: Increases protein and meal frequency, enhances recovery, and repairs damaged muscles.
- Examples: MRPs from reputable manufacturers: Myoplex (Regular and Deluxe), RTDs and bars, Precision Protein, and Simply Whey
- Notes: You can use similar products from reputable manufacturers. Remember, many meals may require additional carbohydrates and fiber.

Creatine

- Usage: Three to ten grams post-exercise. Be sure to drink eight to ten 12-ounce glasses of water per day.
- Benefits: Enhances recovery and ATP replenishment
- Examples: Phosphagen HP, Synthevol HP, or RiboForce HP
- Notes: Products with d-Ribose should be used right before or during exercise. You can use similar products from reputable manufacturers, but remember to ingest ample carbohydrates according to meal plan.

Glutamine

- Usage: Two to three grams post-exercise plus one to two grams with one to two other meals
- Benefits: Enhances recovery and glycogen and glutamine replenishment
- Examples: CytoVol, glutamine powder
- Notes: Check to see if ample glutamine is included in your creatine product. If so, you're covered. You can use similar products from reputable manufacturers.

Beta-ecdysterone plus Methoxy-isoflavone

- Usage: Two times per day (post-exercise and nighttime with a protein meal)
- Benefits: Reduces muscle-protein breakdown
- Examples: MethoxyFactor HP
- Notes: You can use similar products from reputable manufacturers. Dosage is usually 25-40 mg of ecdysterone plus 200-400 mg of methoxyisoflavone.

Essential Fatty Acids (EFAs)

- Usage: With meals when essential fatty acids are needed
- Benefits: Maintain healthy hormone levels
- Examples: EFAs, flaxseed oil, hemp oil, and olive oil
- Notes: Check label to calculate needs

High-End $$$ Foundation Phase Supplementation

Meal Supplements—meal-replacement powders (MRPs), bars, ready-to-drink shakes (RTDs) and protein powders
- Usage: Use MRPs and protein powders to create two to four supplemental meals. Use RTDs and bars for convenience.
- Benefits: Increases protein and meal frequency, enhances recovery, and repairs damaged muscles.
- Examples: MRPs from reputable manufacturers: Myoplex (Regular and Deluxe), RTDs and bars, Precision Protein, and Simply Whey
- Notes: You can use similar products from reputable manufacturers. Remember, many meals may require additional carbohydrates and fiber.

Creatine
- Usage: Three to ten grams post-exercise. Be sure to drink eight to ten 12-ounce glasses of water per day.
- Benefits: Enhances recovery and ATP replenishment
- Examples: Phosphagen HP, Synthevol HP, or RiboForce HP
- Notes: Products with d-Ribose should be used right before or during exercise. You can use similar products from reputable manufacturers, but remember to ingest ample carbohydrates according to meal plan.

Glutamine
- Usage: Four to five grams post-exercise plus one to two grams with two to three other meals
- Benefits: Enhances recovery and glycogen and glutamine replenishment
- Examples: CytoVol, glutamine powder
- Notes: Check to see if ample glutamine is included in your creatine product, If so, you're covered. You can use similar products from reputable manufacturers.

Beta-ecdysterone plus Methoxy-isoflavone
- Usage: Three times per day (breakfast, post-exercise, and nighttime with a protein meal)
- Benefits: Reduces muscle-protein breakdown
- Examples: MethoxyFactor HP
- Notes: You can use similar products from reputable manufacturers. Dosage is usually 25-40 mg of ecdysterone plus 200-400 mg of methoxyisoflavone.

Essential Fatty Acids (EFAs)
- Usage: With meals where essential fatty acids are needed
- Benefits: Maintain healthy hormone levels
- Examples: EFAs, flaxseed oil, hemp oil, and olive oil
- Notes: Check label to calculate needs

Glucose Disposal Cocktail
- Usage: Post-exercise meal
- Benefits: Glycogen, glutamine, and creatine storage
- Examples: 50-100 mg d-pinitol, 200-400 mg alpha-lipoic acid, 24-28 mg colosolic acid
- Notes: Some nutrients may be included in

your creatine product. Add others as needed.

Antioxidant
- Usage: Take with two meals and after training
- Benefits: Muscle repair/recovery and supports immune system
- Examples: ACE, AAB, NAC, Vitamin E
- Notes: You can use similar products from reputable manufacturers. Dosage is dependent on the company.

d-Ribose
- Usage: Three to ten grams immediately before or during training
- Benefits: Enhances anaerobic peak power output
- Examples: RiboForce HP, straight d-ribose
- Notes: You can use similar products from reputable manufacturers.

Supplement Rotation for Maximum Benefits

The options listed in the previous text will make creating your personal supplement program easier and more effective. Keep in mind that the "core concept" behind the Periodized Bodybuilding and Nutrition Programs in this book is to keep your body responding by systematically making changes in both your diet and exercise regimen. For this reason, don't allow yourself to choose exactly the same supplements each and every time you are in a particular phase. The best strategy is to mix it up. For example, there are several types of products that are designed to decrease muscle-protein breakdown, but for maximum results you should rotate them in a cyclical manner. You may want to use specific combinations such as using ecdysterone plus methoxyisoflavone for one cycle and HMB plus extra glutamine in the next. The bottom line is don't stay on any one compound for more than 12 weeks. Keeping track of the supplements you take and in what quantities will allow you to systematically give your body the change it needs by rotating them in and out.

References Cited

[1]Kleiner, S. M., et al., "Nutritional status of nationally ranked elite body-builders." *Int J Sport Nutr* 4.1 (1994) : 54-69.

[2]Wolfe, B. M., et al, "Replacement of carbohydrate by protein in a conventional-fat diet reduces cholesterol and triglyceride concentrations in healthy normolipodemic subjects." *Clinical and Investigative Medicine* 22.4 (1999) : 140-148.

*"It's lack of faith that makes
people afraid of meeting challenges,
and I believe in myself."*

-Muhammad Ali

Chapter

5

Achieving Maximum Muscularity

Caution: Each module in the Periodized Bodybuilding Nutrition System is designed for specific time intervals. The following chapter contains the latest techniques for attaining maximum muscularity and leanness, but must only be followed after you complete at least one eight-week cycle of the Bodybuilding Foundation Diet outlined in the previous chapter. In addition, this chapter will only make sense after you have grasped the information that is presented in the Bodybuilding Foundation Diet.

Fat Loss & the State of the Art

There are literally hundreds of products on the market that claim to be able to transform your body into what you've always wanted. Some work, some don't. The reality of the situation is that scientists who study the mechanisms of fat loss have found some very interesting "rules" of the game you need to get a grip on. The first rule is that your body releases stored fat to supply energy that is not provided in your diet. Therefore, aside from exercising more, the best way to incur this energy deficit is to reduce the number of calories you consume. This self-imposed calorie deficit is our first rule of fat loss. With this in mind, we must carefully adjust our macronutrient levels in a way that accomplishes the above **and** poses less of a threat to your existing muscle mass. To initiate the initial stage of fat loss, we will use a diet called the Muscularity Diet.

The advanced bodybuilder or athlete who follows the guidelines of the Muscularity Diet usually sees incredible results without the undue stress that would otherwise force him or her to sacrifice valuable muscle tissue. During this phase, the athlete reduces carbs per meal to a number equivalent to 35% less than protein. For instance, an athlete with the 200-lb desired lean bodyweight (DLB) goal would consume approximately 35 grams of carbs for every 50 grams of protein per meal. This is our second rule of fat loss, which simply implies that when energy calories go down, a higher **proportion of calories from protein** must be in the diet to offset muscle protein breakdown (see Figure 3).

Bodyfat Sleight of Hand

Your body doesn't know that when you go on a fat-loss regimen, it shouldn't use amino acids from body protein to make up the energy deficit. Weight-loss programs often fail because the person on the diet loses both fat and muscle tissue during this process, and therefore winds up with the same or worse percentage of bodyfat, just in a smaller body. You've probably seen an example of this at the gym in the form of a "skinny fat" person; you know, someone that's rather small but carries a higher percentage of bodyfat.

Supplying protein at optimum levels also provides another benefit, which is described as an increased "thermic" effect. This is the heat generated due to the food we eat, and can account for anywhere from 5 to 20% of our daily caloric intake. The process of digesting, absorbing, and assimilating the various nutrients actually requires energy from calories. It is thought that protein produces the highest thermic effect (up to 20%) when compared to carbohydrates (8%) or fat (2%). Additionally, researchers have noted that people fed meals with proportionately higher protein have a greater sense of appetite satisfaction.

The Slow Meltdown

The Muscularity Diet is designed to slowly adjust a bodybuilder or athlete to use stored bodyfat for fuel. The slight energy deficit and

Figure 3

Desired Lean Bodyweight Multiplier 200 lbs.			
Muscularity Diet (non-training days)	Protein	Carbs	Fat
Meal A	45	33.33	8.33
Meal B	45	33.33	8.33
Meal C	45	33.33	8.33
Meal D	45	33.33	8.33
Meal E	45	33.33	8.33
Meal F (Post-exercise example)	45	33.33	8.33
Total Grams per Macronutrient	270	200	50
Calories per Macronutrient	1080	800	450
% Calories per Macronutrient + or - 1%	46%	34%	19%
Total Calories	2330		
Post-Exercise Meal Percentages (Example is Meal F)	17%	17%	17%

adjustment of macronutrients signals greater amounts of fat to be burned, and more lean mass will be retained than on super restrictive programs. If you feel you are not losing fat quickly enough (1 to 2 lbs per week), then slightly increase the amount of calories you burn each week. This can be accomplished by simply adding two or three 20-minute aerobic training sessions per week. This program should be followed for six weeks, at which time you may want to take your fat-loss program to the highest level, which we can accomplish with the Maximum Muscularity Diet, explained below. Follow the Muscularity Diet on non-training days and the Maximum Recovery version (Figure 4) on training days. This phase of the diet works extremely well, and does not cause undue "shock" to your system. A quick review shows that we have covered our metabolic bases to maximize the benefits of this program, which are:

- To offset muscle-protein breakdown, protein as a percentage of calories goes from 41% on the Bodybuilding Foundation Diet to 46% on the Muscularity Diet.

- To create an energy deficit, calories on the Muscularity Diet are approximately 10% less than on the Bodybuilding Foundation Diet. This reduction comes solely from carbohydrates.

- To avoid a reduction in fat-burning enzymes, fat intake as a percentage of calories goes from 17% on the Standard Foundation Diet to 19% on the Muscularity Diet.

Figure 4

Desired Lean Bodyweight Multiplier 200 lbs.

High-Performance Recovery Muscularity Diet (training days)	Protein	Carbs	Fat
Meal A	45	25	12
Meal B	45	25	12
Meal C	45	3	8
Post-Exercise Primer (Immediately after training)	4	21	0
Post-Exercise Meal A (1 hour after training)	65	65	8
Post-Exercise Meal B (3 hours after training)	65	65	10
Total Grams per Macronutrient	269	204	50
Calories per Macronutrient	1076	816	450
% Calories per Macronutrient + or - 1%	45.94%	34.84%	19.21%
Total Calories	2342		
Post-Exercise Meal Percentages	48%	63.73%	36%

THE MUSCULARITY DIET NOTES

Protein Intake Calculations:

Your DLB goal multiplied by 1.35 grams of protein per day equals 270 grams. And 270 grams of protein per day divided into 6 meals equals 45 grams per meal for non-training days, and will be adjusted for training days to make your post-exercise meals more effective (Figure 4).

> "Popular media has been promoting a concept for weight loss that may confuse even the most advanced athlete."

Carbohydrate Intake Calculations:

Your DLB goal multiplied by 1 gram of carbohydrate per day equals 200 grams. And 200 grams of carbohydrate per day divided into 6 meals equals 30 to 35 grams per meal for non-training days, and will be adjusted for training days to make your post-exercise meals more effective (Figure 4).

Fat Intake Calculations:

Your DLB goal multiplied .25 grams of fat per day equals 50 grams. And 50 grams of fat per day divided into 6 meals equals 8 to 9 grams per meal on non-training days, and will be adjusted for training days to make your post-exercise meals more effective (Figure 4).

The Maximum Muscularity Diet—The Bodybuilder's Low-Carb Diet

Popular media has been promoting a concept for weight loss that may confuse even the most advanced athlete. The belief is one where fitness enthusiasts and anyone looking to radically improve body composition often follows a high-protein, very low-carbohydrate diet (HP-VLC Diet) in order to intensify fat loss. While I have personally worked with larger athletes who can achieve a desirable fat-burning state by ingesting about 200 carb grams per day (see the Muscularity Diet above), the standard protocol for a HP-VLC Diet is to limit daily carbohydrate intake to less than 100 grams. The remainder of your daily calories must come from protein and fat. Nevertheless, the scientific community calls these very rigid diets "ketogenic," while the media has sometimes referred to them by their "brand" names such Protein Power, The Carbohydrate Addict's Diet, Anabolic Diet, or Atkins. It is no secret that when training intensity is high (and of course intensity and some sort of volume is key to keeping or increasing muscle size), even 200 grams of carbohydrates per day for larger athletes is tremendously meager. That's why I never recommend this type of diet to athletes for the long term, nor do I ever see or recommend any top athlete to follow this regimen for more than six to eight weeks. In fact, our program is more of a low-carb "sprint," because it only last four weeks.

How the Maximum Muscularity Diet Works

First, when you deprive your body of glucose and thus insulin (all carbohydrates eventually become blood glucose), it becomes necessary for your body to use alternate energy sources (ketones). This can be a very good strategy, because stored bodyfat is an abundant alternate energy source. In fact, our ancestors did not have an endless supply of carbohydrate foodstuffs at their disposal. This "shortage" of glucose-producing foods is what many researchers feel prompted our bodies to store additional bodyfat for use as energy at times of "glucose insufficiency."

Athletes should know that the other readily available fuel source is your own skeletal muscle proteins, and if you don't do your homework, your body will tear them down to make more glucose. Regardless, tapping into your fat stores provides a virtually endless supply of energy, since I cannot recall anyone who is fat free. Anyway, second on the list of low-carb diet attributes is that when carbohydrate intake is decreased, so is your body's secretion of the hormone insulin. The dieting benefit associated with reduced insulin secretion lies in the fact that when it is over-secreted, it can inhibit enzymes that promote fat burning, and upgrade the activity of other enzymes that promote fat accumulation. Indeed, insulin secretion seems to be highest during sleep, making more sense of the notion that carbs at bedtime are counterproductive to fat loss. True to form, many of the popular low-carb weight-loss diets such as The Zone, Protein Power, Atkins, and others, regard controlling insulin and carbohydrate intake as equally vital parts of their success equation. The important thing to note is that any diet can work on a short-term basis. The trick is in knowing the mechanisms by which they work and short-circuiting the downside.

What to Watch for on Low-Carb Diets

On the flip side, the HP-VLC Diet creates a metabolic environment called ketosis, which is not conducive to high-intensity weight training. Moreover, you should also consider the fact that these diets suppress insulin secretion, a regulator of muscle-protein synthesis. Normal, moderate carbohydrate intake at each meal stimulates the proper insulin levels needed for maximum muscle-protein synthesis. Over time, this depressed insulin secretion may halt any additional muscular progress.

However, this macronutrient profile can be useful when it is necessary for the athlete to accelerate fat burning, but it must be closely engineered (more on that later), and used in four-week sprints. Individuals who follow a low-carb diet periodically need to understand how they work, so that muscle tissue is spared at the expense of fat loss. In the end, periodically lowering carb intake to the levels outlined in the Maximum Muscularity Diet (see Figure 5 for example) can work to reduce bodyfat to the extreme. Here are some of the changes from the last diet that make accelerated fat loss while conserving lean tissue on the Maximum Muscularity Diet possible:

To offset muscle protein breakdown, protein as a percentage of calories goes from 46% on the Muscularity Diet to 58% on the Maximum Muscularity Diet.

Figure 5

Desired Lean Bodyweight Multiplier 200 lbs.			
Maximum Muscularity Diet (non-training days)	Protein	Carbs	Fat
Meal A	45	10	10
Meal B	45	10	10
Meal C	45	10	10
Meal D	45	10	10
Meal E	45	10	10
Meal F (Post-exercise example)	45	10	10
Total Grams per Macronutrient	270	60	60
Calories per Macronutrient	1080	240	540
% Calories per Macronutrient +or- 1%	58%	13%	29%
Total Calories	1860		
Post-Exercise Meal Percentages (Example is Meal F)	17%	17%	17%

To create an energy deficit, calories on the Maximum Muscularity Diet are approximately 20% less than on the Muscularity Diet. This reduction comes solely from carbs, while calories from fat go up slightly.

To avoid a reduction in fat-burning enzymes, fat as a percentage of calories goes from 19% on the Muscularity Diet to 29% on the Maximum Muscularity Diet.

THE MAXIMUM MUSCULARITY DIET NOTES

Protein Intake Calculations:

A 200-lb DLB goal multiplied by 1.35 grams of protein per day equals 270 grams. And 270 grams of protein per day divided into 6 meals equals 45 grams per meal.

Carbohydrate Intake Calculations:

A 200-lb DLB goal multiplied by .30 grams of carbs per day equals 60 grams. And 60 grams of carbohydrate per day divided into 6 meals equals about 10 grams per meal.

Fat Intake Calculations:

A 200-lb DLB goal multiplied by .30 grams of fat per day equals 60 grams. And 60 grams of fat per day divided into 6 meals equals about 10 grams per meal.

Targeted Recovery on the Maximum Muscularity Diet

Most of the popular HP-VLC Diets are marketed to inactive or sedentary people. This poses a problem for athletes, because if you've ever taken carbohydrate intake levels to between 50 and 100 grams per day, you know your muscles can start looking extremely small and flat. The reason for this is that your muscle stores become severely depleted of several key components, thus reducing their overall cell volume. For those of you restricting carbs, the most likely missing nutrient in your muscle cells is stored glycogen! Glycogen is the storage form of glucose (blood sugar), of which two third of total glycogen stores are found in skeletal muscle (the other one third is found in the liver). The glycogen found in muscle is generally used for the muscle only and not to maintain blood sugar levels. Several movement studies have shown that anaerobic threshold and power output are markedly decreased in muscles that are glycogen depleted. In addition, each particle of stored glycogen dramatically increases water content inside your muscle cells, which researchers believe is part of a water-balance (osmotic) mechanism to regulate whole body protein metabolism. This section discusses the special concerns necessary for weight trainers to complete a successful Maximum Muscularity Diet or HP-VLC Diet cycle.

Glutamine, Glycogen Storage, and Muscle-Protein Breakdown

The most problematic and overlooked area is that of cellular hydration while on a low-carb diet. This is a vital part of the equation if your goal is to maintain muscle size while achieving ultra low levels of bodyfat. Since glycogen is an essential component for muscular performance and cell volume, the question arises as to how can we get more inside our muscles without resorting to eating more carbs. The solution here is glutamine and pre- and post-exercise carbohydrate feedings. Researchers have been looking into the stimulatory effects of diets high in glutamine as a zero-carbohydrate means to increase glycogen storage. Although the mechanism is not fully understood, initial work suggests that after exercise, the increased availability of glutamine promotes muscle glycogen accumulation by mechanisms possibly including the diversion of glutamine to glycogen. In addition, low glutamine status is quite common for anyone on low-carb diets due to its use as an important biochemical fuel. When energy stores are depleted, glutamine is released by skeletal muscle and fulfills several functions in human metabolism, making this nutrient even more vital. This may be why researchers theorize that the size of the glutamine pool (intracellular glutamine stores) may determine whole body protein metabolism.

Carbohydrate Timing

The timing of ingested carbohydrates is of great importance when trying to improve glycogen stores while staying in a desirable fat-burning mode. Research again shows us that pre- and post-exercise meals can contain liberal amounts of carbohydrates without spilling carbohydrate calories over into our fat cells. This is due to the fact that for up to two hours after intense training, muscle glycogen re-synthesis takes precedence over liver and other storage sites, such as our fat cells. Several studies have shown that creatine and insulin-producing carbohydrates taken post-exercise will improve glycogen stores up to 18% more than when taking carbs alone. In addition, there is a net energy cost of about 10% (of the carbohydrate calories) in creating ATP out of glycogen. In that sense, it is even wiser to ingest carbs post-exercise. I have also discussed this topic with Lyle McDonald, the author of "The Ketogenic Diet," which is an excellent reference tool for athletes on low-carb diets. He has devised a simple option for low-carb dieters who train with weights called Targeted Ketogenic Dieting or TKD. Basically, his work

> "The timing of ingested carbohydrates is of great importance when trying to improve glycogen storage."

validates the fact that carbs taken around 30 to 60 minutes before or immediately after exercise will not lessen the fat-burning effects of the diet. I have engineered a targeted recovery system of eating on the Maximum Muscularity Diet (Figure 6) below, and I suggest you use it on training days, because it not only makes good sense scientifically, but your workouts will be much more intense.

TARGETED RECOVERY ON THE MAXIMUM MUSCULARITY DIET NOTES

Protein Intake Calculations:

A 200-lb DLB goal multiplied by 1.35 grams

of protein per day equals 270 grams. And 270 grams of protein per day divided into 5 meals equals 45 grams per meal for 3 meals and over 65 grams per meal for the 2 post-exercise meals.

Carbohydrate Intake Calculations:

A 200-lb DLB goal multiplied by .50 grams of carbohydrate per day equals about 100 grams. And 100 grams of carbohydrate per day should be centered on the meals prior to and after training and not divided into 5 or 6 equal portions.

Fat Intake Calculations:

A 200-lb DLB goal multiplied by .30 grams of fat per day equals 60 grams. And 60 grams of fat per day should not be centered on the meals prior to and after training. A good rule of thumb is to use more fat in the very low-carb meals as seen in the example (Figure 5). This provides greater appetite satisfaction and helps you burn ketones.

How Long Do I Stay on the Muscularity Diets?

Here again, each module in the Periodized Bodybuilding Nutrition System should be used for specific intervals. With that said, the Muscularity Diet must be followed by the Bodybuilding Foundation Diet so that you do not lose too much muscle on the program. And the Maximum Muscularity Diet must be followed by the Muscularity Diet for the same reasons as above. Once you complete eight weeks on the Bodybuilding Foundation Diet, you can move to the six-week Muscularity Diet and then the four-week sprint on the

Figure 6

Desired Lean Bodyweight Multiplier 200 lbs.

Targeted Recovery Maximum Muscularity Diet (weight-training days)	Protein	Carbs	Fat
Meal A	45	3.15	13.33
Meal B	45	3.15	13.33
Meal C	30	3.15	13.33
Pre-Exercise Meal	25	2	0
Post-Exercise Primer (Immediately after training)	4	21	0
Post-Exercise Meal A (1 hour after training)	60	50	10
Post-Exercise Meal B (3 hours after training)	60	25	10
Total Grams per Macronutrient	269	107.45	60
Calories per Macronutrient	1076	429.8	540
% Calories per Macronutrient + or - 1%	53%	21%	26%
Total Calories	2045.8		
Targeted Pre- & Post-Exercise Meal Percentages	55%	91%	33%

Maximum Muscularity Diet. Once you have gone through all of these phases, I suggest a break by going back to the meal plans outlined in the Bodybuilding Foundation Diet. Once you complete another eight weeks on the Bodybuilding Foundation Diet and give your body a rest, you may re-evaluate your progress and repeat the Muscularity Diet cycles again.

SUPPLEMENTATION FOR THE MUSCULARITY DIET

Just as we did in the Foundation Diet, here is a table that has recommended supplements for the Muscularity Diet. Here again, there are three programs to choose from—economy, mid-range, and high-end depending on your supplement budget. You should already be familiar with your protein needs from the previous diet, so start your meal planning from that perspective. The next area of concern during this stage will be to consume adequate quantities of nutrients that may help you protect lean muscle tissue—glutamine, ecdysterone, HMB, and methoxy-isoflavone.

Economy $ Muscularity Phase Supplementation

Meal Supplements—meal-replacement powders (MRPs), bars, ready-to-drink shakes (RTDs) and protein powders

- Usage: Use MRPs and protein powders to create two to four supplemental meals. Use RTDs and bars for convenience.
- Benefits: Increases protein and meal frequency, enhances recovery, and repairs damaged muscles.
- Examples: MRPs from reputable manufacturers: Myoplex (Regular and Deluxe), RTDs and bars, Precision Protein, and Simply Whey
- Notes: You can use similar products from reputable manufacturers. Remember, many meals may require additional carbohydrates and fiber.

Creatine

- Usage: Three to ten grams post-exercise. Be sure to drink eight to ten 12-ounce glasses of water per day.
- Benefits: Enhances recovery and ATP replenishment
- Examples: Phosphagen HP, Synthevol HP, or RiboForce HP
- Notes: Products with d-Ribose should be used right before or during exercise. You can use similar products from reputable manufacturers, but remember to ingest ample carbohydrates according to meal plan.

HMB (Beta-hydroxy beta-methylbutyrate)

- Usage: Three grams per day

- Benefits: Decreases muscle-protein breakdown
- Examples: BetaGen, HMB capsules
- Notes: You can use similar products from reputable manufacturers.

Thermogenic

- Usage: Consult with your physician first and foremost. Use as directed on packaging, and read all warning statements carefully.
- Benefits: Increases caloric expenditure and energy
- Examples: BetaLean HP
- Notes: You can use similar products from reputable manufacturers. Remember to consult with your physician first and foremost. Use as directed on packaging, and read all warning statements carefully.

Mid-Range $$ Muscularity Phase Supplementation

Meal Supplements—meal-replacement powders (MRPs), bars, ready-to-drink shakes (RTDs) and protein powders
- Usage: Use MRPs and protein powders to create two to four supplemental meals. Use RTDs and bars for convenience.
- Benefits: Increases protein and meal frequency, enhances recovery, and repairs damaged muscles.
- Examples: MRPs from reputable manufacturers: Myoplex (Regular and Deluxe), RTDs and bars, Precision Protein, and Simply Whey
- Notes: You can use similar products from reputable manufacturers. Remember, many meals may require additional carbohydrates and fiber.

Creatine
- Usage: Three to ten grams post-exercise. Be sure to drink eight to ten 12-ounce glasses of water per day.
- Benefits: Enhances recovery and ATP replenishment
- Examples: Phosphagen HP, Synthevol HP, or RiboForce HP
- Notes: Products with d-Ribose should be used right before or during exercise. You can use similar products from reputable manufacturers, but remember to ingest ample carbohydrates according to meal plan.

Glutamine
- Usage: Four to five grams post-exercise

- Benefits: Enhances recovery and glycogen and glutamine replenishment
- Examples: CytoVol, glutamine powder
- Notes: Check to see if ample glutamine is included in your creatine product. If so, you're covered. You can use similar products from reputable manufacturers.

HMB (Beta-hydroxy beta-methylbutyrate)
- Usage: Three grams per day
- Benefits: Decreases muscle-protein breakdown
- Examples: BetaGen, HMB capsules
- Notes: You can use similar products from reputable manufacturers.

Thermogenic
- Usage: Consult with your physician first and foremost. Use as directed on packaging, and read all warning statements carefully.
- Benefits: Increases caloric expenditure and energy
- Examples: BetaLean HP
- Notes: You can use similar products from reputable manufacturers. Remember to consult with your physician first and foremost. Use as directed on packaging, and read all warning statements carefully.

Beta-ecdysterone plus Methoxy-isoflavone
- Usage: Two times per day (post-exercise and nighttime with protein meal)
- Benefits: Reduces muscle protein breakdown
- Examples: MethoxyFactor HP
- Notes: You can use similar products from reputable manufacturers. Dosage is usually 25-40 mg of ecdysterone plus 200-400 mg of methoxyisoflavone.

Essential Fatty Acids (EFAs)

- Usage: With meals when essential fatty acids are needed
- Benefits: Maintain healthy hormone levels
- Examples: EFA's, flaxseed oil, hemp oil, and olive oil
- Notes: Check label to calculate needs

High-End $$$ Muscularity Phase Supplementation

Meal Supplements—meal-replacement powders (MRPs), bars, ready-to-drink shakes (RTDs) and protein powders

- Usage: Use MRPs and protein powders to create two to four supplemental meals. Use RTDs and bars for convenience.
- Benefits: Increases protein and meal frequency, enhances recovery, and repairs damaged muscles.
- Examples: MRPs from reputable manufacturers: Myoplex (Regular and Deluxe), RTDs and bars, Precision Protein, and Simply Whey
- Notes: You can use similar products from reputable manufacturers. Remember, many meals may require additional carbohydrates and fiber.

Creatine

- Usage: Three to ten grams post-exercise. Be sure to drink eight to ten 12-ounce glasses of water per day.
- Benefits: Enhances recovery and ATP replenishment
- Examples: Phosphagen HP, Synthevol HP, or RiboForce HP
- Notes: Products with d-Ribose should be used right before or during exercise. You can use similar products from reputable manufacturers, but remember to ingest ample carbohydrates according to meal plan.

Glutamine

- Usage: Four to five grams post-exercise plus

four to five grams with two to three other meals
- Benefits: Enhances recovery and glycogen and glutamine replenishment
- Examples: CytoVol, glutamine powder
- Notes: Check to see if ample glutamine is included in your creatine product. If so, you're covered. You can use similar products from reputable manufacturers.

HMB (Beta-hydroxy beta-methylbutyrate)
- Usage: Three grams per day
- Benefits: Decreases muscle-protein breakdown
- Examples: BetaGen, HMB capsules
- Notes: You can use similar products from reputable manufacturers.

Thermogenic
- Usage: Consult with your physician first and foremost. Use as directed on packaging, and read all warning statements carefully.
- Benefits: Increases caloric expenditure, energy
- Examples: BetaLean HP
- Notes: You can use similar products from reputable manufacturer. Remember to consult with your physician first and foremost. Use as directed on packaging, and read all warning statements carefully.

Beta-ecdysterone plus Methoxy-isoflavone
- Usage: Three times per day (breakfast, post-exercise, and nighttime with a protein meal)

- Benefits: Reduces muscle-protein breakdown
- Examples: MethoxyFactor HP
- Notes: You can use similar products from reputable manufacturers. Dosage is usually 25-40 mg of ecdysterone plus 200-400 mg of methoxyisoflavone.

Essential Fatty Acids (EFAs)
- Usage: With meals where essential fatty acids are needed
- Benefits: Maintain healthy hormone levels
- Examples: EFAs, flaxseed oil, hemp oil, and olive oil
- Notes: Check label to calculate needs

Glucose Disposal Cocktail
- Usage: Post-exercise meal
- Benefits: Glycogen, glutamine, and creatine storage
- Examples: 50-100 mg d-pinitol, 200-400 mg alpha-lipoic acid, 24-28 mg colosolic acid
- Notes: Some nutrients may be included in your creatine product. Add others as needed

Antioxidant
- Usage: Take with two meals and after training
- Benefits: Muscle repair/recovery and supports immune system
- Examples: ACE, AAB, NAC, Vitamin E
- Notes: You can use similar products from reputable manufacturers. Dosage is dependent on the company.

SUPPLEMENTATION FOR THE MAXIMUM MUSCULARITY DIET

The supplement guidelines for the Maximum Muscularity Diet places a tighter focus on lower carbohydrate versions of MRPs, bars and ready-to-drink shakes. Here again, there are three programs to choose from—economy, mid-range, and high-end depending on your supplement budget. You should already be familiar with your protein needs from the previous diets, so start your meal planning from that perspective. Just like the Muscularity Diet, this stage is a more critical time to be supplementing with nutrients that may help you protect lean muscle tissue—glutamine, ecdysterone, HMB, and methoxyisoflavone.

Economy $ Maximum Muscularity Phase Supplementation

Meal Supplements—meal-replacement powders (MRPs), bars, ready-to-drink shakes (RTDs) and protein powders

• Usage: Use MRPs and protein powders to create two to four supplemental meals. Use RTDs and bars for convenience.

• Benefits: Increases protein and meal frequency, enhances recovery, and repairs damaged muscles.

• Examples: MRPs from reputable manufacturers: Myoplex (Regular and Deluxe), RTDs and bars, Precision Protein, and Simply Whey

• Notes: You can use similar products from reputable manufacturers. Remember, many meals may require additional carbohydrates and fiber.

Creatine

• Usage: Three to ten grams post-exercise. Be sure to drink eight to ten 12-ounce glasses of water per day.

• Benefits: Enhances recovery and ATP replenishment

• Examples: Phosphagen HP, Synthevol HP, or RiboForce HP

• Notes: Products with d-Ribose should be used right before or during exercise. You can use similar products from reputable manufacturers, but remember to ingest ample carbohydrates according to meal plan.

Glutamine

• Usage: Two to three grams post-exercise

plus one to two grams with two other meals

- Benefits: Enhances recovery and glycogen and glutamine replenishment
- Examples: CytoVol, glutamine powder
- Notes: Check to see if ample glutamine is included in your creatine product. If so, you're covered. You can use similar products from reputable manufacturers.

HMB (Beta-hydroxy beta-methylbutyrate)

- Usage: Three grams per day
- Benefits: Decreases muscle protein breakdown
- Examples: BetaGen, HMB capsules
- Notes: You can use similar products from reputable manufacturers.

Thermogenic

- Usage: Consult with your physician first and foremost. Use as directed on packaging, and read all warning statements carefully
- Benefits: Increases caloric expenditure and energy
- Examples: BetaLean HP
- Notes: You can use similar products from reputable manufacturer. Remember to consult with your physician first and foremost. Use as directed on packaging, and read all warning statements carefully.

Mid-Range $$ Maximum Muscularity Phase Supplementation

Meal Supplements—meal-replacement powders (MRPs), bars, ready-to-drink shakes (RTDs) and protein powders

- Usage: Use MRPs and protein powders to create two to four supplemental meals. Use RTDs and bars for convenience.
- Benefits: Increases protein and meal frequency, enhances recovery, and repairs damaged muscles.
- Examples: MRPs from reputable manufacturers: Myoplex (Regular and Deluxe), RTDs and bars, Precision Protein, and Simply Whey
- Notes: You can use similar products from reputable manufacturers. Remember, many meals may require additional carbohydrates and fiber.

Creatine

- Usage: Three to ten grams post-exercise. Be sure to drink eight to ten 12-ounce glasses of water per day.
- Benefits: Enhances recovery and ATP replenishment
- Examples: Phosphagen HP, Synthevol HP, or RiboForce HP
- Notes: Products with d-Ribose should be used right before or during exercise. You can use similar products from reputable manufacturers, but remember to ingest ample carbohydrates according to meal plan.

Glutamine

- Usage: Three to four grams post-exercise

plus two to three grams with two other meals
- Benefits: Enhances recovery and glycogen and glutamine replenishment
- Examples: CytoVol, glutamine powder
- Notes: Check to see if ample glutamine is included in your creatine product. If so, you're covered. You can use similar products from reputable manufacturers.

HMB (Beta-hydroxy beta-methylbutyrate)
- Usage: Three grams per day
- Benefits: Decreases muscle protein breakdown
- Examples: BetaGen, HMB capsules
- Notes: You can use similar products from reputable manufacturer.

Thermogenic
- Usage: Consult with your physician first and foremost. Use as directed on packaging, and read all warning statements carefully
- Benefits: Increases caloric expenditure and energy
- Examples: BetaLean HP
- Notes: You can use similar products from reputable manufacturer. Remember to consult with your physician first and foremost. Use as directed on packaging, and read all warning statements carefully.

Beta-ecdysterone plus Methoxyisoflavone
- Usage: Two times per day (post-exercise and nighttime with a protein meal)
- Benefits: Reduces muscle-protein break-

down
- Examples: MethoxyFactor HP
- Notes: You can use similar products from reputable manufacturers. Dosage is usually 25-40 mg of ecdysterone plus 200-400 mg of methoxyisoflavone.

Essential Fatty Acids (EFAs)
- Usage: With meals where essential fatty acids are needed
- Benefits: Maintain healthy hormone levels
- Examples: EFAs, flaxseed oil, hemp oil, and olive oil
- Notes: Check label to calculate needs

High-End $$$ Maximum Muscularity Phase Supplementation

Meal Supplements—meal-replacement powders (MRPs), bars, ready-to-drink shakes (RTDs) and protein powders

- Usage: Use MRPs and protein powders to create two to four supplemental meals. Use RTDs and bars for convenience.
- Benefits: Increases protein and meal frequency, enhances recovery, and repairs damaged muscles.
- Examples: MRPs from reputable manufacturers: Myoplex (Regular and Deluxe), RTDs and bars, Precision Protein, and Simply Whey
- Notes: You can use similar products from reputable manufacturers. Remember, many meals may require additional carbohydrates and fiber.

Creatine

- Usage: Three to ten grams post-exercise. Be sure to drink eight to ten 12-ounce glasses of water per day.
- Benefits: Enhances recovery and ATP replenishment
- Examples: Phosphagen HP, Synthevol HP, or RiboForce HP
- Notes: Products with d-Ribose should be used right before or during exercise. You can use similar products from reputable manufacturers, but remember to ingest ample carbohydrates according to meal plan.

Glutamine

- Usage: Four to five grams post-exercise plus four to five grams with two to three other meals
- Benefits: Enhances recovery and glycogen and glutamine replenishment
- Examples: CytoVol, glutamine powder
- Notes: Check to see if ample glutamine is included in your creatine product. If so, you're covered. You can use similar products from reputable manufacturers.

HMB (Beta-hydroxy beta-methylbutyrate)

- Usage: Three grams per day
- Benefits: Decreases muscle-protein breakdown
- Examples: BetaGen, HMB capsules
- Notes: You can use similar products from reputable manufacturers.

Thermogenic

- Usage: Consult with your physician first and foremost. Use as directed on packaging, and read all warning statements carefully.
- Benefits: Increases caloric expenditure, energy
- Examples: BetaLean HP
- Notes: You can use similar products from reputable manufacturer. Remember to consult with your physician first and foremost. Use as directed on packaging, and read all warning statements carefully.

Beta-ecdysterone plus Methoxy-isoflavone

- Usage: Three times per day (breakfast, post-exercise, and nighttime with a protein meal)

- Benefits: Reduces muscle-protein break-down
- Examples: MethoxyFactor HP
- Notes: You can use similar products from reputable manufacturers. Dosage is usually 25-40 mg of ecdysterone plus 200-400 mg of methoxyisoflavone.

Essential Fatty Acids (EFAs)
- Usage: With meals where essential fatty acids are needed
- Benefits: Maintain healthy hormone levels
- Examples: EFAs, flaxseed oil, hemp oil, and olive oil
- Notes: Check label to calculate needs

Glucose Disposal Cocktail
- Usage: Post-exercise meal
- Benefits: Glycogen, glutamine, and creatine storage
- Examples: 50-100 mg d-pinitol, 200-400 mg alpha-lipoic acid, 24-28 mg colosolic acid
- Notes: Some nutrients may be included in your creatine product. Add others as needed

d-Ribose
- Usage: Three to ten grams immediately before or during training
- Benefits: Enhances anaerobic peak power output
- Examples: RiboForce HP, straight d-ribose
- Notes: You can use similar products from reputable manufacturers.

Antioxidant
- Usage: Take with two meals and after training
- Benefits: Muscle repair/recovery and sup-
- ports immune system
- Examples: ACE, AAB, NAC, Vitamin E
- Notes: You can use similar products from reputable manufacturers. Dosage is dependent on the company.

Supplement Rotation for Maximum Benefits

The options listed in the previous text will make creating your personal supplement program easier and more effective. Keep in mind that the "core concept" behind the Periodized Bodybuilding and Nutrition Programs in this book is to keep your body responding by systematically making changes in both your diet and exercise regimen. For this reason, don't allow yourself to choose exactly the same supplements each and every time you are in a particular phase. The best strategy is to mix it up. For example, there are several types of products that are designed to decrease muscle protein breakdown, but for maximum results you should rotate them in a cyclical manner. You may want to use specific combinations such as using ecdysterone plus methoxyisoflavone for one cycle and HMB plus extra glutamine in the next. The bottom line is don't stay on any one compound for more than 12 weeks. Keeping track of the supplements you take and in what quantities will allow you to systematically give your body the change it needs by rotating them in and out.

"Winning is something that builds physically and mentally every day you train and every night that you dream."

-Emmitt Smith

Chapter

6

Defining the Hardgainer—Providing Solutions

The following chapter contains the latest techniques for attaining maximum muscle size for the hardgainer, but must only be followed after you complete at least one eight-week cycle of the Bodybuilding Foundation Diet outlined in the previous chapter. This chapter will only make sense after you have grasped the information that is presented in the Bodybuilding Foundation Diet.

Are You a Hardgainer?

The most common problem many people have is losing the fat, not gaining muscle. But if you find it difficult to put on solid muscle mass, you might be a hardgainer. In the real world, the true hardgainer is hard to define because there are so many variables that may affect your ability to put on muscle. One method is that of using Somatypes (body-type classification). This system defines three distinct categories of human bodies: the endomorph, characterized by a prevalence of bodyfat; the mesomorph, discernible by a well-developed musculature; and the ectomorph, distinguished by a lack of either much bodyfat or muscle tissue.

In the 1940s, William H. Sheldon introduced this theory of Somatypes in two main works, *The Varieties of Human Physique* (1940) and *The Varieties of Human Temperament: A Psychology of Constitutional Differences* (1941). His hypothesis projected the above-mentioned three basic body types, and connected them with sets of personality traits. In the present day, Sheldon's explanation of three body types is common when speaking about weight loss, exercise, and bodybuilding. Nevertheless, this basic classification of body types is less precise when you realize you might not always fall neatly into one category. On the next page is Sheldon's basic body-type classification chart.

As you can see, it is not easy to cast yourself into one category exclusively. Virtually all of

Body-Type Characteristics

ECTOMORPH	MESOMORPH	ENDOMORPH
▪ Thin	▪ Hard, muscular body	▪ Soft body
▪ Flat chest	▪ Overly mature appearance	▪ Underdeveloped muscles
▪ Delicate build	▪ Rectangular shaped	▪ Round shaped
▪ Young appearance	▪ Thick skin	▪ Over-developed digestive system
▪ Tall	▪ Upright posture	▪ Trouble losing weight
▪ Lightly muscled	▪ Gains or loses weight easily	▪ Generally gains muscle easily
▪ Crouched shoulders	▪ Grows muscle quickly	
▪ Large brain		
▪ Has trouble gaining weight		
▪ Muscle growth takes longer		

us have some characteristics that we would like to see improved, or better yet, wish we could change all together. If you can determine which of these body types you are most like, you may be on your way to unlocking the keys to gaining lean muscle mass. For example, if you think you are an ectomorph, the likely candidate for true hardgainer status, exploit the fact that you may be taller than average, have trouble gaining bodyfat, and may even look younger than your years! Vince Gironda, one of the greatest bodybuilding "gurus" ever, often stated that the hallmark of the athlete with an impressive physique is that they are not worriers, have a happy outlook on life, and think positively.

Overcoming Hardgainer "Neurosis"

One of the most interesting parallels in Sheldon's work is the body-type personality connection. His work reveals that there are personality traits that have strong links to body type. Here are a few examples: Extreme mesomorphs, the guys in the gym who seem to just look at the weights and grow muscles, are likely to be self-sufficient, resourceful, decisive, assertive, aggressive, and stubborn. The qualities of an endomorph, or those who have trouble losing fat, tend to be warm-hearted, easygoing, participating, enthusiastic, and happy-go-lucky. Finally, the ectomorph, which is the likely candidate for being a hardgainer, tends to be shy, timid, and anxious, with a myriad of nervous habits.

The moral of the story is that if you are a true hardgainer, part of the problem may be ingrained in your nervous system. You can alter this by consciously slowing down, worrying and obsessing less, and being more methodical in your diet and training. Of course, another integral piece to the puzzle is how to eat and train, which we will discuss.

The Hardgainer "Syndrome"

If you were to search for "bodybuilding hardgainers" on the Internet, you would find web sites and newsgroups that are full of information that implies nearly everyone in the gym who makes gains are genetic abnormalities or are on some sort European pharmaceutical combination for animals. The rest of us normal guys or girls are doomed because we have hardgainer syndrome. Now, from personal experience, I agree we are all hardgainers to some degree. After all, being skinny is the reason many athletes get into bodybuilding in the first place!

I am naturally an ectomorph and have a skinny body, so I have had plenty of experience with being a hardgainer. First, I believe that the biggest problem for any of you who thinks you are in this category is **knowledge**. More specifically, knowledge of daily caloric needs, proper nutrition, holistic training, recovery, and yes, supplementation. The next biggest problem is assessing your strong and weak points and making the best of them. I've seen lack of focus and not knowing your limitations wreck even the most gifted athletes.

A very close friend recently demonstrated this example to me. Here was a guy who was by all means small-boned, yet who had very good muscularity. However, he always resented the fact that he could have been mistaken for a male model. I don't mean a skinny model for some men's cologne either; this guy had great symmetry and surely enough muscle to attract his share of women. But for some reason he wanted to pursue power lifting, which seemed to be something that was totally against his genetic makeup. When I confronted him about this, he admitted that he really did not want to lose the look of his current physique, he was only depressed that his lifts were not off the charts! To me, this is a classic case of not knowing what you want to achieve, or utilizing your genetic gifts.

> "Many hardgainers believe sports supplements and the companies that market them are full of hot air."

More Hardgainer Beliefs

The last factor related to the hardgainer syndrome is that many of these athletes have already given up on making impressive gains, and have either lost interest or are searching for excuses not to succeed. This educated guess is based on the following observation: Ironically, many dyed-in-the-wool hardgainers believe sports supplements and the companies that market them are all full of hot air. They think "none of that stuff really works," and that it is all just a bunch of marketing hype. I agree there are good and bad companies in this industry, but a generalized statement like this, in light of all the recent scientific data to support many of these products, almost guarantees ignorance. This is especially ridiculous since the most cynical hardgainers usually want to cut training down to just one high-intensity workout every seven to ten days. This type of training suggests an abnormally low amount of sets per workout and workouts per week, and is called H.I.T. or high-intensity training. Now don't get me wrong, I know that intensity is one key component to turning on your muscle-building machinery. Nevertheless, any experienced weight-training coach will tell you that this is only part of the "muscle-size" puzzle. And the purpose of this chapter is to fit all the pieces of the puzzle together so you can gain the muscle mass you've always wanted as a hardgainer.

The True Hardgainer's Biggest Problem

Is there any difference between a good base diet such as the Bodybuilding Foundation Diet and a lean-mass-gaining diet for the hardgainer? The answer is an emphatic YES. As I stated in Chapter 3, the power of the Periodized Bodybuilding Nutrition System is harnessed only by continually manipulating your macronutrient ratios to trigger different metabolic responses. If you're a true hardgainer, you must address several vital factors so that gaining lean mass is a reality. Number one is "maximizing" your body's natural growth-promoting anabolic hormones, insulin and testosterone. Second, your diet must minimize catabolic hormones such as cortisol and glucagon, muscle-destroying demons that can literally "chew" up hard-earned muscle tissue. Last but not least, your diet must have enough energy substrates available to allow glycogen storage to take place. The Hardgainer Diet is designed with these factors in mind, and if

you follow this regimen, I am confident you will see dramatic improvements over other mass-gaining programs.

Depressing the Muscle-Destroying Demons

There are several attributes that are common among athletes and bodybuilders who are true "hardgainers." One of the most significant, and that which has the most validity in the scientific community, is fuel metabo-

> "There are several attributes that are common among athletes and bodybuilders who are true 'hardgainers.'"

lism. Scientific evidence shows that a true hardgainer likely has a higher metabolism than ordinary athletes do. By analyzing the problem, it becomes clear that the goal of the hardgainer's diet regimen is to modify the energy balance in a way that does not totally interrupt fat metabolism. Since you already have a constant number of protein grams in the Bodybuilding Foundation Diet, the logical macronutrients for you to modify are carbohydrates and fats. The truth of the matter is that while frequent dieters or endomorphs often suffer from an over-abundance of glucose, which can hinder the fat-burning process, hardgainers suffer from glucose insufficiency, which makes gaining lean muscle size very difficult. Here's why.

Hardwired for Glucose Insufficiency— The Hardgainer Dilemma

We established in the Bodybuilding Foundation Diet that your basic carbohydrate intake should be equal to your daily protein intake. However, we are assuming that if you are a true hardgainer, you tend to suffer from anxiousness and nervous habits, so you will need to calculate an increased number of carbs in your diet to offset this. Numerous studies show that adequate carbs in the diet can improve muscle glycogen stores and quench catabolic hormones such as cortisol. If you are looking to gain size, you need to also be aware that glycogen stores can account for a large increase in overall muscle cell volume. Muscle glycogen, which is the storage form of glucose (all carbs eventually become glucose), is an important aspect in how a bodybuilder's muscles look. My personal belief is that hardgainers never "top off" their glycogen stores because of their high metabolisms, which in turn makes their muscles look flat and impairs their performance to a larger degree than other body types.

Therefore, carbohydrates on the Hardgainer Diet should equal 1.6 grams per pound of lean bodyweight. For example, an athlete striving for a desired lean bodyweight (DLB) of 200 lbs would use the following formula: 200 lbs multiplied by the goal of 1.6 grams of carbohydrate per day equals 320 grams. As with protein, your goal should be to strive for 5 to 6 meals, with the carbohydrate content per meal at 54 to 64 grams. This example is illustrated in Figure 7, and will serve as your carb-per-meal guide on non-training days. For training days, you should follow the Maximum Recovery Hardgainer Diet seen in Figure 8. By following these guidelines, you can start to enjoy muscles that are bigger, fuller, and rounder.

The Glycemic Index—The Hardgainer's Secret Weapon

If you are a hardgainer, carbohydrate selection becomes even trickier, since you not only have an increased need for energy, but likely also want to stay lean while gaining mass. As you've already learned, the glycemic index of a carbohydrate affects your insulin levels. On the Bodybuilding Foundation Diet, I recommended consuming foods that elicit a small response in insulin levels during normal meals, and foods that elicit an amplified insulin response after your workout. Well, this application has even more relevance if you are on the Hardgainer Diet. Why? Simply put, the main problem with the higher carbohydrate diets that were in vogue in the late '80s is that many athletes created too much insulin, which put the brakes on the fat-burning process. This may confuse many of you, because as a hardgainer, you may not care that much about burning fat—but there is a critical reason why you should. Hardgainers still need to keep the fat-burning flame running high, because if your body stops using this fuel source, it will start using glucose from carbs to make up the difference. When this cycle starts, it will be even harder to fill up your glycogen stores, and you may gain excess fat to boot.

The secret to layering on lean mass while eluding bodyfat accumulation on the Hardgainer Diet is making sure every meal that is not eaten after your workout has a minimum of 1 gram of fiber for every 7 to 10 grams of carbs. Using this strategy, you can limit the amount of insulin produced after each meal, giving you a better chance to keep the fat-burning flame cranking, thus sparing carbs for muscle glycogen. In addition, by somewhat blunting the insulin response to carbs for regular meals, your body may actually overcompensate by cranking out additional insulin for post-exercise meals—which is the exact time you need it. Remember, it is after exercise, when your body has become depleted of glycogen and other energy stores, that insulin can best be utilized as an anabolic mechanism for enhancing growth and recovery. If you're still not familiar with the glycemic index, I suggest you go back to the Bodybuilding Foundation Diet in Chapter 4. Here again, understanding how to amplify insulin and manage the glycemic response to ingested carbs is truly one of the hottest areas in sports supplements today. I have more detailed explanations in Chapter 9, called "The Next Wave of Bodybuilding Supplementation." For a comprehensive list of foods and their glycemic index, as well as additional information, go to www.glycemic.com.

Fat Intake for Hardgainers

Due to the relationship with so many hormonal and nerve functions, your best bet is to increase the percentage of fat in your diet. Consuming more fat also makes sense because it can spare carbohydrates stored as muscle glycogen. Fat intake at 40% of your lean bodyweight multiplier is a perfect number to shoot for. For example, using the same 200-lb DLB goal, this would mean a fat intake of 80 grams divided into 6 meals (200 lbs multiplied by the 40% multiplier of grams of fat per day equals 80 grams). As with all the periodized nutrition plans, the best sources of fats are high in unsaturated fats and low in saturated fats. Most animal sources like ground beef, pork chops, and sausages contain saturated fats and should be avoided. Look for sources like flax, sunflower, and olive oils, salmon, black olives, avocados, and others. If you are used to eating a low-fat diet and find it difficult to get to these levels, I suggest using a good essential fatty acid supplement such as flaxseed, hemp oil, or an EPA blend for insurance.

THE HARDGAINER DIET NOTES

Protein Intake Calculations:

Take your DLB goal multiplied by 1.35 grams of protein per day. In the example, this equals 270 grams. And 270 grams of protein per day divided into 6 meals equals 45 grams per meal for non-training days (Figure 7), and will be adjusted for training days to make your post-exercise meals more effective (Figure 8).

Carbohydrate Intake Calculations:

Take your DLB multiplied by 1.6 grams of carbohydrate per day. In the example, this equals 320 grams. And 320 grams of carbohydrate per day divided into 6 meals equals

Figure 7

Desired Lean Bodyweight Multiplier 200 lbs.

Standard Hardgainer Diet	Protein	Carbs	Fat
Meal A	45	53.33	13.33
Meal B	45	53.33	13.33
Meal C	45	53.33	13.33
Meal D	45	53.33	13.33
Meal E	45	53.33	13.33
Meal F (Post-exercise example)	45	53.33	13.33
Total Grams per Macronutrient	270	320	80
Calories per Macronutrient	1080	1280	720
% Calories per Macronutrient + or - 1%	35%	42%	23%
Total Calories	3080		
Post-Exercise Meal Percentages (Example is Meal F)	17%	17%	17%

Figure 8

Desired Lean Bodyweight Multiplier 200 lbs.

Maximum Recovery Hardgainer Diet	Protein	Carbs	Fat
Meal A	36	40	18
Meal B	36	40	18
Meal C	36	40	18
Post-Exercise Primer (Immediately after training)	4	21	0
Post-Exercise Meal A (1 hour after training)	78.75	100	10
Post-Exercise Meal B (3 hours after training)	78.75	78.75	15
Total Grams per Macronutrient	269.5	319.75	79
Calories per Macronutrient	1078	1279	711
% Calories per Macronutrient + or - 1%	35%	42%	23%
Total Calories	3068		
Post-Exercise Meal Percentages	58%	56%	32%

about 55 grams per meal for non-training days (Figure 7), and will be adjusted for training days to make your post-exercise meals more effective (Figure 8).

Fat Intake Calculations:

Take your DLB multiplied by .40 grams of fat per day. In the example, this equals 80 grams. And 80 grams of fat per day divided into 6 meals equals 12 to 14 grams per meal on non-training days (Figure 7), and will be adjusted for training days to make your post-exercise meals more effective (Figure 8).

How Long Do I Stay on the Hardgainer Diet?

The Hardgainer Diet and training plan is designed for eight-week intervals. Once you complete eight weeks on the program, re-evaluate your progress and either repeat the cycle again, revert back to the Bodybuilding Foundation Diet and training, or move on to the fat-loss programs in the previous chapters. Remember, the cycling effect of each diet and their respective training regimen makes every module work better. Therefore, don't stay in a rut. Change is not only good, it's necessary.

SUPPLEMENTATION FOR THE HARDGAINER DIET

The supplement guidelines for the Hardgainer Diet takes into consideration that you will be consuming additional carbohydrates. Therefore, you will have more options available when choosing MRPs, bars, and ready-to-drink shakes. Increased carbohydrate intake is also why fiber intake is critically important in this phase—don't neglect this key piece of the nutrition puzzle. Remember your protein needs from the Foundation Diet and start your meal planning from there. This stage is a critical time to be supplementing with nutrients that may help you increase protein retention—glutamine, ecdysterone, HMB, and methoxyisoflavone. Of course, like

the previous diets, there are three programs to choose from—economy, mid-range and high-end depending on your supplement budget.

Economy $ Hardgainer Phase Supplementation

Meal Supplements—meal-replacement powders (MRPs), bars, ready-to-drink shakes (RTDs) and protein powders

- Usage: Use MRPs and protein powders to create two to four supplemental meals. Use RTDs and bars for convenience.
- Benefits: Increases protein and meal frequency, enhances recovery, and repairs damaged muscles.
- Examples: MRPs from reputable manufacturers: Myoplex (Regular and Deluxe), RTDs and bars, Precision Protein, and Simply Whey
- Notes: You can use similar products from reputable manufacturers. Remember, many meals may require additional carbohydrates and fiber.

Creatine

- Usage: Three to ten grams post-exercise. Be sure to drink eight to ten 12-ounce glasses of water per day.
- Benefits: Enhances recovery and ATP replenishment
- Examples: Phosphagen HP, Synthevol HP, or RiboForce HP
- Notes: Products with d-Ribose should be used right before or during exercise. You can use similar products from reputable manufacturers, but remember to ingest ample carbohydrates according to meal plan.

Glutamine

- Usage: Two to three grams post-exercise

- Benefits: Enhances recovery and glycogen and glutamine replenishment
- Examples: CytoVol and glutamine powder
- Notes: Check to see if ample glutamine is included in your creatine product. If so, you're covered. You can use similar products from reputable manufacturers.

Fiber Supplement

- Usage: As needed for fiber needs
- Benefits: Maintains proper glycemic environment
- Examples: Bran, syllium seed husks, guar gum, and apple pectin
- Notes: Cereals such as All Bran work well. Also check your local health food store.

Mid-Range $$ Hardgainer Phase Supplementation

Meal Supplements—meal-replacement powders (MRPs), bars, ready-to-drink shakes (RTDs) and protein powders

- Usage: Use MRPs and protein powders to create two to four supplemental meals. Use RTDs and bars for convenience.
- Benefits: Increases protein and meal frequency, enhances recovery, and repairs damaged muscles.
- Examples: MRPs from reputable manufacturers: Myoplex (Regular and Deluxe), RTDs and bars, Precision Protein, and Simply Whey
- Notes: You can use similar products from reputable manufacturers. Remember, many meals may require additional carbohydrates and fiber.

Creatine

- Usage: Three to ten grams post-exercise. Be sure to drink eight to ten 12-ounce glasses of water per day.
- Benefits: Enhances recovery and ATP replenishment
- Examples: Phosphagen HP, Synthevol HP, or RiboForce HP
- Notes: Products with d-Ribose should be used right before or during exercise. You can use similar products from reputable manufacturers, but remember to ingest ample carbohydrates according to meal plan.

Glutamine

- Usage: Two to three grams post-exercise plus one to two grams with one to two other meals

- Benefits: Enhances recovery and glycogen and glutamine replenishment
- Examples: CytoVol and glutamine powder
- Notes: Check to see if ample glutamine is included in your creatine product. If so, you're covered. You can use similar products from reputable manufacturers.

Fiber Supplement

- Usage: As needed for fiber needs
- Benefits: Maintains proper glycemic environment
- Examples: Bran, psyllium seed husks, guar gum, and apple pectin
- Notes: Cereals such as All Bran work well. Also check your local health food store.

Beta-ecdysterone plus Methoxy-isoflavone

- Usage: Two times per day (post-exercise and nighttime with protein meal)
- Benefits: Reduce muscle protein breakdown
- Examples: MethoxyFactor HP
- Notes: You can use similar products from reputable manufacturers. Dosage is usually 25-40 mg of ecdysterone plus 200-400 mg of methoxyisoflavone.

Essential Fatty Acids

- Usage: With meals when essential fatty acids are needed
- Benefits: Maintain healthy hormone levels
- Examples: EFA's, flaxseed oil, hemp oil, and olive oil
- Notes: Check label to calculate needs

High-End $$$ Hardgainer Phase Supplementation

Meal Supplements—meal-replacement powders (MRPs), bars, ready-to-drink shakes (RTDs) and protein powders

- Usage: Use MRPs and protein powders to create two to four supplemental meals. Use RTDs and bars for convenience.
- Benefits: Increases protein and meal frequency, enhances recovery, and repairs damaged muscles.
- Examples: MRPs from reputable manufacturers: Myoplex (Regular and Deluxe), RTDs and bars, Precision Protein, and Simply Whey
- Notes: You can use similar products from reputable manufacturers. Remember, many meals may require additional carbohydrates and fiber.

Creatine

- Usage: Three to ten grams post-exercise. Be sure to drink eight to ten 12-ounce glasses of water per day.
- Benefits: Enhances recovery and ATP replenishment
- Examples: Phosphagen HP, Synthevol HP, or RiboForce HP
- Notes: Products with d-Ribose should be used right before or during exercise. You can use similar products from reputable manufacturers, but remember to ingest ample carbohydrates according to meal plan.

Glutamine

- Usage: Four to five grams post-exercise plus four to five grams with two to three other meals

- Benefits: Enhances recovery and glycogen and glutamine replenishment
- Examples: CytoVol and glutamine powder
- Notes: Check to see if ample glutamine is included in your creatine product. If so, you're covered. You can use similar products from reputable manufacturers.

Fiber Supplement

- Usage: As needed for fiber needs
- Benefits: Maintains proper glycemic environment
- Examples: Bran, psyllium seed husks, guar gum, and apple pectin
- Notes: Cereals such as All Bran work well. Also check your local health food store.

Beta-ecdysterone plus Methoxy-isoflavone

- Usage: Three times per day (breakfast, post-exercise, and nighttime with a protein meal)
- Benefits: Reduces muscle protein breakdown
- Examples: MethoxyFactor HP
- Notes: You can use similar products from reputable manufacturers. Dosage is usually 25-40 mg of ecdysterone plus 200-400 mg of methoxyisoflavone.

Essential Fatty Acids (EFAs)

- Usage: With meals when essential fatty acids are needed
- Benefits: Maintain healthy hormone levels
- Examples: EFAs, flaxseed oil, hemp oil, and olive oil
- Notes: Check label to calculate needs

Glucose Disposal Cocktail

- Usage: Post-exercise meal

- Benefits: Glycogen, glutamine, and creatine storage
- Examples: 50-100 mg d-pinitol, 200-400 mg alpha-lipoic acid, 24-28 mg colosolic acid
- Notes: Some nutrients may be included in your creatine product. You can add others as needed.

Antioxidant
- Usage: Take with two meals and after training
- Benefits: Muscle repair/recovery and supports immune system
- Examples: ACE, AAB, NAC, Vitamin E
- Notes: You can use similar products from reputable manufacturers. The dosage is dependent on the company.

d-Ribose
- Usage: Three to ten grams immediately before or during training
- Benefits: Enhances anaerobic peak power output
- Examples: RiboForce HP, straight d-ribose
- Notes: You can use similar products from reputable manufacturers.

Supplement Rotation for Maximum Benefits

The options listed in the previous text will make creating your personal supplement program easier and more effective. Keep in mind that the "core concept" behind the Periodized Bodybuilding and Nutrition Programs in this book is to keep your body responding by systematically making changes in both your diet and exercise regimen. For this reason, don't allow yourself to choose exactly the same supplements each and every time you are in a particular phase. The best strategy is to mix it up. For example, there are several types of products that are designed to decrease muscle-protein breakdown, but for maximum results you should rotate them in a cyclical manner. You may want to use specific combinations such as using ecdysterone plus methoxyisoflavone for one cycle and HMB plus extra glutamine in the next. The bottom line is don't stay on any one compound for more than 12 weeks. Keeping track of the supplements you take and in what quantities will allow you to systematically give your body the change it needs by rotating them in and out.

"The only yardstick for success our society has is being a champion. No one remembers anything else."

-John Madden

Chapter

7

The Standard-Issue Supplements

When we talk about supplements, there are always several that instantly come to mind. These items occupy prominent space in our noodles because they are either totally bogus or because they actually work. We will keep our discussion to the supplements that work—in fact, we're going to center this particular discussion around products that should be considered "standard issue" for every hard-training athlete.

We'll first discuss the biological impetus driving us to seek these convenient meals like meal-replacement powders (MRPs), nutrition bars, and ready-to-drink beverages. I will then discuss how to incorporate these "gems" as the foundation of your nutritional structure. Then, in addition to these "foundation" items, we'll review the key supplements science has elevated to the dependable status of "standard issue" (meaning essential) for serious bodybuilders. Now that you know what we'll cover in this chapter, let's get after it.

Energy Collection

Our metabolic demands come from our need to survive. Simple enough, right? We are unique biological machinery that is in constant need of "service." Tissue breakdown and repair are part of the cycle, and require energy. And how do we consistently supply this energy without contributing to the unwanted storage of excess energy (i.e. body-fat)? We're oversimplifying, but you get the picture.

As we mentioned, your body's tissues must be repaired, and sometimes they must grow (or at least we force them into growing). This growth is stimulated by intense and deliberate exercise. If the muscle stimulation is significant, then we are rewarded with growth. These series of events are incessantly pursued by bodybuilders and fitness enthusiasts alike. But again, these events require energy.

Immediately usable sources of energy are not available to humans—we're not plants that can just grow on air, sunlight, and water. That is, we can't collect that precise energy "currency" our cells deal with when fueling their various forms of work. But evolution has been good to us. No longer are we forced to hunt in the wilderness, looking for energy sources for ourselves. For better or for worse, our current "environment" is abundant with supermarkets, convenience stores, and drive-thru grease peddlers.

> "...it can be quite the strenuous activity selecting convenient meals that are in line with our health and physique goals."

The collection of food is always thwarted by the fact that we, as humans, can never get the energy mix right. We'll choose the wrong types of food for the wrong moment in time. I mean, even when we're given a nutrient "map," as we outlined in Chapters 4 through 6, we still get off track. And further bugger-ing up the process is that a lot of us don't know the precise nutrient breakdown of the foodstuffs we pull out of our environment. Sometimes we provide our bodies with too much energy (overfeeding), and sometimes too little (underfeeding). Oftentimes, we give our bodies a different form of energy than they were hoping for.

Now I don't want to take us on a tangent, but hopefully it becomes obvious why we dis-cussed the significance of energy—and keep-ing energy on your side in the battle for a bet-ter physique. We were very particular about setting up the caloric values in the preceding chapters. So let's move forward into the dis-cussion of convenient meals, which are the tools that will help us stick to our goals.

Convenient Meals

I'm sure many of you reading this will attest that convenience plays an integral part in your everyday life. Let's face it; in our fast-paced world, we all need convenience. For bodybuilders and fitness enthusiasts alike, it can be quite the strenuous activity selecting convenient meals that are in line with our health and physique goals. I mean, a value meal consisting of a burger and fries can def-initely be considered a convenient "meal," but it surely doesn't come close to meeting the goals of someone concerned about losing fat and putting on muscle!

We just mapped out several diet plans that can help you achieve your particular goals, but oftentimes it is hard to find quick, easy, and efficient foods that fulfill our needs. This convenience "answer" we seek lies in the form of packets, bars, and ready-to-drink bev-erages that populate the health food and sports nutrition stores throughout the land. Besides the chronic lack of time on our hands, there is something else driving this need for convenient meals. As you'll remember from the preceding chapters, the metabolic signifi-cance of multiple feedings is great. And in this chapter, we'll lightly brush over the different types of meals that are available with respect to their strengths and weaknesses, as well as which products are best suited for your particular regimen.

Gaining muscle and stripping away bodyfat is a war, and the following are your military-issue strategic supplements. Strap 'em on, soldier! Don't go into battle without them.

Meal-Replacement Powders (MRPs)

The original meal replacement, the aptly named MRP, came on the scene in the early 1990s. Now, of course, there will be arguments about who pioneered the category, so we'll steer clear of that trap and concern ourselves with the attributes that make an MRP.

MRPs typically carry all the nutrients that the FDA recognizes as part of a balanced meal. Protein, carbohydrates, fat, fiber, vitamins, and minerals are all usual suspects in a true MRP. The most common MRP, and most suited for everyone's needs, are those products that tote around 45 to 50% of calories from protein, 35 to 40% calories from carbohydrate, with the remaining calories coming from fat. They range anywhere from 190 to 300 calories per serving, and adding to their convenience factor, most come in pre-portioned, highly portable packets.

MRPs are typically considered to be the best choice for nutrition when selecting a convenient meal. It earns this bragging right due to their consistent and predictable macronutrient profile. MRPs have become the foundation meal for use on all the previously described diets over the other convenient products because they (bars and ready-to-drink meals), have processing restraints that typically cause the powders to win the side-by-side nutritional comparison. Unfortunately, where they win in nutrition, they lose out in total convenience. After all, you still need to have access to water and a blender or shaker cup; and then there's the clean-up factor. All in all, MRPs are still the way to go, considering that there are so many on the market today. Whether you're a hardgainer or someone trying to strip away unwanted bodyfat, there is an MRP out there that meets your needs.

Ready-to-Drink Beverages (RTDs)

As you move down the convenience continuum, the next item is the ready-to-drink beverages (RTDs). The basic premise behind these beverages is to develop a more convenient form of the MRP or protein powder. There are several types of RTDs available. Everything from high-protein, bodybuilding-specific formulas to the ill-conceived "sugar in a can" approach by some popular, mainstream products.

Keep in mind that there are several processing techniques that may limit the functionality of some of these products. There have been a lot of recent advances in the processing techniques that allow formulators to get closer and closer to both the taste and nutritional value of MRPs. RTDs either come in plastic bottles, glass bottles, cans, or composite materials designed for aseptic processing (Tetra®). Here's what to look for when selecting the RTD for you:

Plastic Bottles—These products were the first to really impact the sports market. They typically have a low pH (acidic) and a fair amount of preservatives to keep the micro-organisms at bay. These items are shelf-stable, but are only good for about nine months. Due to the low pH, these beverages only come in fruit-based flavors (sorry, chocoholics). These beverages can have very solid nutritional profiles; they are low in fat (most have none), and their process allows them to use artificial sweeteners like aspartame or the increasingly popular sucralose. And I hope you like whey protein, because due to the processing techniques, whey protein is the only form of protein you'll find in these products.

Glass Bottles—The discussion around glass bottles is usually short, especially when you're talking about products that you can take with you to the gym. Glass is a huge "no way, dude" in the gym. And currently, outside of some of the pedestrian beverages, there are no serious RTDs that come in glass bottles. But glass does have some advantages. You can get away with using little or no preservatives, and the formulas can contain other milk proteins like casein.

Retort Cans—Through a process called retort, the product is literally cooked in the can. This is a sort of pasteurization process used to remove all the undesirable little critters. And fans of traditional shake flavors can rejoice. Milk proteins can be used, and the product pH is hovering around the neutral mark, so chocolate, vanilla, and strawberry are the typical flavor offerings. As with plastic bottles, most retort cans can deliver high marks in nutrition, with low fat content, little

or no sugar, and no preservatives. There are still some drawbacks to a can. Due to the cooking process, delicate proteins still get destroyed, and sometimes the product actually gets cooked to the bottom of the can, making it a struggle to get the muscle-nourishing nectar out of the penny-sized hole in the top.

Tetra—Tetra boxes have been around for a long time, but are just now finding their application relevant to the health and fitness market. You might recognize these "boxes" from the grocery stores as juice boxes or cartons of soymilk. Basically what you get with these packs is an aseptic process (similar to what goes on with glass packaging) that allows for a shelf-stable, milk-based product that isn't cooked in its container. The end results are usually a better-tasting, more user-friendly product.

Nutrition Bars

As you move down the convenience continuum toward the simplest form, you'll bump into the biggest and fastest growing market—nutrition bars. These bars are a familiar sight in any grocery, convenience, and health food store. There's no doubt that nutrition bars represent the ultimate in convenience, but do they really represent the ultimate in nutrition?

Be sure to read the labels on all your favorite bars. Oftentimes you'll find them loaded with sugar and fat. The so-called low-carb bars represent the latest trend. They offer anyone on the Muscularity Diet a chance to eliminate some of the carbohydrates from their daily intake. But watch out for these. Low-carbohydrate bars use glycerin to maintain moisture in the bar, a job usually reserved for high-fructose corn syrup or some other type of sugar syrup.

Now is removing sugar and replacing it with glycerin a bad thing? No, it's not necessarily a bad thing. However, keep in mind that glycerin yields about 4 calories per gram, and with many of these bars packed with 15 grams or greater of glycerin, it still means there is caloric significance. So you may be under your daily amount of carbohydrates, and right on with your protein and fat, but still be overboard on calories! Glycerin can be advantageous because of the simple fact that it does not trigger an immediate rise in circulating glucose as do the sugar syrups that glycerin replaces. As far as these glycerin-based bars parading around as low-carbohydrate bars... well, the FDA has reviewed the glycerin loophole, and may soon mandate that the glycerin be declared as a carbohydrate.

The Need for a Meal-Replacement

The need for convenient meal-replacement supplements are the product of our evolutionary shortcomings and our evolving "lifestyle" demands. Sure, whole foods can provide the basic nutrients you require, but they seldom address the simultaneous needs of convenience and nutritive quality. Not to mention, when was the last time you picked up a chicken dinner and could immediately ascertain the total protein, carbohydrates, fat, and calories in a single glance?

In addition, you can imagine how incredibly difficult it would be to provide day after day, meal after meal, a source of protein and energy

capable of conveniently addressing all of your needs. Incredibly difficult, that is, if you are intending to rely on "regular" food.

But as you can see, there are food alternatives. They are engineered to deliver a predictable amount of nutrition to enhance your training. Tear open an envelope, mix the contents with water, and dramatically bolster your productivity. Or pop the cap or tear open a wrapper, revealing a highly usable nutritional shortcut. A shortcut to convenience that doesn't leave your body feeling shortchanged.

> "...pop the cap or tear open a wrapper, revealing a highly usable nutritional shortcut."

Protein Powder—Adjunctive Adjustment

One note about protein powders: These can easily be added to your MRPs to get you the amount of protein that has been predetermined by your particular goals. Protein powders are extremely versatile, and can easily round out your daily protein needs. Each protein powder has about 20 to 25 grams of protein per ounce, with little to no carbohydrates and minimal fat. For more on the differences in individual proteins, please see Chapter 8, called "Protein, the Bedrock of Bodybuilding."

Creatine

Unless you have been in a hole for the last decade, you've heard of the effectiveness of creatine. Creatine has become probably the most popular supplement ever—and rightly so.

Creatine in its phosphocreatine form is used in muscle cells to store energy for explosive movements—movements that chew up ATP storage quickly—like sprinting, jumping, and, of course, weightlifting. When faced with an intense and acute workload, phosphocreatine is cracked into creatine and phosphate. The phosphate group is then used to regenerate the cellular energy currency, ATP. When ATP stores get depleted (and they do), output power drops and workouts suffer. So, the trick to keep your ATP clipping is to hypersaturate the available phosphocreatine. The easiest way to do this is through creatine supplementation.

But is it that easy? Do you just need to take a wad of creatine, and then the bounty of effects is yours for the taking? Well, it's a little more sophisticated than that, but not much. The debate has raged on about what is the ideal way to deliver creatine; here are some points of interest.

Creatine is typically administered in a loading phase, and then maintained through a maintenance phase. The loading phase is necessary to quickly elevate the cellular storage of creatine. The loading phase usually calls for a daily dose of 20 grams or more spread out over 3 to 4 doses. This ritual is usually carried on for a week, and then shifts into maintenance mode. While most people agree on the loading phase amount, when discussing maintenance amounts, the opinions start to differ. Several researchers have investigated daily doses ranging from 2.5 to 25 grams to facilitate creatine upkeep. But the bottom line is that the stuff works even at moderate doses.

The delivery of creatine is a whole different story. While most camps will concur that insulin is a driving factor in creatine uptake, recent research has determined that 50 grams of protein plus 50 grams of carbohydrate augments creatine retention to the same extent as ~90 grams of carbohydrates.[27] The latter protein/carbohydrate/creatine mixture just may be a better way to deliver creatine since not only does it supply amino acids, but it also reduces the amount of simple carbs required for an insulin effect into a range that is more in line with low-carb diets. In addition, several new compounds are being studied for their ability to amplify insulin secretion without resorting to ingesting huge amounts of simple sugars.

Indeed, new research is coming in every year that will surely change the way we look at creatine transport and delivery. We'll delve into the details in later chapters. As you progress through the chapters, you'll find that depending on your particular goals, your creatine use, dose, and delivery vehicle will vary.

Glutamine

Glutamine has been a hot supplement for quite some time now. Although this important amino acid can't deliver the feel-able effects like creatine or caffeine and ephedra, glutamine is a must-have for anyone pursuing a better physique.

Glutamine, traditionally considered a non-essential amino acid, often finds itself classified under the "conditionally essential" column—especially when strenuous exercise is the condition. After a bout of strenuous exercise, the metabolic activity of your body changes (as you might have guessed), triggering a cascade of events that warrant glutamine to give up its non-essential status.

Glutamine is the most abundant amino acid in the muscle, but it isn't necessarily in the muscle where glutamine works its wonders. In fact, the muscle cell does not possess an import mechanism for glutamine, instead intramuscular glutamine, synthesized from ammonia and glutamic acid, serves as a storehouse for more important biological functions than muscle building (yes, I hate to break it to you, there are more important functions). Glutamine plays a vital role in gut integrity and in the immune system.

Most quality MRPs contain ample amounts of glutamine, plus this popular amino acid is finding its way into everything from protein powders to creatine formulas. Here again, for those that are interested, the research on glutamine has demonstrated this amino acid's ability to support protein synthesis, muscle cell hydration, and immune function while limiting muscle catabolism and sparing glycogen.[23,24,25,26]

Ephedra and Caffeine

These two supplements have become the "gruesome twosome" of the industry. More controversy has surrounded this fat-burning dynamic duo than any other supplement on the market. So what gives? Why am I talking to you about controversial products? First, because they shouldn't be that controversial, and second, there is no other more potent supplement combination on the market for increasing caloric expenditure. And an increase in caloric expenditure is the road to an increase in bodyfat loss—end of story.

The Nitty Gritty on Caffeine and Ephedra's Fat-Burning Effects

This potent supplement combination essentially gives your metabolic rate a "tune up" that increases the fat-burning process. For those who can tolerate a little science tutorial, let me give you the background on lipolysis, commonly known as the fat-burning process.

> "...there is no other more potent supplement combination on the market for increasing caloric expenditure."

Lipolysis is the process of breaking down triglyceride molecules into one 3-carbon glycerol and three fatty acids. To complete this process, an enzyme called hormone-sensitive lipase or HSL is required. Compounds like ephedrine act to increase this process, thus increase fat burning. Ephedrine directly stimulates the central nervous system, causing the release of norepinephrine, and a subsequent rise in circulating epinephrine levels. These two work to trigger certain receptors, namely alpha and beta-adrenergic receptors, to initiate a complex sequence of events to increase lipolysis.

This sequence of events is rather complex, but here is a brief rundown. Ephedrine first stimulates the release of norepinephrine, and increases circulating levels of epinephrine. These then bind to the alpha and beta-receptors. As these bind, a subsequent rise is seen in levels of the enzyme adenylate cyclase. Adenylate cyclase is responsible for converting ATP or adenosine triphosphate into cyclic adenosine monophophate (cAMP). cAMP is what is known as a second messenger, due to the fact that it works indirectly, triggering another sequence of events to attain a certain outcome. cAMP binds to the regulatory protein kinase, which subsequently frees up its catalytic subunit. This catalytic subunit is what then phophorylates HSL to its active form. HSL then catalyses another sequence of events that breaks the bonds of a triglyceride molecule, exposing the free fatty acids for utilization as ATP or energy.

> "...it's not just about protein, carbs, and fat— vitamins and minerals play vital roles as well."

Caffeine, on the other hand, takes a more direct route at increasing the rate of fat burning. Caffeine works by two main functions. It increases circulating levels of norepinephrine, which then works by the above mechanisms to increase fat burning. In addition, caffeine also inhibits an enzyme called phophodiesterase or PDE. PDE works to decrease the amount of cAMP by catalyzing a reaction that renders cAMP as useless linear AMP. By inhibiting this negative feedback loop, it essentially allows this sequence of events to run without hindrance, thus increasing the rate of fat burning, and reducing the fat-storing effects of adenosine, a compound with multiple functions in the human body, while promoting the lipolytic and fat-burning effects of other agents in the body.

When used in combination, caffeine and ephedrine act synergistically to produce greater benefits than the sum of each taken on its own. But are they safe?

Again the issue of safety keeps coming up. Here are some direct quotes from the top researchers in the field with reference to ephedrine and caffeine for weight loss:

"During the last two years, defined doses daily of the E+C [ephedrine + caffeine] combination have been used in Denmark, but only 86 adverse drug reactions have been reported to the health authorities..." Breum et al. (1994)

"...most, if not all of the undesirable side-effects of ephedrine exhibit tachyphylaxis [disappearance with time], whereas the thermogenic [increased calorie/fat-burning] effects are preserved, or even enhanced

[(Astrup et al., 1985)] with chronic treatment." Dulloo and Stock (1993)

"Over-the-counter pharmaceutical preparations capable of stimulating metabolic [calorie/fat-burning] rate offer a relatively safe and already extensively tested range of drugs which may prove of use in the treatment of obesity." Horton and Geissler (1991).

The list of research to support this tag-team supplement mixture as a potent fat burner, energy, and workout-enhancer is as exhaustive as it is impressive.[9,10, 11,12,13,14,15,16,17,18,19,20,21,22] However, if you are still curious, just type in the references above in the Internet search engine at the National Library of Medicine, www.ncbi.nlm.nih.gov/PubMed , and you will no doubt become a believer that caffeine and ephedra deserve the rating as "standard issue."

One important precaution is even though I feel that these compounds are completely safe, you should check with your physician and completely read all package-warning labels before using this potent combination. Also be sure to read the extensive warning at the end of this chapter. Other than that, caffeine and ephedra can help you get that extra advantage in the war against bodyfat.

HMB

EAS pioneered supplemental HMB use beginning around 1996, and since then, an ever-increasing body of scientific research has shown that supplementing with HMB can improve lean body mass, endurance, strength, and even decrease muscle soreness.[1,2,3,4,5,6,7,8] With all of this solid science data, I feel that HMB should join the elite status of "standard issue."

The branched-chain amino acid (BCAA) metabolite ß-hydroxy ß-methylbutyrate monohydrate (HMB) has been shown to support the body's ability to minimize protein (i.e., muscle) breakdown and damage to muscle cells, which can occur after intense resistance exercise. In my personal experience, HMB is especially important on low-carb diets, therefore anyone on the Muscularity Diets should take note. By reducing muscle-tissue breakdown, HMB may tip the scales of protein turnover in favor of new muscle growth.

Vitamins and Minerals

For optimal performance of the human body, it's not just about protein, carbs, and fat—vitamins and minerals play vital roles as well.

As bodybuilders and athletes, we often get too focused on the macronutrients, and don't pay attention to micronutrients. Luckily for us, most of the meal replacements we consume are chock full of essential vitamins and minerals. Healthy eating habits don't hurt either. But we can't neglect the fact that some of these unsung vitamin heroes can help us stay in the saddle while we're desperately trying to reach our fitness goals. Here I'll refer you to Chapter 12, where you should familiarize yourself with all the vitamins and minerals—especially antioxidants and minerals.

Conclusion

There you have it. These are the essentials of any bodybuilder's tool chest. Meal-replacement powders, bars, and drinks to build the foundation. Protein powder for fine-tuning protein requirements. And the gizmos and gadgets that can augment all your hard work and efforts. Be sure to read Chapter 9, called "The Next Wave of Bodybuilding Supplementation," because you're bound to find out about the next amazing nutritional assault in the never-ending battle for the ultimate physique.

EPHEDRA AND CAFFEINE WARNING: NOT FOR USE BY INDIVIDUALS UNDER THE AGE OF 18. DO NOT USE IF PREGNANT OR NURSING. CONSULT A PHYSICIAN OR LICENSED QUALIFIED HEALTH CARE PROFESSIONAL BEFORE USING THIS PRODUCT IF YOU HAVE, OR HAVE A FAMILY HISTORY OF, HEART DISEASE, THYROID DISEASE, DIABETES, HIGH BLOOD PRESSURE, RECURRENT HEADACHES, DEPRESSION OR OTHER PSYCHIATRIC CONDITION, GLAUCOMA, DIFFICULTY IN URINATING, PROSTATE ENLARGEMENT, OR SEIZURE DISORDER, IF YOU ARE USING A MONOAMINE OXIDASE INHIBITOR (MAOI) OR ANY OTHER DIETARY SUPPLEMENT, PRESCRIPTION DRUG OR OVER-THE-COUNTER DRUG CONTAINING EPHEDRINE, PSEUDOEPHEDRINE OR PHENYLPROPANOLAMINE (INGREDIENTS FOUND IN CERTAIN ALLERGY, ASTHMA, COUGH/COLD, AND WEIGHT CONTROL PRODUCTS). EXCEEDING RECOMMENDED SERVING MAY CAUSE SERIOUS ADVERSE HEALTH EFFECTS INCLUDING HEART ATTACK AND STROKE. DISCONTINUE USE AND CALL A PHYSICIAN OR LICENSED QUALIFIED HEALTH CARE PROFESSIONAL IMMEDIATELY IF YOU EXPERIENCE RAPID HEARTBEAT, DIZZINESS, SEVERE HEADACHE, SHORTNESS OF BREATH, OR OTHER SIMILAR SYMPTOMS. INDIVIDUALS WHO CONSUME CAFFEINE, OR OTHER STIMULANTS, WITH THIS PRODUCT MAY EXPERIENCE SERIOUS ADVERSE HEALTH EFFECTS. KEEP OUT OF REACH OF CHILDREN.

References Cited

1 Panton, L.B., et al., "Nutritional supplementation of the leucine metabolite ß-hydroxy- ß-methylbutyrate (HMB) during resistance training" *Nutrition* 16 (2000) :734-739.

2 Knitter, A., et al., "Effects of ß-hydroxy- ß-methyl butyrate on muscle damage following a prolonged run." *J. Appl. Physiol.* 89 : 1340-1344.

3 Gallagher, P., J et. al, "Beta-hydroxy-beta-methylbutyrate ingestion, Part I: effects on strength and fat free mass. *Med. Sci. Sports Exer.* 32.12 (2000): 2109-2115

4 Byrd, P.L., et al., "Changes in muscle soreness and strength following downhill running: Effects of creatine, HMB, and Betagen supplementation." *Med. Sci. Sports Exer.* 31 : S263.

5 Vukovich, M.D., et al., "The effect of ß-hydroxy-ß-methylbutyrate (HMB) on VO2 peak and lactate threshold in endurance trained cyclists. *J. Strength and Conditioning.* In press.

6 Cohen, D.D., "The effect of ß-hydroxy-ß-methylbutyrate (HMB) and resistance training on changes in body composition during positive and negative energy balance - a randomized double-blind study." M.Sc. Thesis, St. Bartholomew's and Royal London School of Medicine and Dentistry, Queen Mary and Westfield College, University of London, London.

7 Nissen, S.L., Panton, J. Fuller, Jr., Rice, D., and Sharp, R., "Effect of feeding ß-hydroxy- ß-methyl butyrate (HMB) on body composition and strength of women. *FASEB J.* 11 (1997) : A150.

8 Vukovich, M.D. and Adams, G.D., "Effect of ß-hydroxy- ß-methyl butyrate (HMB) on VO2 peak and maximal lactate in endurance trained cyclists." *Med. Sci. Sports Exer.* 29 (1997) : S252.

9 Dulloo, A.G., Miller, D.S., "The thermogenic properties of ephedrine/methylxanthine mixtures: human studies." *Int J Obesity* 10 (1986) : 467-481.

10 Pasquali, R., Cesari, M.P., Besteghi, L., Melchionda, N., Balestra, V., "Thermogenic agents in the treatment of human obesity: preliminary results." *Int J Obesity* 11.3 (1987) : 23-26.

11 Astrup, A., Buemann, B., Christensen, N.J., Toubro, J., Thorbek, G., Victor, O.J., Quaade, F., "The effect of ephedrine/caffeine mixture on energy expenditure and body composition in obese women." *Metabolism* 41.7 (1992) : 686-688.

12 Astrup, A., Bruem, L., Toubro, S., Hein, P., Quaade, F., "The effect and safety of an ephedrine/caffeine compound compared to ephedrine, caffeine and placebo in obese subjects on an energy restricted diet. A double blind trial." *Int J Obesity* 16 (1992) : 269-277.

13 Toubro, S., Astrup, A., Breum, L., Quaade, F., "The acute and chronic effects of ephedrine/caffeine mixtures on energy expenditure and glucose metabolism in humans." *Int J Obesity* 17.3 (1993) : S73-S77.

14 Breum, L., Pedersen, J.K., Ahlstrom, F., Frimodt-Moller, J., "Comparison of an ephedrine/caffeine combination and dexfenfluramine in the treatment of obesity. A double-blind multi-centre trial in general practice." *Int J Obesity* 18 (1994) : 99-102.

15 Horton, T.J., Geissler, C.A., "Aspirin potentiates the effect of ephedrine on the thermogenic response to a meal in obese but not lean women." *Int J Obesity* 15 (1991) : 359-366.

16 Daly, P.A., Krieger, D.R., Dulloo, A.G., Young, J.B., Landsberg, L., "Ephedrine, caffeine and aspirin: safety and efficacy for treatment of human obesity." *Int J Obesity* 17.3 (1993) : S73-S78.

17 Colker, C.M., Kalman, D.S., Minsch, A., "Ephedrine, caffeine, and aspirin enhance fat loss under nonexercising conditions." *J Am Coll Nutr* 16.5 (1995) : 501.

18 Krieger, D.R., Daly, P.A., Dulloo, A.G., Ransil, B.J., Young, J.B., Landsberg, L., "Ephedrine, caffeine and aspirin promote weight loss in obese subjects." *Trans Assoc Am Phys* 103 (1990) : 306-312.

19 Dulloo, A.G. and Miller, D.S., "Aspirin as a promoter of ephedrine-induced thermogenesis: potential use in the treatment of obesity." *Am J Clin Nutr* 45 (1987) : 564-569.

20 Dulloo, A.G., "Ephedrine, xanthines and prostaglandin-inhibitors: actions and interactions in the stimulation of thermogenesis." *Int J Obesity* 17.3 (1993) : S35-S40.

21 Dulloo, A.G., Seydoux J, Girardier L, "Potentiation of the thermogenic antiobesity effects of ephedrine by dietary methylxanthines: adenosine antagonism or phosphodiesterase inhibition?" *Metabolism* 41.11 (1992) : 1233-1241.

22 Dulloo, A.G. and Miller, D.S., "Ephedrine, caffeine and aspirin: 'over-the-counter' drugs that interact to stimulate thermogenesis in the obese." *Nutrition* 5.1 (1989) : 7-9.

23 Rowbottom, D.G., Keast, D., Morton, A.R., "The emerging role of gluta-mine as an indicator of exercise stress and overtraining." *Sports Med* 21.2 (1996) : 80-97.

24 Jepson, M.M., Boles, P.C., Broadbent, P., Pell, J.M., Millward, D.J., "Relationship between glutamine concentration and protein synthesis in rat skeletal muscle." *Am J Physiol* 255 (1988 : E166-E172.

25 Rennie, M.J., Tadros, L., Khogali, S., Ahmed, A., Taylor, P.M., "Glutamine transport and its metabolic effects." *J Nutr* 124.8 (1994) : 1503S-1508S.

26 Varnier, M., Leese, G.P., Thompson, J., Rennie, M.J., "Stimulatory effect of glutamine on glycogen accumulation in human skeletal muscle." *Am J Physiol* 269 (1995) : 309-315.

27 Steegne, G.R., Simpson, E.J., Greenhaff, P.L., "Protein- and carbohydrate-induced augmentation of whole body creatine retention." *J Appl. Phys.* 89 (2000) :1165-1171.

"Knowing is not enough;
we must apply.
Willing is not enough;
we must do."

-Bruce Lee

Chapter
8

Protein—The Bedrock of BodyBuilding

As you read through this book, the chapters on diet and supplementation will all speak of one reoccurring element. In fact, this element links together just about all the written pieces on bodybuilding nutrition. This element is, of course, protein intake — huge, heroic protein intake. There is not one esoteric gadget or supplement on this planet that can have more impact on your physique than protein. It's no wonder that the word "protein" was derived over 150 years ago from the Greek word proteios, which means "of prime importance."

But with all this talk about protein, unanswered questions still remain. What type of protein is the best and why? In this section, I will give you an overview of the different types of popular physique augmenting proteins, as well as the positives and negatives of each. I will also discuss some of the processing techniques that can make a definite difference in both the quality and function of the end product.

"Obsession in Pursuit of Dream is Not a Vice"-unknown

I am not sure where I heard the above statement, but when it comes to bodybuilders' obsession with protein intake, it couldn't be more fitting. Bodybuilders realize that muscles need protein to repair, rebuild, and most of all, GROW! Thus, various protein powders have been considered "must-use" supplements for over 40 years (see the chapter on standard-issue supplements). The issue of protein intake and protein sources is multifaceted and is being continually updated and redefined as the science of sports nutrition moves forward. As a matter of fact, the science surrounding new protein technologies is moving so quickly that no one in the market seems to be able to keep up. The focus on protein supplements (especially among bodybuilders and other athletes) has become quite one-sided. Currently, there is one protein that has become the "belle of the ball" for bodybuilders. This, of course, is whey protein.

The previous statement should not be misconstrued. I do believe whey protein proponents are one-sided in their view AND I do believe that whey protein is a great source of protein. However, I feel that proper attention has been withheld from other quality proteins—namely certain milk proteins—because nutritional science rolls on. Just think, if scientists had stopped researching proteins back in the 1960s after they determined egg protein to be the "gold standard" protein for humans—we'd all still be choking down a glassful of egg whites every morning.

Understanding the "Bodybuilding Value" of Different Proteins

There are certain "absolutes" where protein intake is concerned. Almost every bodybuilder knows he/she needs to consume a minimum amount of protein every day (as you probably noticed, I recommend 1.35 grams per pound of lean body mass) in order to supply the amino acid building blocks necessary to support muscle growth. Bodybuilders also know the quality of protein is important (complete proteins versus incomplete proteins). However, we see a slight decrease in the need for quality as the absolute number of grams (and total calories) increases. However, the higher the protein quality, the easier it is for the body to use the amino acids, and the more likely one's going to meet your body's demands. Therefore, it is best to concern yourself with getting quality proteins most of the time and aim for your target amount—this will help to eliminate the guesswork. Does this protein have the right amino acid profile? Is this the best form of whey protein? What is the best form of milk protein?

In this chapter, I'll give you an overview on the latest science behind a number of quality protein sources—their functional properties, their strengths and weaknesses, and special uses for each, either alone or in combinations. For the most part I will talk about real-world benefits—some authors are calling it BV. But BV is not an acronym for the traditional (albeit uncertain) "Biological Value" but for the more relevant **Bodybuilding Value.**

One important note: As you learn about the different types and processes of certain proteins, you may notice that your favorite protein supplement or meal-replacement shake (MRP) does not disclose all the fine details about the protein it contains. Typically ingredient lists will give you a breakdown of the multiple proteins in descending order, but no details are available about whether the protein is a 90% concentrate or 30% concentrate—it may be just list whey protein concentrate. Hopefully that will change.

WHEY PROTEIN—Top of the Heap or Top of the Hype?

As I mentioned earlier, whey proteins have been crowned as the ultimate bodybuilder protein. This accolade was bestowed upon whey based on its essential amino acid composition, its branched-chain amino acid content, and its rapid absorption, as well as its physical properties like taste, solubility, and processing resilience. All these attributes, fueled by page after page of advertisements and editorial, have set whey protein at the top of the heap.

The origin of today's high-quality whey proteins is kind of an interesting story. You see, whey is one of the two major types of protein found in milk (casein is the other—and interestingly the casein to whey ratio is 4:1). It was originally isolated as a byproduct of cheese production. When cheese is made, the milk is "curdled," separating the curd from the whey. The curd initially looks like (and is) cottage cheese and contains mostly casein, while the whey is a syrupy sweet liquid that contains a variety of other proteins and large amounts of lactose. Up until not too long ago, it was thought that whey was worthless, and it was simply thrown out as a waste product.

> "There are certain 'absolutes' where protein intake is concerned."

Necessity is the Mother of Invention

Pressured by the Environmental Protection Agency (EPA), cheese producers had to stop dumping the whey into nearby waterways, and eventually someone got the bright idea to figure out a way to get rid of the waste product while recouping some of the costs associated with the disposal. When the cheese makers started looking closely, they found that whey was a substance loaded with a variety of proteins. Upon further investigation, it was discovered these proteins were of very high quality. Not only did they dissolve well in water; they were also highly digestible and contained a better amino acid profile than even the highly regarded egg white.

From that point, attention has turned to separating these high-quality proteins from the undesirable lactose, fat, and cholesterol components of whey. Over the years, many processes were developed, including high-heat drying and acid-treatment extractions. Unfortunately, both of these processes were destructive to the proteins, changing their characteristics and ruining their quality (as far as protein supplementation was concerned). Keep in mind, traditional food manufacturers were the first to benefit from the use of whey. Whey protein was an excellent addition to low-fat foods and worked wonders in baked goods and salad dressings (read the ingredients sometime for kicks).

So what became of all this poking and prodding? What did the whey protein mavericks come up with? Well, basically the trick was to refine the liquid whey — which is about 0.6% protein and 93% water, with lactose, ash, and milk fat rounding out the difference. Initially the whey protein was "washed" with acid to precipitate the protein, but this process destroyed all the acid-sensitive goodies. Washed away or destroyed in the acid bath were important microfractions like glyco-macropeptides, alpha-lactalbumin, immuno-globins, and lactoferrin. These "goodies" are what breathe life into whey protein's special characteristics. The details of their specific functions are too voluminous to explore in this chapter, but I'll tell you this, these microfractions play important roles in areas such as immune response and possibly, in an indirect way, muscle growth.

But recently a couple of processes were perfected that have the ability to extract the proteins from whey while preserving their "integrity." These processes are micro-filtration (where the proteins are physically separated by a microscopic filter) and ion exchange (where proteins are extracted by taking advantage of their specific electronic charges). Both of these processes yield a high-quality, low-lactose, low-fat whey protein. Upon further examination, microfiltrating whey protein isolate has the highest potential for preserving the best parts of the whey (whey fractions). I say "potential" because no matter how the whey is processed, if the initial cheese-producing method destroyed whey's treasures (and it often does), then there is no way of being certain that the whey protein isolate that you are buying contains the valuable microfractions. However, it may be prudent to combine both ion-exchange and microfiltered whey protein in order to take advantage of each protein's special nuances.

There you have it—everything that you didn't want to know about whey protein and its history. So let's summarize with pros and cons. Where does whey protein shine, and where does it fall short?

Strengths

Whole whey-protein isolates could contain approximately 10% intact immunoglobulin proteins (a class of proteins that consists of two pairs of polypeptide chains). This content, among other properties, helps support the body's immune system, placing whey protein at the top of the list for immuno-enhancing potential. This is one of the main functional properties provided by whey.[5,6]

Whey protein contains the highest concentration (23-25%) of branched-chain amino acids (BCAA) of any single protein source. This BCAA content is important to bodybuilders because BCAAs are an integral part of muscle metabolism and are the first aminos sacrificed during muscle catabolism.[15]

Another functional property of whey is its ability to enhance endogenous (occurring naturally in the body) glutathione production.[5] Glutathione is the body's most powerful naturally-occurring antioxidant and also plays a role in immune system support.

One of the more interesting functional properties of whey protein to bodybuilders is its reported ability to stimulate IGF-1 (insulin-like growth factor-1) production.[13]

Weaknesses

Whey protein is highly soluble, which leads to its rapid absorption. Now you might think that this is a good thing, but I will list it under weaknesses for the following reason. When whey protein is rapidly absorbed, it leads to a huge influx of amino acids, and science has recently demonstrated that this rapid influx causes insulin response to rise and also causes many of those rapidly absorbed aminos to be oxidized for fuel —not used for muscle growth.[14]

Quality whey proteins, isolated from one of the processes mentioned above (especially cross-flow microfiltration), are some of the more expensive proteins on the market. They can be up to ten times the cost of other protein sources, and even four to five times more expensive than a quality whey-protein concentrate. For some, this makes usage in heroic amounts cost prohibitive. This price factor has obviously created a huge market for the oversized containers of whey-protein concentrates, which are the most cost effective for athletes with massive protein needs.

Relatively speaking, whey protein is a bit low in the essential amino acid phenylalanine, and therefore might functionally limit the biological value of the protein in some regards.

Whey protein is also lower in both arginine and natural glutamine (both are conditionally essential amino acids) than some other protein powders.

CASEIN — An Unsung Hero

I talked about whey protein being crowned king of all proteins. But how many times throughout history has there been a leader that has had the support of every individual under his or her rule? Now, this isn't another shot at whey. This is just an analogy that illustrates that there might be more than one person or protein that can function effectively as the "king."

When we talk about typical milk proteins—outside the context of whey—casein is the center of discussion. Caseins exist with phosphate in a unique spherical structure known as a micelle. This specialized characteristic has generated a lot of recent discussion. More on that later. It is these micelles that permit the separation of casein from whey in milk. The separation process is typically done through heating, acid precipitation, or enzymes (as when making cheese). Washing and solubilizing with sodium, potassium, or calcium, and then drying, yields what we commonly refer to as caseinates. The common caseinates available in most supplements are derived using acid, and are labeled as sodium, potassium, or calcium caseinates. These each have protein concentrations over 90%.

> "...there might be more than one person or protein that can function effectively as the 'king'."

In contrast to caseinates are the micellular caseins (I told you that you would see that word again). These are typically very expensive and in short supply. They are produced using enzymes, cold processing, and nanofiltration. This "no-heat, no-acid" processing yields the ultimate form of casein. The end product is undenatured with its natural minerals (potassium, calcium, magnesium, and phosphorus) chelated to the micelles.

Initially, most of you probably thought that casein would not be incredibly exciting. The bottom line is that casein is a high-quality protein that possesses some unique and beneficial functional properties. And if you didn't know the reason casein is a major protein component of the most popular meal supplements on the market, you do now. Here's how it stacks up:

Strengths

Casein may help regulate transit time of proteins through the gut because it tends to form a "gel." This slowing of transit time may help increase absorption of amino acids, peptides, and whole proteins from the gut due to extended exposure of the proteins in the intestinal tract. Greater protein absorption may also help bodybuilders more easily meet their amino acid requirements. This is particularly apparent in micellular caseins. This "gelling effect" may be one reason why athletes usually feel more "satisfied" after a protein meal that contains casein over that of a meal containing whey protein. In fact, a recent study found that casein-enriched (70 to 75 grams from a casein supplement) diets containing 1.5 grams protein per kilogram bodyweight per day produced a greater increase in lean mass, and a decrease in fat mass during **resistance training** than did a whey-protein-enriched diet (70 to 75 grams from a whey protein supplement).[17] This study, which thankfully was performed on exercising subjects, may prove to be the beginning of casein protein being viewed in a totally different light—as a valuable dieting tool.

In addition, a recent study suggests that "slow" proteins like casein are better than a "fast" protein like whey with respect to post—meal protein retention.[19]

Casein has a very high glutamine content. At 20.5%, it is higher than whey, soy, or egg. Supplying high concentrations of this amino acid, especially in peptide form—such as that found in casein—can help spare muscle mass during intense training or periods of dieting.[16]

Casein also boasts a high proportion of glucogenic aminos, which include threonine, glutamine, and arginine. The glucogenic aminos lend themselves to glucose production for energy during exercise, and have been shown to possibly help defer muscle breakdown. Large doses of glucogenic aminos have also been shown to increase feed efficiency in animals.[8]

> "...casein-enriched diets... produce a greater increase in lean mass, and a decrease in fat mass during resistance training."

Weaknesses

Commercially available casein products can be quite inconsistent in quality. It is very difficult to assess the quality of a casein protein. A variety of methods are used for isolating casein, and as we discussed, some are better than others. Unfortunately, the method is rarely disclosed on the product label. The only way to be sure of receiving a quality product is to find a supplier you trust, and stick with them.

MILK-PROTEIN ISOLATE—Best of Both Worlds?

A milk-protein isolate is a mixture of all of the proteins found in milk (namely, casein and whey proteins in a 4:1 ratio). This type of protein is quite good due to its strong amino acid composition derived from both its whey and casein components. It probably does retain some of the functional properties of both casein and whey. I won't go into great detail on its pros and cons, as they are well outlined in the whey and casein sections. Overall, I think this is a very good protein, but I would really like to see more research determining its functional properties.

SOY PROTEIN—Full of Beans or Power Plant?

Soy protein has never been big in the bodybuilding community, and it has never been considered a high-quality protein. Because it is derived from a plant source, it has always been looked upon as inferior. And to a certain extent, I agree (or shall I say I used to agree) with this perception. My thoughts on the subject are evolving as the soy-protein industry evolves. Especially when you look at the evidence that suggests females may obtain a greater benefit from soy than their male counterparts.

Soy protein is derived from soybeans by water extraction, followed by precipitation, washing, and drying procedures to produce either a soy-protein concentrate (approximately 70% protein) or soy-protein isolates (90% protein). Some extractions use ethanol/water mixtures, which removes isoflavones. Different soy proteins, depending on quality and degree of concentration, have varying taste and mixability characteristics. Fortunately many of the initial objections to soy—gastrointestinal disturbances, gas, poor taste, and poor mixability—were associated with the relatively low purity of soy proteins from years past.

Due to the fact that soy protein has been unable to play ball with the top-selling bodybuilding proteins such as whey and casein, big research has been sponsored designed to prove soy's worth for the bodybuilder and other top athletes. The folks at Protein Technologies wasted no time throwing their high-end soy isolate into the ring.

First they submitted the soy isolate to be tested against milk, egg, and beef proteins on a scale of protein quality. The most advanced protein-quality measurement scale available today is the Protein Digestibility Corrected Amino Acid Score (PDCAAS) developed by the World Health Organization (WHO). A PDCAAS tops out at a score of 1.0, so any protein with a rating of 1.0 is considered complete for humans. Soy-protein isolate, along with casein and egg proteins, scored a perfect 1.0. Interestingly, beef scored only 0.92.

To further bolster these findings, a clinical trial was undertaken to determine the effects of soy-protein isolate versus beef protein on nitrogen (tissue protein) retention in healthy young men. During this long-term study, subjects were fed 0.8 grams per kilogram of bodyweight per day of either soy or beef protein (only 72 grams for a 200-lb man). This was their only protein source. It was found that body nitrogen balances were similar between groups, and body cell mass showed no deterioration.[12] The authors of the study summarized their findings by stating, "The nutritional quality of isolated soy protein is high, and this plant protein can serve as the sole source of essential amino acids and nitrogen for protein maintenance in adults." But only time will tell if the bodybuilding community will embrace soy protein with open arms—let alone rely on soy as the sole source of daily protein.

So, now that we have established that soy-protein isolates have potential, let me summarize a few key concepts.

Strengths

Soy-protein isolate boasts the highest concentration of amino acids in what is referred to as the "critical cluster." Included in this critical cluster of aminos are the three BCAAs, and glutamine and arginine. These 5 amino acids make up 36.2% of high-quality soy-protein isolates. Glutamine alone accounts for 19.1%—just a hair behind casein. This concentrated source of critical aminos may help a bodybuilder spare muscle during a diet phase.

A variety of studies have shown that consistent intakes of soy-protein isolate may have a positive impact on the endogenous production of thyroxin (T4), triiodothyronine (T3), and even insulin over various other types of protein,

such as casein and fish proteins.[1,3,4,7,9] Thyroxin is a major player in regulation of metabolic rate.

Possibly secondary to the effects mentioned above, animal research indicates soy-protein isolate and peptides may help reduce nitrogen loss and enhance fat loss during low-calorie dieting when compared with casein.[11]

> "...the FDA approved a health claim for soy protein. 'soy protein may reduce cholesterol and the risk of heart disease.'"

Some animal research suggests that one soy isoflavone (daidzein) may have a gender-specific normalizing effect on sex-hormone production. Male lab animals experienced greater testosterone and growth-hormone excretion as well as muscle growth, while female lab animals actually lost weight and showed a decrease in testosterone and growth hormone.[10]

There are also a number of studies supporting the cholesterol- and triglyceride-lowering effects of soy.[2]

Relatively speaking, even the highest quality soy-protein isolates are less than half the price of a quality whey protein.

In October of 1999, the FDA approved a health claim for soy protein. "Soy protein may reduce cholesterol and the risk of heart disease." Specific health claim requirements include 4 servings per day at 6.25 grams per serving.

Weaknesses

Many soy-protein products on the market contain soy-protein concentrates that do not offer the high-quality nutritional profile of soy-protein isolates and lack the unique beneficial functional properties.

Soy-protein isolate has a relatively low level of the essential amino acid methionine, which acts as its limiting amino as far as protein bioavailability goes.

Raw soy products contain substances known as "phytoestrogens." These are plant chemicals that have some of the same biological activity as estrogen. For some, this is a positive attribute. Soy foods are used in the Orient to help control symptoms of menopause in middle-aged women.

EGG PROTEIN—The Old-School Standby

As I alluded to previously in this chapter, egg protein has been considered one of the highest quality proteins available for over 30 years. A few decades ago, it was even crowned by food scientists as the "gold standard" protein for human consumption. This recognition bestowed upon egg protein was due exclusively to its very strong amino acid profile. At the time it was given the title of "gold standard," amino acid profile was the only criteria by which proteins were judged and very little was known about whey protein

or soy-protein isolates back then.

Today, however, it is probably best to think of egg protein as having been honorably discharged from the front lines of the protein supplement fight. It's a good soldier, with plenty of punch, and can still get the job done, but there are younger, stronger, more specialized contenders in the game now.

In summary, here are the ups and downs of egg protein as I see it:

Strengths

Provides an outstanding amino acid profile with sulfur-bearing amino acids.

Provides an excellent, high-quality, whole-food protein source.

The new mix-and-cook powders make solid, whole-food egg-protein intake that much more convenient and transportable—not to mention it works great as an ingredient in baked goods.

Weaknesses

Beyond its strong amino acid profile, egg protein does not really offer any beneficial functional properties.

Eggs are not as inexpensive as they used to be. Egg protein was once the bargain quality protein source; now it ranks up there among the more expensive.

PROTEIN UTILIZATION "GADGETS"

As I mentioned earlier, nutritional science continues to roll. And with this progression, we are discovering new ways to get more bang out of our protein. Just like fuel additives that give gasoline a little more octane, new protein gadgets are being implemented to help further our results from existing protein.

Every trick from manipulating insulin secretion to influencing the rate of protein absorption has been used to affect a positive change in protein utilization efficiency. Some are here now, some are on the horizon (actually they're already here). Some of these protein gizmos are familiar, some may not be. Let's check 'em out.

20-Beta-Hydroxyecdysterone

This phytochemical compound has been researched in many Soviet Union studies and since it can now be extracted in high concentrations, it gets my vote for **"New Bodybuilding Supplement of the Year."** Around 1988, researchers hypothesized that this compound may help to increase hepatic protein synthesis and subsequently positive nitrogen balance! These are two critical factors for anyone trying to add lean mass. The more nitrogen your body maintains and the greater the rate of protein synthesis, the more mass, period.

Other data indicates that this compound possessed effects that help prevent the loss of muscle mass and promote the growth of contractile fibers. Yet other research concentrated on ecdysterone's effects on fatigue, work capacity, fat loss, and immune function. A protein turbo charger to say the least. For more on ecdysterone's powerful effects when combined with protein, see Chapter 9, called "The Next Wave of Bodybuilding Supplementation."

Glutamine and Glutamine Peptide

I believe that the inclusion of glutamine in protein products is an absolute. Glutamine's unique properties that affect everything from improved glycogen storage and gut integrity to the immune system make it a perfect addition to protein powders and meal replacements. For more on glutamine, and its valuable effects see Chapter 7, called "Standard Issue."

Creatine

As you may have noticed, creatine has been added to protein powders since Phosphagain was released in 1994. Now creatine is being added to whey protein, to enhance its protein utilization efficiency. I think creatine, coupled with protein and carbs, will produce the best results, but I'm not sure about adding it to a pure protein product. This may not be a bad idea if you can increase insulin without causing a decrease in blood glucose.

HMB

I've always thought HMB was a good high-protein, low-carb supplement—like during the Maximum Muscularity Diet. The mechanism makes sense especially under the physiological climate created by a diet like the Max Muscularity. And there are some studies that show enhanced protein synthesis due to HMB supplementation.[18]

Methoxyisoflavone

This powerful flavone was issued a patent in the '70s as an anabolic agent. A Hungarian company filed the main patent in 1977 as an animal feed additive, but for some reason no one ever marketed it for humans. I can only speculate that during that time the availability and reputation of effective pharmaceutical anabolics kept 7-Methoxy from making the cut. It wasn't until the early '80s that the cattle industry picked up on this compound to increase lean muscle. When 5-Methy-7-Methoxyisoflavone was approved for animals, this new compound became a favorite among livestock producers.

The human studies and results weren't too shabby either. Methoxyisoflavone demonstrated an increase in protein utilization. After a few weeks, 4.4- to 6.6-lb increases of lean muscle were reported. Furthermore, these anabolic effects also increased calcium, phosphorous, potassium, and nitrogen retention to a significant degree.

In other experiments, the catabolic effects of cortisone were partially suppressed, and the research concluded that identical doses of anabolic steroids do not exert anabolic effects stronger than the effects of Methoxyisoflavone. One of the best-discovered benefits is that Methoxyisoflavone does not exhibit androgenic or liver-damaging effects. For more on Methoxyisoflavone, see Chapter 9, called "The Next Wave of Bodybuilding Supplementation."

ZMA (Zinc Magnesium Aspartate)

This is not exactly a protein booster due to its sensitivity to calcium, since there is usually a significant amount of calcium in protein. So why are some manufacturers adding ZMA to their calcium-containing protein powders?

Beats me. It makes absolutely no sense.

ZMA should be taken on an empty stomach before bed. Clinical studies strongly suggest that ZMA, when taken as recommended, produces positive results such as maintaining normal serum testosterone ranges and improving the quality of sleep. Both important factors facilitating exercise recovery.

Carbohydrates

You might think that this is an odd addition to our line-up, and I would tend to agree, since it is not really a gadget. But the importance of carbohydrates with regard to protein utilization should be briefly addressed. Carbohydrates have a sparing effect on amino acids. Carbohydrates jump in the line of fire (your energy requirements), leaving amino acids to do more important functions like contribute to muscle growth. I believe that it is this intricate relationship that has made MRPs so popular. Now, I'm not suggesting that if you take a boatload of carbs, you'll grow gigantic muscles, but you'd be surprised how much further your protein will go with just the right amount of carbohydrates watching its back.

References Cited

1. Y. Akiba and L.S. Jensen, "Temporal Effect of Change in Diet Composition on Plasma Estradiol and Thyroxine Concentrations and Hepatic Lipogenesis in Laying Hens." *J. Nutr.* 113.10 (1983) : 2178-2184.

2. J.W. Anderson, et al., "Meta-Analysis of the Effects of Soy Protein Intake on Serum Lipids." *N. Engl. J. Med.* 333 (1995) : 276-282.

3. C.A. Barth, et al., "Difference of Plasma Amino Acids Following Casein or Soy Protein Intake: Significance for Differences of Serum Lipid Concentrations." *J. Nutr. Sci. Vitaminol.* 36.II (1990) : S111-S117.

4. C.A. Barth and M. Pfeuffer, "Dietary Protein and Atherogenesis." *Klin.*

Wochenschr. 66.4 (1988) :135-143.

5. G. Bounous and P. Gold, "The Biological Activity of Undenatured Dietary Whey Proteins: Role of Glutathione." *Clin. Invest. Med.* 14.4 (1991) : 296-309.

6. G. Bounous and P.L. Kongshavn, "Differential Effect of Dietary Protein Type on the B-Cell and T-Cell Immune Responses in Mice." *J. Nutr.* 115.11 (1985) :1403-1408.

7. W. Forsythe, et al., "Plasma Thyroxine and Cholesterol Changes Over Time as Affected by Dietary Protein Source." *FASEB J.* 5.5 (1991) : A947.

8.P.A. Geraert, et al., "Effects of Dietary Glucogenic Amino Acid Supplementation on Growth Performance, Body Composition, and Plasma-Free Amino Acid Levels in Genetically Lean and Fat Chickens." *Reprod. Nutr. Dev.* 27.6 (1987) : 1041-1051.

9.V. Stroescul, et al., "Metabolic and Hormonal Responses in Elite Female Gymnasts Undergoing Strenuous Training And Supplementation With Supro® Brand Isolated Soy Protein." (Brussels, Belgium: Second International Symposium on the Role of Soy in Preventing and Treating Chronic Disease,1996) 38.

10. J. Wang and Z.K. Han, "Effects of Daidzein on Muscle Growth and Some Endogenous Hormone Levels in Rats." (Brussels, Belgium: Second International Symposium on the Role of Soy in Preventing and Treating Chronic Disease, 1996) 45.

11. T. Yamamoto, et al., "Soy Protein and Its Hydrolysate Reduce Bodyfat of Dietary Obese Rats." (Brussels, Belgium: Second International Symposium on the Role of Soy in Preventing and Treating Chronic Disease, 1996) 55-56.

12.R. Young, et al., "A Long-Term Metabolic Balance Study in Young Men to Assess the Nutritional Quality of an Isolated Soy Protein and Beef Proteins." *Am J Clin Nutr* 39.1 (1984) : 8-15

13. Keys JE, et al., "Bovine mammary explant versus primary cell cultures: effect of bovine somatotropin and insulin-like growth factor-I on DNA content and protein synthesis." *In Vitro Cell Dev Biol Anim* 33.3 (1997) : 206-11. USDA-ARS, Milk Secretion and Mastitis Laboratory, Beltsville, Maryland 20705, USA.

14 Boire Y. et al., "Slow and fast dietary proteins differently modulate post-prandial protein accretion." *Proc. Natl. Acad. Sci. USA,* 94 (1997) :14930-14935.

15. Wagenmakers AJ, "Muscle amino acid metabolism at rest and during exercise: role in human physiology and metabolism." *Exerc Sport Sci Rev* 26 (1998) : 287-314.

16. Rowbottom DG, et al., "The emerging role of glutamine as an indicator of exercise stress and overtraining." *Sports Med* 21.2 (1996) : 80-97.

17. Robert Demling, M.D., "Effect of a hypocaloric diet, increased protein intake and resistance training on lean mass gains and fat loss in overweight police officers." *Annals of Nutrition & Metabolism,* 44 (2000) :21-29.

18. Kreider RB, "Dietary supplements and the promotion of muscle growth with resistance exercise." *Sports Med* 27.2 (1999) : 97-110.

19. Dangin, M. et al., "The digestion rate of protein is on independent regulating factor of postprandial protein retention." *Am J Physiol Endocinol Metab,* 280 (2001): E340-E348

Chapter

9

The Next Wave of BodyBuilding Supplementation

I'm assuming most of you who are reading this book have seen the 1997 issue of the *Sports Supplement Review*. You might also regularly read the popular fitness magazines such as *Muscle Media*, *Muscle & Fitness*, *Flex*, *Muscular Development* or *Ironman* or visit websites such as www.eas.com. My guess is you probably know a thing or two about supplements; maybe you are even an expert. Given that, this chapter may be one of your favorites because it addresses what's new in the world of bodybuilding supplements and what you need to know about them. The information presented here may change your views on what works and what does not for years to come. After you read this chapter, you may be able to fast-forward your supplement program into the future and with a bit of luck save literally hundreds of dollars in cash you might otherwise spend on over-hyped products and the flimsy concepts they are based on.

Where My Opinions Come From...

You may be wondering about the basis for my opinions and suggestions that are contained in this book. In other words, where do I get my information? That's why I want to make it clear that my opinions in this chapter come directly from a considerable amount of "in-the-trenches" body-building experience and scientific research that I have come across during the last several months. My suggestions in this chapter may or may not stand the test of time, and there is a chance some of my opinions will turn out to be mere supplement fads and nothing more. But I suspect you are reading this chapter with an open mind to get the real skinny on the hottest supplements and trends. You probably want cutting-edge information surrounding the latest sports supplements that the "regular" media just doesn't give you.

An Exciting Time for Athletes

For sure, we are moving into an exciting era for bodybuilders who want to use legitimate supplements to maximize their physique development. Why? Well, I have a few thoughts as to why this is area is becoming more and more progressive. One thought is that we have more classically trained scientists than ever before working with guys who are actually passionate about the muscle-building business. In the past, most successful sports nutrition companies were run by "street wise" bodybuilding experts who had few, if any, researchers that took the sport and products seriously.

Today, the sub-group of sports nutrition and diet aids now totals over $5 billion in annual sales. Talk about an improved labor force. Now genuine performance-based companies have a combination of "in-the-trenches" bodybuilding and sports performance experts on staff who can run their "theories" by a whole host of reliable researchers, and who analyze the actual biological, chemical, and physiological pieces of the puzzle. As I said before, I am the guy who has the "in-the-trenches" bodybuilding experience (usually through trial and error), and my time in the industry has allowed me to ask researchers a lot of questions over the years regarding performance and supplementation. If we look back a year or two from now, who knows whether or not my thoughts on new supplement trends will have been proven to work in the real world. It could go either way. However, I think there is a chance that some of the trends you will learn about in this chapter will stand the test of time (otherwise I wouldn't have even put them in the book).

The New Breed of Natural Anabolic Supplements

Let's start with a topic I am sure avid weight trainers are interested in—Natural Anabolic Supplements. If you tend to be skeptical, you might be saying "no way, natural products that are actually anabolic don't exist." Well, I'm probably as skeptical as you are, but I think you'll find the data in this section very promising to say the least. So let's get on with the Next Wave of Supplementation and a discussion on how to promote an anabolic environment NATURALLY.

20-Beta-Hydroxyecdysterone

Now here's where I really go out on a limb and make my **biggest prediction** for 2001. The prediction is this; if I could only bet on **one new supplement** that in the very near future would become "standard issue" or a "can't miss" compound for bodybuilders, athletes, and even fitness enthusiasts, it would be 20-Beta-Hydroxyecdysterone or as some refer to it, ecdysone. Here's the story: the compound I am talking about can be isolated from a couple of herbs, namely Rhaponticum/Leuzeae and Cyanotis vaga—which means they are phytochemicals or derived from plants in nature. Since the active ingredient ecdysone originates from plants, the compound is definitely natural (I briefly cover both of these plants in the herb section) but as you will soon see, the scientific data that has been collected on this ingredient is truly amazing.

Now, let me tell you why the active ingredient has me predicting such a great future for it.

If you read the last issue of the *SSR,* which was over three years ago, you know that at that time the common belief was that ecdysterone was not a valuable supplement for bodybuilders or athletes. Much of the disregard for this compound was based on the fact that up until last year there weren't any solid raw material suppliers that could produce high-potency ecdysterone. Today, however, raw material suppliers that specialize in standardizing herbs have changed the market for ecdysterone considerably. Back then, there was an issue with standardizing particular herbs for the active ingredient, which we now know, is ecdysterone. During the last 12 months, researchers that work on standardizing special herbs have discovered a methodology to "concentrate" the ecdysterone in raw Rhaponticum/Leuzeae and Cyanotis vaga herbs **up to 97%**. To put this in perspective, if you could get a 5% extract for ecdysterone in 1997, you would have had to pay an enormous amount of money and literally have to go on a waiting list to get the stuff. This is big news for athletes, because as I said before there is an impressive list of scientific studies on ecdysterone performed in healthy athletes that demonstrate gains in lean muscle size and enhanced performance but only when the compound is **very pure and concentrated**. Many of these studies were done in the Soviet Union around 1988, and the researchers hypothesized that the mechanism of action for this compound is that it may help to increase hepatic protein synthesis and subsequently promote positive nitrogen balance! These are two critical factors for anyone trying to add lean mass, since the more nitrogen your body maintains and the greater the rate of protein synthesis, the more mass, **period**.

Putting Ecdysterone to the Test

So how does this stuff work? Well, the basic effect from the consumption of ecdysone seems to positively regulate the protein balance of the organism. Researcher V. Smetanin from the Smolenk State Medical Institute in Russia speculates that a decrease in bodily urea and an increase in hemoglobin levels stimulate the anabolic process in protein metabolism.[22] Other data indicates that of an adaptogenic trait where the compound allows an organism to rapidly adapt to an environment and the stresses placed upon it. In any case, data firmly shows that this compound possessed effects that prevent the loss of muscle mass and promote the growth of contractile fibers.

Highlights of Research
Performed on Ecdysterone:

"If I could bet on one new supplement that will become 'standard issue,' it would be 20-Beta-Hydroxyecdysterone."

Research on ecdysone has looked at many different variables including, work capacity, immune function, lean body mass, fat loss, and many others. Most of this research points to a direct effect on increasing lean mass, especially when combined with some form of protein.

In a study by Simakin, 78 highly trained athletes were assessed for muscle tissue mass and fat mass while consuming either a placebo, protein, or ecdysone with a protein supplement.[23] Results were greatest in the group consuming both ecdysone and protein. In this group, a **6-7%** increase in lean muscle tissue after **10 days** of the test was observed. In addition, in this same test, **fat content was reduced by an average of ~10%** for males and females in the same time frame (see chart ECD-1). Additionally, this study assessed different safety parameters and hormonal markers, which yielded no differences between groups.

In addition to these effects, a study by Fadeev, B.G. et al., performed with 112 athletes revealed that 89% of those receiving ecdysone reported less fatigue, improved performance, less apathy, and greater speed-strength qualities.[24] Furthermore, these effects were noted no later than the fifth day after administration of the compound and lasted until the end of the protocol! Here again, the best news of all is that this study reported no side effects.

B.Ya. Smetanin, 1986, performed a trial using 117 highly qualified speed skaters aged 18-28, tests for work capacity, body-weight, lung capacity, and VO_2 max were measured. Results from the data showed an increase in all of the above parameters.[25] Also, a tendency toward an increase in the exhalation of CO_2 and O_2 pulse max was seen.

By now, you should realize that this stuff works, but is it safe? Well, for starters, a complete material safety data sheet and LD50 test (12/31/98) has been done on ecdysone, performed by ICN Biochemicals, showing a very low toxicity level. The LD50 data obtained showed a toxic dose to be 6400 mg/kg. This data would equate to 494,528 mg for a 170lb person, a factor of 4,121 beyond that of which a person should consume. Furthermore, several studies address human endocrine data regarding this compound's effect. *The data shows that this compound does not exert any effect on the hormonal system in mammals, namely humans.* To assess these data, various parameters have been measured including, insulin, testosterone, cortisol, ACTH, growth hormone, and leutinizing hormone. The following is just the start of studies, which address this topic and show no affect on hormonal balance.

- The Influence of Ecdisten, Prime Plus and Prime 1 on the Hormonal Balance of the Organism. (Review)[26]

- Report-Regarding the Pharmacological Attributes of "Ecdisten" (Review)[27]

- Mechanism of Thymolytic Action of Anabolic Steroids. (Semeykin A.V. et al)[28]

- The Combined Use of Ecdisten and the Product Bodrost during Training in Cyclical Types of Sports. (Simakin, VV et al)[23]

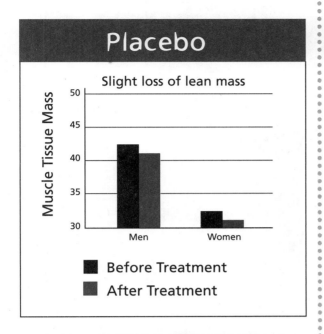

Placebo

Slight loss of lean mass

Muscle Tissue Mass

Men   Women

■ Before Treatment
■ After Treatment

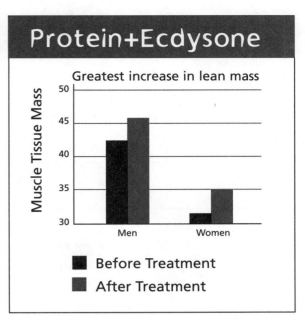

Protein+Ecdysone

Greatest increase in lean mass

Muscle Tissue Mass

Men   Women

■ Before Treatment
■ After Treatment

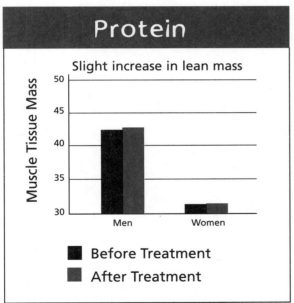

Protein

Slight increase in lean mass

Muscle Tissue Mass

Men   Women

■ Before Treatment
■ After Treatment

Real World Results with Ecdysterone

I don't know about you, but with all of these data and more coming in, I'm putting beta-ecdysterone on the top of my supplement list. In fact, I already started taking this compound right after I reviewed the material

safety data sheets and lab analysis confirmed an ultra-high potency for the ecdysterone samples we ordered at EAS (actually right before the final edits of this book). My first "test drive" was for four weeks while I was also on the second meso-cycle of the Foundation Diet and exercise phase. Remember during this phase the program calls for adequate protein, carbs, and fats, plus a significant amount of training volume, which in and of itself should cause even an experienced lifter to make good gains. From my experience, I took about 30-40 mg three times per day during the first two weeks, and my bodyweight shot up from about 199 to 203.5 lbs. I regret that during this time I did not check my bodyfat, but I can say without hesitation that I was stronger, had much more tolerance to the physical demands of my training volume, and got noticeably much better pumps in the gym. When I asked other guys in the gym to tell me if I was getting

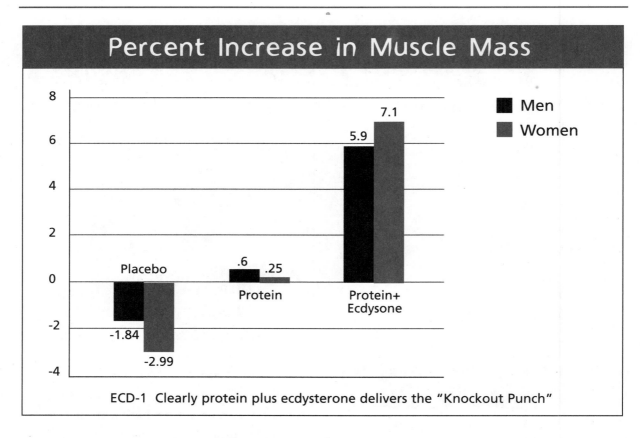

Percent Increase in Muscle Mass

Men
Women

Placebo
-1.84
-2.99

Protein
.6
.25

Protein+
Ecdysone
5.9
7.1

ECD-1 Clearly protein plus ecdysterone delivers the "Knockout Punch"

smooth (I only asked the guys who wouldn't sugar coat their answers and really tell me the truth). The only thing I ever heard was "do you have any of that beta-ecdy stuff for me?" Hardly scientific information, but I think you get the idea, especially since I've been training for 20-plus years! During my second two weeks, I continued to make gains in overall performance and my bodyweight stabilized at 204.5 lbs. By the time you read this, I am sure that I'll be into another EAS Periodized Bodybuilding and Nutrition program outlined in this book, but no doubt ecdysterones will be part of my supplement regimen. This stuff appears to me to have the most potential of any of the "new" supplements on the market.

To study this unique compound further, EAS will be funding research in humans, and we will be the first to let you know the results. In any case, I am convinced that ecdysterone is definitely worth a try for any serious athlete or bodybuilder.

Methoxyisoflavone

Now here is a compound that I really wasn't so sure of when I first read about it a year and a half ago, but since then I am starting to come around. My initial lack of confidence was probably because so many marketers early on were over-hyping the compound 5-Methyl-7-methoxyisoflavone or Methoxy-isoflavone to be some sort of super anabolic compound. This type of advertising nearly always makes me skeptical. In this instance however, 7-Methoxy had already gone through the patent process (U.S. patent

4,163,746) in the '70s and was issued for use as an effective anabolic compound for the pharmaceutical industry or as use as a feed additive for animals. A Hungarian company filed the main patent in 1977 as an animal feed additive, but for some reason no one ever marketed it for humans. My guess is that during that time the availability and reputation of effective pharmaceutical anabolics kept 7-Methoxy from making the cut. It wasn't until the early '80s that the cattle industry picked up on this compound by getting past the USDA regulations that governed hormones and drugs to increase lean muscle. When 5-Methy-7-Methoxyisoflavone was approved for animals, this new compound became a favorite among livestock producers.

The Scientific Data Regarding 7-Methoxy

In standard rat tests using anabolic steroids vs. 5-Methyl-7-MethoxyIsoflavone, it was determined that 7-Methoxy was indeed highly anabolic, yet free of any hormonal characteristics such as testosterone. No kidding, this was a pharmaceutical-to-supplement comparison that was for real! Now, with livestock, after 30 days on 7-Methoxy, the following bodyweight increases were recorded time and time again:

8 to 15% in calves
7 to 10% in cattle
7 to 10% in hogs
8 to 20% in poultry
10 to 20% in rabbits
8 to 12% in guinea pigs

This research is a little dated (the late '70s),

but the data suggest the increases were mainly lean tissue and were accompanied by an increase in vitality. The best part of this work was that the researchers found no alteration of endocrine function, which indicates that gains were non-hormonal in origin.

The human studies and results were as exciting: Methoxyisoflavone demonstrated an increase in protein utilization, happening in half the usual time. After a few weeks, 4.4- to 6.6-lb increases of lean muscle were reported. Furthermore, these anabolic effects also increased calcium, phosphorous, potassium, and nitrogen retention to a significant degree.[30]

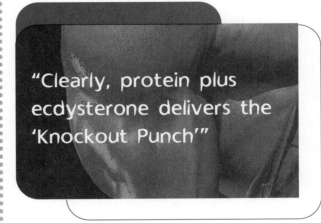

"Clearly, protein plus ecdysterone delivers the 'Knockout Punch'"

In other experiments, the catabolic effects of cortisone were partially suppressed, and the research concluded that identical doses of anabolic steroids do not exert anabolic effects stronger than those of these compounds. One of the best-discovered benefits is that Methoxyisoflavone does not exhibit androgenic or liver-damaging effects. It actually decreases oxygen consumption of tissues and lowers cholesterol. Looking at the research, most of it is done in animals, or some sort of animal tissue, which is a good start.

Personally, I'm going to take Methoxy-isoflavone plus beta-ecdysterone in hopes of getting even bigger and leaner in the months ahead. The anecdotal evidence makes me want to give it a try. The safety data looks good, too. I like the potential for Methoxy-isoflavone, but one study is not sufficient enough detail for me to render my final decision. In fact, we may even fund a study here at EAS just to find out the "real deal."

Insulin Manipulation—The Future is in the Details

Now let's discuss how to manipulate the positive and negative effects of insulin. As you probably know with insulin, we're dealing with a hormone that can promote gains in lean mass yet, on the other hand, hinder our quest for a muscular body. Talk about a double-edged sword! I suggest that you learn how to master this hormone if you want to create the ideal physique in this world of processed foods. Insulin management has great health implications, especially for any athlete who wants to be active later in life, when many of the debilitating side effects of this hormone come into play. I have divided this section into three integral parts: glucose disposal agents, insulin amplifiers, and glycemic response modifiers. Don't worry if you've never heard of these terms. You will soon.

Glucose Disposal Agents

One category of sports supplements that you may not be aware of is called glucose disposal agents. This category describes products or compounds that allow your body to direct glucose into the tissues that need it most, and help to maintain proper overall blood sugar levels. While many products have touched on the subject of glucose transport and blood sugar management, never before has this nutritional topic been so hot within the scientific community. One reason for this newly found interest might be because of the book "Syndrome X", by Burton Berkson, M.D. According to him, glucose intolerance and insulin resistance may affect more than half the U.S. population. In other words, any nutrient that affects glucose (any carbohydrate we ingest eventually becomes glucose) and insulin metabolism is becoming very important for the supplement and drug companies because it carries a high revenue potential.

"One category of sports supplements that you may not be aware of is called glucose disposal agents."

For those of us who exercise regularly, especially weight trainers, preferentially "disposing" more nutrients into muscle, but not fat cells, makes perfect sense. In fact, a key benefit to weight training is that it creates a need for glucose to be directed into muscle storage sites, and not into your fat cells. Glucose disposal agents enhance the effects of insulin. The main anabolic properties of insulin come from stimulating muscle cells to take up glucose. Insulin is an integral part of your body's "shuttle system." When optimized, it may allow muscle cells to accept more nutrients like glucose, amino acids, protein, and creatine. Most glucose disposal agents increase insulin sensitivity. In laymen's terms, this means that glucose disposal agents allow your body to use the insulin your body produces more efficiently. On the other side of the equation, we have insulin resistance, which is associated with decreased whole-body glucose disposal and reduced glucose metabolism. In the past, sports nutrition consumers hailed chromium and vanadium supplements as "kings of the hill," so to speak, for increasing insulin sensitivity and glucose metabolism. However, most recently some newer compounds have emerged and the clinical data supporting their use is growing rapidly. Here is a review of the best and latest compounds in the category.

Alpha-Lipoic Acid (ALA)

Known by a few different names (lipoic acid, alpha-lipoic acid, and thioctic acid), this compound acts as a coenzyme for several reactions in your body, one of which is called "glycolysis," which is the process of converting blood sugar to energy. Alpha-lipoic acid does this by supporting the activity of mitochondria, tiny organelle "powerhouses" that produce energy and are found in every muscle cell. Alpha-lipoic acid is a nutrient your body can produce, so it is not considered "essential."

However, multiple studies done on Type-II diabetics (those with decreased insulin sensi-

tivity) lead me to believe that alpha-lipoic acid may benefit athletes, bodybuilders, and pretty much everyone trying to build muscle and lose fat. Let me explain.[1] As I mentioned before, it is estimated that over 50% of the U.S. population may have a problem with the utilization of blood glucose, otherwise known as insulin insensitivity. Why? Well, one of the reasons may be because the typical American diet is full of "JUNK FOOD." Yes, you heard me right; processed foods, refined sugars, saturated fats, fast food, and so on may be negatively influencing one of our body's insulin levels and insulin sensitivity. In fact, alpha-lipoic acid supplementation may even help decrease recovery time, increase glycogen storage, and even help people trying to reduce bodyfat on ketogenic diets or other diets.

How Does ALA Work?

Muscle represents the primary site of glucose disposal. Therefore it is likely that alpha-lipoic acid aids in the muscular uptake of glucose, possibly leading to greater glycogen synthesis. In one study, diabetics using 1 gram of intravenous lipoic acid per day increased their metabolic clearance rate of glucose by 30%. While this research was done in diabetics and not healthy athletes, it may be a hint as to how a supplement can enhance energy production in muscles and possibly decrease bodyfat storage.

Alpha-lipoic acid is also a very powerful antioxidant. Numerous studies to date indicate that alpha-lipoic acid is extremely beneficial at combating free-radical damage.

Specifically, alpha-lipoic acid has been studied for its effects on metal chelating capacity, its ability to scavenge reactive oxygen species (ROS), its ability to regenerate endogenous antioxidants, and its ability to repair oxidative damage.[2,3] As you can see, alpha-lipoic acid happens to be a very diverse antioxidant.

So far, clinical studies show alpha-lipoic acid is quite safe. However, any time you're experimenting with a supplement that may act as an insulin mimicker, you should proceed very cautiously. As a matter of fact, alpha-lipoic acid has a reputation for being a rather potent agent, and if you take too much of it all at once, you could experience low blood sugar levels, which include symptoms such as fatigue, anxiety, jitteriness, confusion, frustration, etc. If you decide to try alpha-lipoic acid, start with a small dosage of approximately 100 - 200 mg with a meal. Eventually, a dose of 600 mg per day, taken in divided doses with meals (for example, 200 mg with 3 separate meals), could produce very nice results. I don't think athletes would need to take more than 600 mg per day. Apparently, for antioxidant purposes, an effective dose of alpha-lipoic acid could be as low as 200 - 300 mg per day.

Alpha-lipoic acid supplements have been on the market for quite a while. They are used frequently by those trying to control blood sugar and there is some evidence ALA supplementation may help enhance the anabolic and fat-burning effects of insulin, which could benefit anyone looking to build mass or lose fat. In addition, alpha-lipoic acid may help you protect your body against free-radical damage by working as an all- around antioxidant.

d-Pinitol

Pinitol, d-Pinitol, Inzitol™, or D-chiro-inositol all relate to the same compound, the latest in the lineup of glucose disposal agents geared to enhance performance and complement your training efforts. Pinitol is a methylated sugar that is showing tremendous potential in the world of glucose disposal and glycogen storage. Pinitol is an isomer of inositol, which is typically extracted from soy and sugar pine heartwood. Pinitol was first researched on its main attribute that showed it possessed hypoglycemic effects or blood-sugar lowering properties.[4,5,6] As with most glucose disposal agents, the initial research was done on people with Type-II diabetes, where it seems to mimic or enhance the effects of insulin in the body.[6] However, unlike most other compounds in its class, Pinitol seems to assist in the clearance of blood glucose without causing a hypoglycemic reaction or extremely low blood sugar.[4]

How d-Pinitol Appears to Work?

Pinitol seems to increase the uptake of glucose into the cell and may also increase glycogen synthesis. If you're an athlete, glycogen storage and the control of blood glucose is extremely important in order to give your muscles the fuel they need to recover and perform at the levels you require. Overall, Pinitol makes a perfect fit with your nutrition program or your everyday creatine supplement, where it can help transport glucose (and possibly even creatine) into your muscle cells. For starters, try using 50 mg of d-Pinitol with meals that contain over 50 grams of carbohydrates. Most products that contain this ingredient usually contain 50 mg of d-Pinitol per serving, which seems to be an effective dose.

Colosolic Acid

If you've read my Sport Supplement Review columns in *Muscle Media*, you've heard about Colosolic acid. I told you I thought there was another interesting glucose disposal agent, which comes from standardizing the herb *Lagerstroemia speciosa*, otherwise known as the banaba tree. Standardized extracts from the leaf of *L. speciosa* have been demonstrated to stimulate glucose transport activity in vitro[7] and lower plasma glucose in both diabetic rodents[8] and humans. I have been aware of this compound for about a year and a half now, and I have had a chance to look at the research. At this point, I have to say Colosolic acid seems to make the grade. From what I can see, it seems that Colosolic acid reduces serum glucose in a dose-response relationship.[9] For example, I reviewed two papers where the researchers studied Colosolic acid intake ranging from 0.16 mg - 0.48 mg taken with meals. The people given higher levels of Colosolic acid showed greater lowering of plasma glucose.[9] Colosolic acid has also been studied for weight loss, and a dose-response relationship was also found.[10] In this study, greater reductions in bodyweight were reported with the 0.32 mg - 0.48 mg doses. This study suggests that Colosolic acid may also prove to be a powerful new weight-loss

supplement. My guess is that it probably won't be long until we get a whole new breed of glucose disposal cocktails that combine alpha-lipoic acid, D-Pinitol, *and* Colosolic acid. If so, the synergy between all of these compounds may allow us to use Colosolic acid in dosages of roughly 0.16 mg, 3 times per day, for weight management and to preferentially direct carbohydrates into muscle tissue and not fat cells!

> "...insulin, when amplified, has the ability to promote muscle-protein synthesis and decrease protein breakdown."

Insulin Amplifiers—The Next Step in Sports Supplementation

Amplifying insulin secretion without ingesting large amounts of simple sugar will become a natural "next step" for sports supplementation. The major reason for this is that athletes realize that insulin, when amplified, has the ability to promote muscle-protein synthesis and decrease protein breakdown.[11] Then again, athletes are getting wise to the fact that excess sugars may impede a muscular physique. So the question for the bodybuilding elite becomes, how can we get the anabolic effects of increased insulin output without gaining excess bodyfat? One approach is to use less simple sugar combined with specific nutritional compounds that may assist in driving insulin levels up for an anabolic effect. Here are the latest individual ingredients that may just do the trick.

Arginine

Arginine is an integral amino acid necessary for wound healing, growth hormone production, and protein metabolism. Arginine is also required for nitrogen transport and storage (i.e. nitrogen balance), and has proven to be extremely useful in treating persons in severe catabolic states such as burn victims. In addition, arginine has a very solid scientific history as an insulinogenic amino acid. In fact, to determine potential abnormalities in beta-cell function after pancreas transplantation (we produce insulin in our pancreas), medical practitioners often use an arginine-induced insulin secretion test. The standard procedure is to give people a dosage of arginine hydrochloride (3-5 grams orally) and chart the insulin response.[12] If during this test insulin is not significantly amplified, doctors often suspect a defect. Another interesting mechanism by which arginine may induce amplified concentrations of insulin is through the production of nitric oxide (NO), which is further explained later in this chapter. Nitric oxide is formed from this amino acid by a family of enzymes, called NO synthases (NOS). Several researchers[13] have noted that NOS activity has been detected in insulin-producing cells. Further findings headed by Fonovich de Schroeder suggest that adequate levels of NO may be necessary for positive modulation of insulin secretion.[14] This 3-5 gram dose of arginine causes small increases in NO, but this

small rise may just be the ticket to new muscle growth and maximum insulin output. On the other hand, the data to support achieving supraphysiological amounts of NO from arginine ingestion using less than 3-5 grams is simply not available. The fact that arginine is in relatively low amounts in typical protein products such as whey makes a very good case for using 3 - 5 grams of supplemental arginine as an insulin amplifier and NO precursor. I give arginine a definite "thumbs up" as an insulin amplifier.

4-Hydroxyisoleucine

Scientists have recently discovered that Fenugreek seeds (*Trigonella foenum graecum*) contain an amino acid that may act as an insulin promoter called 4-hydroxyisoleucine. These same researchers demonstrated that 4-hydroxyisoleucine potentiates insulin secretion in a glucose-dependent manner.[15] This means that although 4-hydroxyisoleucine by itself may not ramp up insulin secretion, you may be able to ingest fewer simple carbs and still get your insulin levels to spike. This could be a real breakthrough for post-exercise recovery nutrition, and of course creatine transport, which is insulin mediated. Most of my colleagues estimate that about 100 mg of the 4-hydroxyisoleucine per dose will do the trick. The problem is, at this point the raw material manufacturers cannot standardize fenugreek to a high enough concentration of 4-hydroxyisoleucine to provide an efficacious dose. One of the industry's seasoned raw material suppliers is working on a very high potency standardized version of fenugreek and has told me that they are extremely close, so be on the watch for this unique compound in the coming months. When they get the process perfected—and I am sure they will—I think we'll see this compound incorporated into a whole new breed of supplements. In the mean time, if you can get your hands on some potent fenugreek that delivers high amounts of 4-hydroxyisoleucine, I suggest you try it. (Make sure to take it with about 10 to 20 grams of simple carbohydrates.)

Caution: The Insulin Balancing Act

By now you can see that science has shown some unique compounds have the ability to drive up insulin levels and increase receptor affinity for insulin without **large amounts of carbohydrates**. This sounds like a perfect scenario for a more anabolic and less fat-storing metabolic environment. But, as with all types of dietary modifications, you must be able to determine when a positive concept is **taken too far**. Let me explain.

When your body is "primed" to produce more insulin without supplying carbohydrates to utilize the elevated concentrations, you can become hypoglycemic. Why? Well, when your insulin levels are pushed high enough to create an anabolic effect without enough carbohydrates, your body wants to make glucose elsewhere. To do this, your body first releases a hormone called glucagon so that you can release glucose from your liver. However, if your liver runs out of glycogen (which may happen on a low-carbohydrate regimen) your body may start the process that dismantles amino acids so they can be used for energy called glucogneogenesis.

This is a normal occurrence during sleep and is not good for bodybuilding and should be minimized as much as possible. During sleep the body relies on liver glycogen and an amino acid pool that it will work on first during glucogneogenesis. In rare instances amino acids from body tissues will be used for energy. This is the main reason why intelligent athletes usually include a meal high in protein such as casein (which deliver amino acids slowly throughout the night) to offset the possibility of using amino acids from muscle tissue. The bottom line is this; if you plan on using compounds that have the ability to drive up insulin levels and increase receptor affinity for insulin sensitivity, make sure you are taking in some carbohydrates, if not you may be wasting your money and putting your muscle tissue at risk. That's why I always recommend ingesting at least a few simple and complex carbohydrates after your workout if you are going to raise insulin for an anabolic effect. By doing so, you can create a "safety net" for the insulin mechanism without the subsequent downside.

Glycemic-Response Modifiers

We have covered the compounds that unlock the gates for insulin to do its best work, plus the ones that amplify this key hormone. Now let's take a look at the other side of the equation. Remember when I told you early on that insulin manipulation holds the KEY to many aspects related to overall health and building a better body? I stressed this point for good reason. The anabolic effects of insulin must be carefully managed because the downside of insulin's role as a storage hormone lies in the fact that excess secretion can inhibit fat burning and promote bodyfat accumulation. Thus, properly managing its secretion is critical to muscle growth and bodyfat regulation.

Actually, insulin should only be amplified post-exercise, while moderate insulin levels and glucose disposal agents should be "in play" after every other meal. This allows you to have both the anabolic benefits of insulin after training and minimal insulin spikes during the day, so you do not potentially interrupt the fat-burning process. The best method to help manage the "dark side" of insulin is to eat mixed meals containing a nice blend of protein, carbs, fats, and fiber, plus limit your carbohydrate choices to those that rate lower on the glycemic index. This is a topic that was briefly discussed in all of the Periodized Nutrition Plans in this book. This is a great concept and, of course, if I were a "normal" nutritionist, I would tell you that this is all you have to do. On the contrary, this healthy and balanced eating plan of attack usually fails when put to the real-world test. Here's why. Nearly everyone in this day and age is tied to some sort of hectic schedule that hinders his or her ability to eat properly. Even with meal-replacement powders and the like, getting fiber with a good dose of carbs seems nearly impossible, at least at every meal. Next, the food industry is consistently milling out the valuable fibers from the carbohydrates in our everyday food supply, leaving us with very limited choices. There is a huge opportunity for the supplement industry to start adding more fiber to their food products, and come up with con-

venient ways for those of us who don't always eat correctly to get the fiber we need. Then again, maybe science will help us discover new ways to put the brakes on insulin spikes. Here are my thoughts on getting the fiber you need, and a little herbal trick that may be all you need to keep insulin in the "healthy range."

> "Dietary fiber can help slow the absorption of glucose from the carbohydrates we eat."

Get the Fiber Right

We've all heard that eating a high-fiber diet is a healthy way to live. However, when we rely on meal-replacement powders and high-protein diets for building and maintaining muscle tissue, this is often difficult. Dietary fiber is the part of a plant that provides and maintains the structure of the plant. Cellulose, hemicellulose, polysaccharides, pectins, gums, mucilages, and lignins are dietary fibers. These all have one thing in common: your body can't digest them. For this reason, they can help slow the absorption of glucose from the carbohydrates we eat, thus allowing more moderate insulin output. Foods high in fiber are called fibrous carbs, of which steel-cut oatmeal, broccoli, lentils, and other beans are good sources.

Recommendations for dietary fiber intake for adults generally fall in the range of 20 to 35 grams per day or 10 to 13 grams of dietary fiber per 1,000 calories. Nutrition Facts labels use 25 grams of dietary fiber per day for a 2,000-calorie diet or 30 grams per day for a 2,500-calorie diet as goals for American intake. However, average dietary fiber intake continues to be at "less-than-recommended" levels in the U.S. population, with usual intakes averaging only 14 to 15 grams per day.[16] One reason for this is that most popular American foods are low in dietary fiber. Servings of commonly consumed grains, fruits, and vegetables contain only 1 to 3 grams of dietary fiber. Legumes and high-fiber cereal products supply more dietary fiber but are not commonly consumed. If you don't get enough fiber in your diet, you may want to add about 10 grams for every 100 grams of carbohydrate you get from food. This way you can moderate the glucose uptake into your bloodstream and avoid wild blood sugar swings.[17]

Of course if you don't want to eat these highly fibrous foods, you can always count on a supplement. My favorite fiber supplement is called Fibersol II, by Matsutani Inc. This is a great source of fiber that not only tastes good, but also dissolves extremely well in water, unlike some of the more popular fiber supplements on grocery store shelves. Other good fiber supplements include BeneFiber, psyllium husks, and oat or wheat bran. Any way you choose to go, I highly recommend anyone, especially those looking to lose fat or limit fat gain, consume 5 to 10 grams of fiber with each meal, especially with meals containing other carbohydrates.

Green Tea—A Glycemic Modifier?

Green tea has been receiving a lot of attention lately due to the growing number of scientific studies verifying its health benefits. Researchers believe that the active ingredients in green tea are flavanols, of which catechins, epicatechins, and epigallocatechins are the most prominent. As for reducing the rise in serum glucose after a meal, green tea was recently shown to reduce glucose by over 23%, which I believe may also cause a blunted insulin response.[18] Further investigation reveals that tea polyphenols may be able to lower serum glucose by inhibiting the activity of a starch-digesting enzyme called amylase.[18] Green tea also inhibits both salivary and intestinal amylase, so that starch is broken down more slowly, and the rise in serum glucose is thus minimized. Therefore, I feel using green tea as a glycemic response modifier may be one of the best non-fiber approaches around. Green tea is also discussed in Chapter 13, which is about herbs.

Nitric Oxide Gadgets

If you've been reading the fitness magazines, you may be wondering whether or not nitric oxide (NO) is a possible muscle-building agent. I know this topic has been one of the most popular supplement questions for me, so it has spurred my interest even more. First of all, nitric oxide is a gas that is derived from the amino acid L-arginine by nitric oxide synthases (NOS). It plays beneficial roles in proper health and functioning of the cardiovascular, immune, and nervous systems. Nitric oxide is also a key regulator of blood flow and pressure, which explains why drugs like Viagra, which act to potentiate the actions of nitric oxide (Viagra does not stimulate the release of nitric oxide), are vital to erectile response.

From a bodybuilding perspective it appears nitric oxide may have the *potential* to increase muscle growth by increasing the wound healing process,[37, 38] blood flow,[39] and nutrient delivery. This is big news for athletes but at this time, we just don't know how to judge these benefits against say simple creatine supplementation. One of the most interesting areas where NO may benefit athletes is in insulin production. As I said when we discussed L-arginine, adequate levels of NO may be necessary for positive modulation of insulin secretion. One of my thoughts is that the nitric oxide-insulin connection may be one reason why L-arginine has shown such remarkable wound-healing properties in severely catabolic burn victims or those recovering from major surgery. Now, for the flip side: too much of a good thing can be bad. Nitric oxide is a pro-oxidant and overproduction may have deleterious side effects.[19] However, there is no reason to be alarmed. Research has never shown that dangerous levels can be attained through supplementation, as some sports nutrition companies would lead you to believe. Bottom line: Stimulating nitric oxide might be achieved with the right nutrients such as L-arginine and others (see sections below), and it may be of tremendous benefit to those looking to add mass. This topic is very interesting, so I'll keep my eyes open for additional research and keep you posted.

Gynostenma Pentaphyllum

Gynostenma is an herb that I have a close eye on because of its incredible ability to ramp up NO. This herb was first brought to my attention by one of EAS' best and brightest product development managers, Peter Miller (he is also one of the contributing editors of this book). Though research on it is rather limited, from what I have seen and discussed with researchers, I see great potential. Gynostenma is an herb in the Panax family, closely related to ginseng. Researchers have isolated a series of compounds known as gypenosides. In fact, one of the most prominent researchers of this herb, Dr. Xin Bu from Vanderbilt, performed an in-vitro study and showed gypenosides caused a dramatic increase in nitric oxide production.[20] In conversations with Dr. Bu, it seems gynostemma has been widely used in many countries for the treatment of heart disease because of its NO-producing properties. This herb is so powerful, that when my colleagues and I got lab samples for our own little in-house testing, even a small 50 mg dose seemed to send our blood pressure down a few notches. The stuff is extremely powerful and when we get a handle on dosing for healthy athletes, we may see NO become an even hotter topic in the bodybuilding world. No doubt NO production has the capability of increasing numerous functions in your body, maybe even some that that can dramatically "open up" blood flow to the point where your ability to pull nutrients into cells and create an anabolic environment for growth are greatly improved.

Steroidal Saponins

These sets of compounds are typically derived from the Panax species of ginseng. It is thought that these compounds possess the ability to increase the production of nitric oxide in your body similar to gynostenma.[21] Since these compounds are so closely related, this makes perfect sense. However, I'd have to say that my bet is on gynostemma as a direct NO precursor.

d-Ribose—Is It a Peak Performer?

Since the introduction of creatine monohydrate, any product, such as d-ribose, when is supposed to increase peak power output certainly has a tough act to follow. After all, for many of us supplementing with creatine for just a week or so delivered results that literally blew our minds. The significant and prompt increases in muscle size and strength were almost too good to be true. But somewhere along the way the instant gratification we received from creatine use made us very "greedy" consumers to be sure. So how does d-ribose, the latest compound promoted to increase peak power output and energy stack up to creatine? Well it appears that with respect to weight trainers, we really don't

"...nitric oxide may have the potential to increase muscle growth by increasing... blood flow and nutrient delivery."

have much data to go by. To date, two studies using high doses of ribose (24-30 grams over a 24-hour period) have given ribose the promise that it can indeed improve muscle performance. On the other hand, doses at this level are very expensive. No studies using "recommended doses" (1-5 grams/day) have yet to be published. As I write this section there are a few university studies that have either just been completed or are under way, with results expected this summer. But with all this "promise," I would like to suggest a different dose/timing program for bodybuilders so they can get the most bang for their d-ribose dollar. Let me explain.

Priming the Human Energy Machine

For most athletes if a supplement doesn't provide building blocks for new muscle tissue, make us stronger *faster*, increase our ability to use more protein, or allow us to shed bodyfat, we're just not interested. Supplements that we don't feel right away or must consume every day to maintain and build muscle mass are the first ones to go when supplement dollars are being budgeted. But an often overlooked aspect of the muscle game is continuous improvements in one area— ENERGY. That's because on the most basic level, every bit of muscle size and strength gains we can possibly make—all the enhancements in athletic performance we can ever hope to realize—are reliant on one elemental thing: ENERGY. With a more topped-off energy reserve at our disposal, we're quite simply capable of performing *more* physical work. And the more work we do (whether it's lifting increasingly heavier weights or running more intense 100-meter sprints), the stronger and faster we become.

The reason I bring this point up when speaking about d-ribose is simply this: High- level athletes need to accept the fact that tolerance of work is indeed a key to greater physical development. In fact, most illegal ergogenic aids usually offer a way to shorten the recovery process during and after exercise so that more overall tonnage can be moved in a given time frame of weeks, months, or years.

What is d-Ribose?

Specifically, the energy source for all cells in the body, including muscle cells, is a compound called adenosine triphosphate, or ATP for short. Simply put, this molecule contains four parts: one "adenosine" molecule and three high-energy phosphate molecules. The adenosine portion of ATP is made up of one molecule each of something called "adenine" and a five-carbon sugar called "ribose." This ribose molecule is known as a "building block" of ATP. d-Ribose is a pentose sugar produced in adequate amounts through normal metabolism. However, ribose, although a sugar by chemical definition, is not like glucose, a sugar that is utilized primarily as a fuel. Rather than being a simple carbohydrate utilized for energy production, ribose is fundamentally a structural element in various enzyme cofactors, RNA (ribonucleic acid), and purine nucleotides like ATP, ADP, AMP, and IMP. Ribose is primarily produced within the tissues using it for purine salvage or de novo synthesis. But all science aside, the bottom line for athletes is if supplemental ribose is to be helpful, it may be due to the fact that its biosynthesis is relatively slow and energy dependent.

Synergy Between d-Ribose and Creatine

OK, now for all of the dyed-in-the-wool instant-gratification junkies, this next bit of

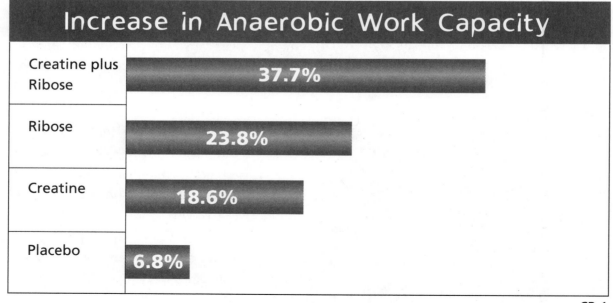

Increase in Anaerobic Work Capacity

Creatine plus Ribose	37.7%
Ribose	23.8%
Creatine	18.6%
Placebo	6.8%

information is for you. It appears that leading researchers and experts in muscle physiology have hypothesized that because ribose is an essential building block of ATP, supplementing it with creatine may produce highly synergistic effects at enhancing the replenishment of muscle energy reserves. The reasoning? Well, it's known that ribose supplies one piece of the puzzle for enhanced ATP generation by furnishing the vital building blocks of ATP, while creatine supplies the other piece by supplying the high-energy nutrients needed to increase ATP turnover. Taken together, we are able to create a situation where ribose is used to *build* the energy engine and creatine is used to *fuel* it. At this time we do not know exactly to what extent supplementing with d-ribose and creatine would affect exercising humans, but the picture is becoming clearer. Recently, a double-blind, placebo-controlled study at a major university conducted by Dr. Jeffrey Stout, indicates that the combination of 5 grams of creatine and 3 grams of ribose (the same combination that is contained in EAS' RiboForce HP) enhances exercise performance to a greater extent than ribose or creatine alone. In this study, 38 subjects, randomly assigned to four groups as shown in figure CR-1, were assessed for anaerobic work capacity (AWC) using cycle ergometry. After two days of supplementation, the ribose/creatine group showed nearly a 40% improvement in work output. Ribose alone also produced significantly greater performance gains than creatine. This study also found that 3 grams of ribose increased exercise performance more than 5 grams of creatine.[36]

Of particular note to weight trainers is the fact that in this study (although unpublished) the addition of ribose **doubled** the performance-enhancing benefits produced by creatine alone.

Want to know what I think about d-ribose? Well, yes, I'm am using it, but my expectations and use occasions are more specific. For example, I put one packet of RiboForce HP (5 g creatine and 3 g ribose) into my water bottle when I'm doing primarily an upper body workout. This is because legs and calves are my strong suit, and by saving this supplement for "specializing" on my core upper body movements (benches and rows), I get more workouts from each box of RiboForce HP, thus saving me money and prioritizing my training at the same time. I stopped adding my usual 3 grams of ribose to my post-exercise protein/carb/glutamine/creatine shake since I feel my supplementation in that area is pretty strong already. Do I think it works? I'm not sure, mainly because I have been having such great workouts using the Periodized Training outlined in this book and to be honest, I'm not willing to stop using all my other key supplements like beta-ecdysterone and methoxyisoflavone to narrow the variables enough to make an intelligent evaluation. I will say that when I made the switch to taking ribose right **before or during training** it made a huge difference for me personally. I think this strategy is cost effective and may allow you to really blast stubborn body parts.

Stress Relief for the Modern-Day Athlete

Another "Next Wave" supplement strategy

that I feel will be hot during the coming year is that of stress relief. Now if you're anything like me you probably set a goal and just use blood, sweat, and tears to achieve it. This "bulldozer" approach works well, but it does have a drawback that obsessed athletes seem to only notice when it's too late. You see, constantly pushing our bodies to do super human feats in the gym, at work, and by altering our diets can create much more stress than can be tolerated for the long term. But, there is a little-known amino acid found in green tea called L-Theanine that may be able to maximize our ability to fully rest, recover, and even relax the most high-strung athletes.

I first learned about the beneficial effects of L-Theanine from Alan Shugarman, M.S., R.D., who is a researcher at Weider. At first I wondered if he was mispronouncing the name L-Threonine as L-Theanine, but he said it was no mistake. It was just a relatively new compound. Now, before you get too excited, you should realize that L-Theanine is not essential to building muscle, but it might just become an essential part of your recovery supplementation plans.

What is L-Theanine?

Though it is not considered an essential or conditionally essential amino acid, L-Theanine is a compound that contains nitrogen like all other amino acids. The key to understanding how L-Theanine works and its benefits lies in the biochemistry and physiology involved. Once ingested, L-Theanine is readily absorbed into the bloodstream, where it crosses the blood-brain barrier via the large neutral amino acid transporter. For an unknown reason at this point, it seems that L-Theanine is preferentially transported across the blood-brain barrier over other amino acids that use the exact same transport mechanism. This is important because if other amino acids were

> "L-Theanine may be able to maximize our ability to fully rest, recover, and even relax the most high-strung athletes."

favored, then L-Theanine might not get into the brain due to competitive blocking. Once in the brain, L-Theanine is converted to Gamma Amino Butyric Acid (GABA), the second-most abundant neurotransmitter found in the brain. If you've been into supplements for a few years, you may recall that a few companies marketed GABA, which is an inhibitory neurotransmitter that reverses the effects of norepinephrine and causes the relaxation of muscle. Many athletes, myself included, found that supplementing with GABA really didn't get the job done, and thus this compound is not such a popular one these days. So, why is L-Theanine better than GABA? The answer lies in the physiology of the blood-brain barrier, where GABA does not readily cross but L-Theanine does. As for the elevation of GABA via L-Theanine, the effects of the elevated GABA were shown physiologically via a study conducted on human subjects looking at brainwave activity. During stress the body puts out brainwaves called beta waves which are associated with an awake and stressed state. During the study, brainwaves were measured and following the consumption of 200 mg of L-Theanine, the formerly stressed subjects showed a shift in brainwaves from beta to alpha. Alpha brainwaves are associated with an awake yet relaxed state of being. So, by entering the brain and being converted to GABA as well as promoting alpha brainwave production, L-Theanine induces a profound state of relaxation. [31,32,33,34,35]

The ability of L-Theanine to produce a relaxed state in someone who was previously stressed has many applications. All of us have stress from work, family, friends, and just driving home in traffic. This is the kind of everyday stress that lowers our immune system, causes irritability, promotes the production of cortisol, makes us tired, and generally screws up our lives. L-Theanine may help alleviate many of these problems by promoting a biochemical shift within the brain. Because of this shift you simply are not as stressed any more, and your body can more effectively fight off the bad stress-related problems. For fitness enthusiasts and bodybuilders, the stress does not stop at the everyday issues that everyone faces; it goes well beyond due to intense weight training, thermogenics, caffeine, and cardiovascular exercise. All of this on top of cortisol production, and you have the recipe for slow to no progress in the gym. In order to recover from your workouts and make progress in

your gym performance and in the mirror, you must plan to give yourself adequate recovery time. That means getting proper relaxation and rest. L-Theanine is able to reverse the elevation in norepinephrine from caffeine and allows you to "come down" following your thermogenic cocktail, as well as relaxing your body after workouts with weights and/or cardiovascular exercise. This in effect opens the door for proper recovery, and therefore, improvements in your physique and life. In short, training is the stimulus for growth, food is the fuel for training and recovery, and relaxation and rest allow the body to adapt by building the muscles and improving their condition in preparation for future training and more improvement.

THERMOGENIC AMPLIFIERS

Coleus Forskohlii

Coleus is a compound quickly gaining popularity in the supplement world. Why? Coleus has many benefits that are quickly becoming recognized by industry experts. Coleus has the unique ability to raise levels of the enzyme adenylate cyclase. This enzyme increases the conversion rate of ATP to cAMP in your body. Since cAMP is a key regulator of the metabolic rate and fat burning, your body can better utilize fatty acids for energy. In fact, it is so powerful, the government issued a patent on this product to the Sabinsa Corporation for use as an agent to increase the ratio of lean mass to fat tissue. I believe coleus would make an excellent additional to almost any thermogenic formula. In studies, coleus is reported to possess extremely positive cardiovascular benefits. It increases the force at which your heart contracts, and it lowers arterial blood pressure. As you well know, caffeine and ephedrine, found in most popular thermogenics, often raise blood pressure. So, by adding coleus, you may be able to burn fat without "jacking" up your blood pressure.

Furthermore, coleus has been shown in some studies to stimulate insulin secretion. This creates a win-win situation, since most thermogenic formulas are taken with a meal, and insulin then can help with the transport of nutrients.

Naringin

Naringin is an interesting compound isolated from grapefruit. Naringin is an inhibitor of the cytochrome p450 liver enzymes. Of particular interest, one of these enzymes (CYP1A2) is responsible for metabolizing caffeine. Furthermore, some of these enzymes may also appear in the intestinal lining, so naringin may alter the absorption of caffeine. In one study, grapefruit juice was administered (1.2 L/day containing 500mg/L of naringin) which decreased the oral clearance of caffeine by 23% and prolonged its half-life by 31%.[29] Therefore, if you are taking any sort of thermogenic compound with caffeine, I highly recommend you look to add this compound to support, and possibly prolong the fat burning effects.

Mucuna Puriens (L-dopa)

Mucuna puriens, otherwise known as velvet bean, has been used in Ayurvedic medicine for centuries in the management of Parkinson's disease. Furthermore, it has been used in formulas to control mental disorders like depression and to improve cognitive function. Among other natural phytochemicals, Mucuna contains L-dopa (L-dihydroxyphenylalanine), the compound believed to yield a therapeutic benefit. In recent years, it has been used as an aphrodisiac and cognitive tonic. Basically L-dopa works to increase levels of dopamine in the brain, which is the reason it is often used for the treatment of Parkinson's disease. Besides this benefit, L-Dopa also causes the secretion of growth hormone from the anterior pituitary gland. Obviously, GH is well known for its beneficial effects as an anti-catabolic agent and for its fat-burning properties. As far as directly increasing lean mass or decreasing bodyfat, very little data exists. What I can tell you though is that, from personal experience I get incredible workouts on this stuff. In using Mucuna bean extract, a little goes a long way so you'll want to start with a small amount. About 100 mg of Macuna puriens standardized for 15% L-dopa, which equates to about 15 mg of the active compound should give you a nice boost mentally and enhance the effect of any good thermogenic formula.

References Cited

1 Jacob S, Henriksen EJ, Tritschler HJ, Augustin HJ, Dietze GJ. Improvement of insulin-stimulated glucose-disposal in type 2 diabetes after repeated parenteral administration of thioctic acid. *Exp Clin Endocrinol Diabetes.* 1996;104(3):284-8.

2 Biewenga GP, Haenen GR, Bast A. The pharmacology of the antioxidant lipoic acid. *Gen Pharmacol.* 1997 Sep;29(3):315-31.

3 Suzuki YJ, Tsuchiya M, Packer L. Thioctic acid and dihydrolipoic acid are novel antioxidants which interact with reactive oxygen species. *Free Radic Res Commun.* 1991;15(5):255-63.

4 Fonteles MC, Huang LC, Larner J. Infusion of pH 2.0 D-chiro-inositol glycan insulin putative mediator normalizes plasma glucose in streptozotocin diabetic rats at a dose equivalent to insulin without inducing hypoglycaemia. *Diabetologia.* 1996 Jun; 39 (6):731-4.

5 Fonteles MC, Almeida MQ, Larner J Antihyperglycemic effects of 3-O-methyl-D-chiro-inositol and D-chiro-inositol associated with manganese in streptozotocin diabetic rats. *Horm Metab* Res. 2000 Apr;32 (4):129-32

6 Bates SH, Jones RB, Bailey CJ. Insulin-like effect of pinitol. *Br J Pharmacol.* 2000 Aug;130(8):1944-8

7 Murakami C, Myoga K, Kasai R, Ohtani K, Kurokawa T, Ishibashi S, Dayrit F, Padolina WG, Yamasaki K. Screening of plant constituents for effect on glucose transport activity in Ehrlich ascites tumour cells. *Chem Pharm Bull* (Tokyo). 1993 Dec;41(12):2129-31.

8 Kakuda T, Sakane I, Takihara T, Ozaki Y, Takeuchi H, Kuroyanagi M. Hypoglycemic effect of extracts from Lagerstroemia speciosa L. leaves in genetically diabetic KK-AY mice. *Biosci Biotechnol Biochem.* 1996 Feb;60(2):204-8.

9 Judy W.V., Southeastern Institute of biomedical research, Brandenton Florida, 1998 in press.

10 Suzuki Y, Unno T, Ushitani M, Hayashi K, Kakuda T. Antiobesity activity of extracts from Lagerstroemia speciosa L. leaves on female KK-Ay mice. *J Nutr Sci Vitaminol* (Tokyo).1999 Dec;45(6):791-5.

11 Di Pasquale, M, Amino Acids and Proteins for the Athlete. CRC Press, 1997.

12 Christiansen E, Tibell A, Vølund A, Rasmussen K, Groth CG, Holst JJ, Pedersen O, Christensen NJ, Madsbad S, Pancreatic endocrine function in recipients of segmental and whole pancreas transplantation. J Clin Endocrinol Metab 1996 Nov 81:11 3972-9M.

13 Flodstrom M, Tyrberg B, Eizirik DL, Sandler S. Reduced sensitivity of inducible nitric oxide synthase-deficient mice to multiple low-dose streptozotocin-induced diabetes. *Diabetes.* 1999 Apr;48(4):706-13.

14 Fonovich de Schroeder TM, Carattino MD, Frontera M, Catanzaro OL. Constitutive nitric oxide synthase (cNOS) activity in Langerhans islets from streptozotocin diabetic rats. *Braz J Med Biol Res.* 1998 May;31(5):625-32.

15 Broca C, Manteghetti M, Gross R, Baissac Y, Jacob M, Petit P, Sauvaire Y, Ribes G. 4- Hydroxyisoleucine: effects of synthetic and natural analogues on insulin secretion. *Eur J Pharmacol.* 2000 Mar 3;390(3):339-45.

16 Toeller M, Buyken AE, Heitkamp G, de Pergola G, Giorgino F, Fuller JH. Fiber intake, serum cholesterol levels, and cardiovascular disease in European individuals with type 1 diabetes. EURODIAB IDDM Complications Study Group. *Diabetes Care.* 1999 Mar;22 Suppl 2:B21-8.

17 Hallfrisch J, Facn, Behall KM. Mechanisms of the effects of grains on insulin and glucose responses. *J Am Coll Nutr.* 2000 Jun;19(3 Suppl):320S-325S. Review.

18 Zhang J, Kashket S. Inhibition of salivary amylase by black and green teas and their effects on the intraoral hydrolysis of starch. *Caries Res.* 1998;32(3):233-8.

19 Hogg N. Free radicals in disease. *Semin Reprod Endocrinol.* 1998;16(4):241-8. Review.

20 Tanner MA, Bu X, Steimle JA, Myers PR. The direct release of nitric oxide by gypenosides derived from the herb Gynostemma pentaphyllum. *Nitric Oxide.* 1999 ct; 3(5):359-65.

21 Gillis CN. Panax ginseng pharmacology: a nitric oxide link? *Biochem Pharmacol.* 1997 Jul 1;54(1):1-8. Review.

22 Smetanin, V. "The Influence of Preparations of Plant Origin on Physical Work Capacity." *The Russian Ministry of public Health.* 1986 (In Press)

23 Simakin, S. Yu., et al. "The Combined Use of Ecdisten and the Product "Bodrost" during Training in Cyclical Types of Sport." *Scientific Sports Bulletin,* No. 2, 1988

24 Fadeev, B.G., et al. "Comments on the Results of Research of Ratibol in the Practice of Athletic Training and Rehabilitation." *National Sports Research Institute.* (In Press)

25 Smetanin, B. Ya., et al. "The Influence of Rehabilitation Remedies on Special Endurance of Speed Skaters." *National Research Institute of Sports.* (In Press).

26 Report: "The Influence of Ecdisten, Prime Plus and Prime 1 on the Hormonal Balance of the Organism."

27 Report: "The Pharmacological Attributes of "Ecdisten".

28 Semeykin, V. A., et al. "Mechanism of Thymolytic action of Anabolic Steroids." *Pharmacology and Toxicology,* 1991, Vol. 54, 4: 37-38

29 Fuhr U, Klittich K, Staib AH. Inhibitory effect of grapefruit juice and its bitter principal, naringenin, on CYP1A2 dependent metabolism of caffeine in man. Br J Clin Pharmacol. 1993 Apr;35(4):431-6.

30 U.S. patent 4,163,746

31 Kitaoka S et al. *Biosci Biotech Biochem* 1996;60(11):1768-1771.

32 Yokogoshi H et al. *Neurochemical Research* 1998;23(5):667-673.

33 Kimura R et al. *Chem Pharm Bull* 1971;19(6):1257-1261.

34 Kimura R et al. *Yakugaku Zasshi* 1975;95(7):892-895.

35 Kobayashi K et al. *Nippon Noegikagaku Kaishi* 1998;72(2):153-157.

36 Results were obtained using patented effervescent technology, owned and patented by FSI Nutrition, U.S. Patent 5,925,378. The use of d-ribose is authorized by Bioenergy, Inc. under patents nos. 4,605,644, 4,719,201, 6,159,942, 6,153,943 and other patents pending.

37 Paulsen SM, Wurster SH, Nanney LB Expression of inducible nitric oxide synthase in human burn wounds. Wound Repair Regen 1998 Mar-Apr;6(2):142-8

38 Schaffer MR, Tantry U, van Wesep RA, Barbul A, Nitric oxide metabolism in wounds. J Surg Res 1997 Jul 15;71(1):25-

39 Kingwell BA Nitric oxide as a metabolic regulator during exercise: effects of training in health and disease. Clin Exp Pharmacol Physiol 2000 Apr;27(4):239-50

"I firmly believe that any man's finest hour is that moment when he has worked his heart out in good cause and lies exhausted on the field of battle, victorious."

-Vince Lombardi

Chapter

10

Supplement Delivery Systems

In the last issue of the *Sport Supplement Review*, we mentioned one of the future supplement trends. We talked of an area of supplement research that was being driven mainly by the pharmaceutical industry, a trend that was taking place behind the scenes. I still believe that the initial predictions are correct—I believe this supplement research could double, if not triple, the effectiveness of numerous existing supplements. The research to which I'm referring has to do with improving the delivery—and thus the effectiveness—of ingredients in dietary supplements.

The Problems

One of the reasons many weight trainers don't realize results from various supplements has to do with the fact that using these products for maximum effectiveness can be complex. As a matter of fact, it can be a royal pain in the butt to consume supplements as recommended. You know the story, forgetting to take your supplements exactly when you're supposed to, missing a dose because you're busy, it happens.

The problem is, most dietary supplements (unlike a lot of drugs) have a very short "half-life"—they're in and out of your system in a matter of hours or your liver "beats" the crap out of the compound by preparing it for excretion. Thus, we find ourselves taking multiple doses throughout the day in order to maintain an elevated level of these nutrients. Now this is not the case with all compounds. Some items like creatine do not need to remain at a constant level to deliver desired effects, and still there are other items that you might not want lingering around all day, like caffeine or ephedra. But for the most part it would be advantageous if we could control the amount and frequency of the supplements that we faithfully gobble down. You simply can't take your entire daily dose of most supplements in one serving, as this

> "There are many existing and emerging supplement delivery systems that I have had a chance to review."

would most likely lead to poor intestinal absorption, fleeting serum elevations, and in some cases, a stomach ache. However, solutions are within reach.

The Solutions

Several solutions to these problems may be right around the corner—or right under our noses. As we have mentioned previously, we have been following the progress of some of the most sophisticated delivery systems developed and used in the pharmaceutical industry.

The pharmaceutical researchers have collaborated with manufacturers in the supplement arena, and have adapted these delivery systems. The various supplement delivery systems allow us to manipulate the supplement dose. The type and duration of the manipulation is dependent on the desired effect of the compound being treated.

There are many existing and emerging supplement delivery systems that I have had a chance to review. The following is a list of supplement drawbacks that may be alleviated by advanced delivery systems that until

recently were only utilized by prominent pharmaceutical manufacturers:

- A supplement's blood concentration should be maintained or peaked at a level and time frame that provides maximum therapeutic benefit

- Many supplements or compounds are quickly destroyed in the stomach/intestine, therefore it is important to protect them long enough to reach the target tissues

- To achieve optimal blood concentrations, it may be necessary to deliver nutrients into precise areas of the digestive tract

- To elicit specific physiological responses, many formulations must be delivered in peak concentrations at very specific time frames

To date, here are the latest supplement delivery systems that may already have or will surely show up in health food stores in the months ahead.

Absorption and Solubility

As we know, the absorption characteristics of various supplements can lead to a more efficient use of those supplements. This is clearly illustrated by recent research about milk proteins. The research shows that whey proteins are rapidly absorbed and promote protein synthesis in the body, but have no significant role in providing vital anti-catabolic effects related to inhibition of protein breakdown. However, the other major milk protein, casein, although absorbed far slower than whey, does provide significant anti-catabolic effects due to its property of gradual amino acid digestion. Thus, the best type of milk protein-based supplement is one that contains both high-quality whey and casein proteins.

The absorption and dissolution or dissolving characteristics of supplements can vastly improve the results obtainable through the use of those supplements. The pharmaceutical industry is acutely aware of the importance of drug absorption, which can significantly affect the therapeutic value of drugs. But more recent developments have led to far more reliable and efficient drug-delivery systems. One such system, known as molecular dispersion, developed by Nutraceutix Inc., has also recently been used in certain specific supplements, markedly increasing the absorption and value of such supplements. This system works to vastly improve the absorption qualities of substances that are normally insoluble or poorly soluble in water.

The system works by creating conditions where such insoluble substances are made soluble, then presented one molecule at a time to biological membranes—such as those lining the intestine—for greatly enhanced uptake and absorption, as much as a 70% increase with certain compounds.

But how does this information relate to bodybuilding supplements? For one thing, the various prohormone supplements, such as androstenediol, norandrostenedione, and norandrostenediol are insoluble in water. Efficient absorption of these supplements into the gastrointestinal tract requires that they are made soluble in water. This increased solubility promotes the dispersion and transport within the gastrointestinal tract to body membranes. When various poorly soluble compounds are presented to biological membranes within the body as individual molecules coated with solubility-enhancing carrier molecules, this increases the bioavailability of the supplements. The process coats the supplement with hydrophilic (water-loving) molecules, thus making them water-soluble and able to pass freely into the membranes.

There are also several processes that can produce an ultra-small particle of the supplement, which allows it to be presented to as individual molecules. This uniform micronization permits compounds to cross body membranes with far greater efficiency. This uniform, single-molecule technique results in considerably greater absorption, and is being used in conjunction with various solubility-enhancing techniques.

Cyclodextrin

What about cyclodextrin? Any discussion of solubility technology systems would be incomplete without mentioning cyclodextrin. Cyclodextrin complexes involve coating any fat-soluble compound (like prohormones) with a carbohydrate that supposedly makes the compound more soluble, particularly in oral mucosa or membranes in the mouth. The idea for this type of delivery is based on recent preliminary studies showing that this type of drug-delivery system may allow a more efficient oral delivery system for testosterone, thereby obviating the need for testosterone injections.

Be aware that not all cyclodextrin products are equal. The process is difficult to pull off and only a fraction of manufacturers know what they are doing. Some ill-conceived cyclodextrin processes tend permit dissociation of the compound from the matrix. And look for Hydroxy-Propyl-Beta-Cyclodextrin—LPJ Research is known as the leader when it comes to cyclodextrin complexes—the stuff that has been proven successful in enhancing solubility.

Liposomes

Liposomes are highly complex microscopic lipid spheres (usually made from lecithin). Liposomes encapsulate water and the active ingredients inside their membranes, which are then released into the bloodstream in a sustained fashion. Originally liposomes were developed for delivering nutrients across the skin membrane in cosmetics.

Typical liposomal delivery is sprayed under the tongue, where the little spheres easily penetrate the mucosal tissue of the mouth and are absorbed into the bloodstream. But liposomes can be used to deliver compounds in a softgel capsule as well. Once in the small intestine, the liposomes are picked up into the lymph system, which allows the compounds to bypass the liver on the first pass.

Some colleagues of mine remember the days of searching for a manufacturer who would create liposomes for use in supplements, and coming up empty. That was in the early '90s, but now the growth of the nutritional industry has attracted the expansion of liposomal technology for use in bodybuilding and other health supplements.

Currently, there are several companies providing liposomal delivery technology—and I expect that number to grow.

In many cases, the goal of some supplements is to provide a steady-state level of absorption, where blood plasma levels are maintained within a specified range. This range in the pharmaceutical industry is considered optimal when the drug provides beneficial effects minus any toxic effects. For supplements, it is definitely not a question of toxicity but more of a question of value—how can a supplement be designed so its users get the best bang for their buck. This requires fine-tuning, and recent advances have made these goals possible. This fine-tuning is further bolstered by advancements made in the timing of the supplement delivery.

Timing

I mentioned at the beginning of this chapter that controlling the release and duration of a supplement could yield very advantageous effects. Now I mention "controlling" the release, and this process is a lot more sophisticated than the generic "timed release" being touted by many supplement manufacturers. Once again, the drug companies have created a high-tech delivery system to increase the effectiveness of certain drugs. And once again, the supplement industry has been quick to follow suit, seeing the immediate impact that controlled release could have in particular applications.

The precise release characteristics are made possible be a series of polymers that liberate the compound in a predetermined rate—the release pattern is not left in the hands of fate. The previous methods often used by our industry were crude by comparison. For instance, so-called "time-release" supplements are designed to release nutrients over an extended time, often eight hours or more. This makes sense, since taking large doses of vitamins often leads to a rapid excretion of such compounds. But if the same dose of vitamins can be gradually released, the absorption levels of those nutrients are increased—this is sound logic. This led to the design of various time-released vitamin preparations often created by using various cellulose matrices and various tableting pressures. But studies have shown disappointing results from many of these primitive time-released systems. Often, such time-released pills don't fully dissolve, and can literally pass through the body. Obviously you can't take the same chances when developing pharmaceuticals—especially those where the precision dosing is of grave importance.

Controlled delivery, or precision release, as it is often called, is a true, efficient patterned-release mechanism for supplement delivery. These pharmaceutical polymer-based systems promote steady-state absorption characteristics of any desired compound. Currently the best success for controlled-release products has been seen in the thermogenic and diet products under the trade names of Controlled Delivery Technology™ and Precision Release Matrix. The precision release of these amplifying compounds can be controlled to give you the benefits of stimulants while minimizing the jitters and other unwanted effects.

The beauty of this type of technology is that it can be "programmed"—meaning that manufacturers can create release patterns based on the desired effects. For instance, in the pharmaceutical world, there are drugs that require around-the-clock serum presence in order to be effective. Instead of taking constant doses—not knowing the particular release of each dose—you can now just take one dose per day that is systematically pulsed into the bloodstream.

> "The precision release of these amplifying compounds... give you the benefits of stimulants while minimizing the jitters..."

Route of Administration

Delivery systems that utilize various routes of administration typically have some of the above-mentioned qualities. But what I'm talking about here isn't so much the actual technology but how that technology is used.

I mentioned cyclodextrin technology to enhance solubility of fat-soluble compounds. The typical cyclodextrin-treated tablet can be delivered through the mucous membranes in the mouth. Incidentally, there are some manufacturers taking the sublingual concept a step further by developing bioadhesive technology that allows the sublingual tablet to "park" itself out of the way, against your gumline. You can keep it in place easily, as it will stick inconspicuously above (or below) your teeth.

And still yet, there are manufacturers who are further exploring other uses of cyclodextrin-treated products. I suppose that if designed properly, you could deliver product through any mucous membrane—ANY mucous membrane. There are even rumors of nasal- and even anal-administered products.

Other tricks that are being perfected are being borrowed from the world of cosmetics. Topical penetration-enhancing formulas have been developed to deliver a variety of compounds—just spray the stuff all over your body, and the escort molecules deliver the desired item past your skin and into your bloodstream.

The Future of Supplement Delivery Systems

Although it is easy to see the benefits associated with advanced supplement delivery systems, the technology necessary to accommodate nutritional products is still in its infancy. Within the next few years, we will likely see some remarkable progress. As we gain more control over the release of supplements, we will see a decrease in supplement side effects, as well as improved efficacy, safety, and consumer convenience. What's more, a number of new nutritional therapies will be possible. We will be able to deliver the complex supplements that are becoming available through scientific research, and we will be more able to target supplements to specific cells. Also important are the potential savings that will accompany the better efficiency and bioavailability of supplements.

Chapter

11

Amino Acids—The Building Blocks

Simply put, amino acids are the building blocks from which proteins can be manufactured in your body. Amino acids are joined together into long strings or peptides known as proteins. Every single cell in your body contains amino acids in some combination. In fact, approximately three-quarters of the dry weight of most cells are made up of amino acids. What separates amino acids and proteins from other macronutrients is that they contain a nitrogen group and a carbon skeleton. The nitrogen group is the point at which other amino acids can link together to become a peptide or protein. Traditionally, we know proteins as something we ingest so that our muscles can grow and recover, but proteins can also take the form of enzymes, hormones, transport mechanisms, and many others you probably don't regularly think of. As previously discussed in Chapters 4 and 8, the importance of protein is so great that it cannot be overlooked. In order to meet and exceed your goals, whether they are to gain muscle or burn fat, you must provide your body with these building blocks.

Over 300 different amino acids exist in nature, but only 20 amino acids make up the backbone of proteins. These 20 include: glycine, alanine, valine, leucine, isoleucine, serine, threonine, tyrosine, cysteine, aspartate, methionine, asparagine, glutamate, glutamine, arginine, lysine, histidine, phenylalanine, tryptophan, and proline. Of primary concern are the "essential" amino acids, which your body cannot manufacture from various carbon and nitrogen precursors. There are eight essential amino acids: leucine, isoleucine, valine, tryptophan, phenylalanine, methionine, threonine, and lysine. For the most part, these eight amino acids are basically all your body needs to function correctly. Well, at least in an ideal world. It is my opinion, and the opinion of many of the world's leading scientific researchers, that active individuals must consume at least three other amino acids for optimum performance. These amino acids, what most call "conditionally essential," are glutamine, taurine, and arginine. Unlike traditional essential amino acids, your body can manufacture these three amino acids, but the demand for them is greatly increased after exercise, and oftentimes your body simply cannot meet this demand. This is why I highly recommend the addition of these three amino acids to the protein you consume on a regular basis.

Aside from these amino acids, there are also non-essential amino acids. These include the remainder of the list above and many others. They are called non-essential because your body has the capability to manufacture them from some combination of essential amino acids and other precursors. However, by no means should you think your body doesn't need them, because they all have their purpose. Luckily, most whole-protein sources like chicken, fish, and whey and milk proteins contain an assortment of essential, conditionally essential, and non-essential amino acids—so for the most part you'll be covered with all of these.

Most likely, the majority of you reading this book have heard the terms "complete" and "incomplete" proteins. A complete protein is one that contains all of the essential amino acids, where an incomplete protein does not. Examples of complete proteins are chicken, fish, eggs, milk, and other meats. Foods that do not contain all the essential amino acids, or incomplete proteins, include many grains and vegetables. On rare occasions, those consuming a vegetarian diet will become deficient in one or more of these amino acids because most vegetable proteins are "incom-

plete." However, for the most part, amino acid deficiencies are very rare, but consuming optimal amounts of the essential, conditionally essential, and non-essential amino acids will aid in your quest to attain the ultimate physique.

ESSENTIAL AMINO ACIDS
Methionine

Sources: Methionine is an essential amino acid found in beef, chicken, fish, pork, egg, soybean, cottage cheese, and yogurt.

General Information: Methionine, along with cysteine, are amino acids that contain a

> "Phenylalanine can trigger the release of a chemical called cholycystokinin (CCK), which induces feelings of fullness."

principal source of sulfur. Methionine is particularly important because it is also a "methyl donor," meaning it gives up terminal methyl groups to choline. This is important, since the methyl group or CH3 (carbon-hydrogen) molecule is imperative in many chemical processes in your body, particularly the synthesis of RNA and DNA.

Methionine is also an important antioxidant, being particularly effective in combating the free radicals caused by alcohol consumption.[1]

Other functions include assisting gall bladder function, detoxifying heavy metals in the body, and even strengthening hair follicles.

Deficiency: Methionine deficiency has been shown to decrease protein synthesis, so consuming enough in your diet is of key importance. Fortunately, this will normally be attained through regular protein sources. Although possible, deficiencies of methionine are very rare.

Effectiveness: I don't really see that methionine supplementation would benefit athletes in any noticeable way. Of course, like any amino acid, sufficient amounts are needed for overall health and optimum athletic performance.

Dosage: Most people require about 200-1,000 mg a day for general health, and can easily obtain this with a normal diet. Methionine supplementation is not necessary.

Phenylalanine

Sources: Phenylalanine is an essential amino acid that's found in cottage cheese, soybeans, fish, meat, poultry, almonds, pecans, Brazil nuts, sesame seeds, chickpeas, and lentils.

General Information: Phenylalanine is a unique amino acid because it's converted into many other amino acids, which are the precursors for other important chemicals. Specifically, phenylalanine is converted into tyrosine, which is the starting point of a variety of neurotransmitters, namely norepinephrine and epinephrine (you adrenalin junkies should know these). These chemicals, in turn, control a variety of processes, such as heart rate and output, arterial blood pressure, oxygen consumption, blood glucose levels, and fat metabolism.

One area of particular interest to us fitness junkies is phenylalanine's alleged role in appetite suppression. Phenylalanine can trigger the release of a chemical called cholycystokinin (CCK), which induces feelings of fullness.[2]

Deficiency: Deficiencies of this amino acid can cause all kinds of personality changes, including depression. Other symptoms of deficiencies include bloodshot eyes and cataracts.

Effectiveness: Phenylalanine is undoubtedly important for overall health, but as far as physique augmentation, I think its most interesting role is that of appetite suppression. Personally, I have tried supplemental phenylalanine, and would grade it a high B for controlling appetite.

Dosage: For appetite suppression, take 300-500 mg before meals.

A cautionary note, however, for people suffering from a genetic condition called phenylketonuria (you might have seen this warning on a product containing aspartame—phenylalanine and aspartic acid form to make aspartame) should never take this supplement. Phenylketonurics lack the enzyme phenylalanine hydroxylase, and can't convert this amino acid into tyrosine. What results are dangerously high levels of phenylalanine in the brain, ultimately causing psychotic or schizophrenic behavior.

Threonine

Sources: Threonine is found in meats, eggs, and various beans. Most grains have little or no threonine.

General Information: The biological roles of this essential amino acid are sketchy at best. Aside from its psychological effects, threonine is said to prevent the liver from storing excess fat. It may also enhance the absorption of other nutrients.

Deficiency: Deficiencies result in irritability, decreased protein synthesis, and a generally difficult personality. Adequate amounts of it in the diet are considered essential in mental illness prevention.

Effectiveness: Although threonine is lacking in most vegetable proteins, I don't think there's any need for non-vegetarian body-builders to take supplemental amounts.

Dosage: The minimum dosage for overall health is about 8 mg per kilogram of body weight, so a 200-lb athlete would need about 720 mg a day.

Tryptophan

Sources: Tryptophan is contained in large amounts in carbohydrate-rich foods, especially bananas, sunflower seeds, milk, and baked potatoes.

General Information: Tryptophan is an essential amino acid that's often been used in the treatment of insomnia, PMS, depression, and obesity. It accomplishes these things because your body converts it into serotonin, a potent neurotransmitter. Serotonin levels can influence your choice of food, specifically, the amount of carbs you eat. For example, if you eat a small amount of carbs before a meal, you'll tend to eat less carbs at the meal.

Tryptophan, along with the amino acid tyrosine, plays a big role in regulating your energy or excitatory levels. Why? Both amino acids compete to cross your blood-brain barrier first. If tryptophan crosses first, you'll be relaxed and ready for a nap. If, however, tyrosine wins the race, you'll be alert and ready to roll.[3] When tryptophan crosses the blood-brain barrier and enters your brain, Vitamins B_3 and B_6 convert it to the sleep-energy regulating transmitter serotonin. What's more, carbohydrates, or more specifically, the insulin surge released when carbs are consumed, are necessary to carry tryptophan across the blood-brain barrier.

Tryptophan is also partly responsible for manufacturing niacin in your body.

Deficiency: As with many other amino acids, a deficiency in tryptophan can lead to edema, liver damage, and weakness, as well as a loss of muscle and fat.

Effectiveness: By now, you're getting the idea that tryptophan can be very useful in controlling your overall energy, sleeping patterns, and even your food cravings. If you want to have more energy, eat a high-protein meal, always making sure to eat a little protein before you dive into your carbs. If you want to relax, consume a lot of carbs and little protein. As far as enhancing performance, well, sleep is important, but you probably wouldn't see anything noticeable from tryptophan.

Dosage: Many of you may remember the tryptophan "scare." In 1989, tryptophan products were pulled from the market because they were thought to have caused a rare disease called eosinophilia-myalgia syndrome. The disease was traced to a contaminated batch of tryptophan manufactured in Japan, but the FDA has yet to reverse its decision and allow the sale of tryptophan because of this and other quality issues with its manufacturing. After this, a variation called 5-Hydoxy-Tryptophan 5-HTP (a hormone) hit the market, which is supposed to perform similar roles, such as helping with sleep, mood, fat loss, and so forth. Personally, I have not tried this stuff, but the feedback I hear is generally positive.

Valine

Sources: Foods that are high in valine include fish, beef, lamb, poultry, soy flour, cottage cheese, brown rice, and various nuts, as well as most good protein powders and meal-replacement powders (MRPs).

General Information: Valine, an essential amino acid, is also known as a branched-chain amino acid or BCAA, which also include leucine and isoleucine. They're called branched-chain amino acids because of the configuration of the molecule: the CH3 (methyl) groups branch out and interlock. Aside from their somewhat unusual molecular configuration, BCAAs play an important role in protein synthesis and/or minimizing protein breakdown.

The trouble is, not much is known about valine or how it works. We do know, however, that intense exercise "eats up" valine. It, along with the other BCAAs, are substrates for two other amino acids, glutamine and alanine. Furthermore, BCAAs are used directly for fuel by muscles, and this task spares other amino acids from being used up during exercise.[4,5]

Research on the amount of valine needed is mixed at this point, but I would recommend somewhere in the neighborhood of 3 to 5 grams daily for active individuals.

Effectiveness: Supplemental valine probably isn't necessary as long as you consume enough protein throughout the day. Most quality MRPs and protein powders contain between 15 to 25% BCAAs.

Dosage: Again, I don't recommend valine supplementation, but it seems that hard-training athletes require between 3 and 5 grams a day to ensure optimum protein synthesis and minimum protein breakdown.

Isoleucine

Sources: Foods that are high in isoleucine include fish, beef, lamb, poultry, soy flour, cottage cheese, and various nuts, as well as most good protein powders and MRPs.

General Information: In many ways, isoleucine is similar to valine: They're both branched-chain amino acids, and neither of them seem to have any specific therapeutic value. Of course, they both serve as a precursor for glutamine and alanine, and they can be used for fuel by muscle cells, thereby sparing other amino acids from being burned up. We do know this though: All three BCAAs play an important role in protein synthesis and minimize protein breakdown.[5]

Effectiveness: I personally get all of the necessary BCAAs I need through a good whey protein powder.

Dosage: I don't recommend taking any isoleucine supplementation other than what you get in a good meal replacement or protein powder, but it seems that hard-training athletes require about 20 mg per kilogram a day (about 1.8 grams for a 200-lb person), to ensure optimum protein synthesis and minimum protein breakdown.[5]

Leucine

Sources: Leucine is contained in every complete protein such as meat, eggs, protein powders, and meal-replacement drinks.

General Information: Together, leucine and the other two BCAAs make up one-third of muscle protein, and leucine is used up at the highest rate of all three. In fact, there's evidence that even sedentary people require much more leucine than the RDA handbook recommends.[19] Like the other BCAAs, leucine is required to ensure high protein synthesis rates and to minimize protein breakdown.

However, a while back, it was discovered that higher amounts of leucine could have a dramatic effect on preventing the kind of protein breakdown typically experienced by intensely training athletes.[20]

Luckily, leucine's beneficial effects were found to be due to one of its downstream metabolic byproducts. After leucine is ingested, it can be broken down in the body into ketoisocaproate (KIC), which can then be converted into another byproduct. This byproduct, of course, is HMB. For more information on this one-of-a-kind sports supplement, be sure to read Chapter 7 for the latest news.

Effectiveness: It seems clear that taking a couple of grams of leucine or KIC, or even 60 grams of either, probably isn't going to have the same protein-sparing effects as taking 3 grams of HMB.

Personally, I prefer to consume 3 grams of HMB a day vs. 60 grams of KIC or leucine. However, in a recent conversation with Dr. Steve Nissen, I found out that HMB and leucine combined may provide an added benefit, beyond that of taking either separately. Why? Well, HMB has been shown to have an anti-catabolic effect (it prevents muscle breakdown), while leucine on the other hand, along with the other BCAAs, tends to increase protein synthesis. So, combining these two or even four in combination before and after exercise may have tremendous potential. I'll be sure to keep you posted when more information arises on this topic.

Dosage: A 200-lb athlete probably requires about 6 grams of leucine a day, and this amount can be obtained through high-quality protein sources. I personally get all I need through my diet and my meal-replacement drink. I do, however, use HMB.

If you want to experiment with the above rationale, I recommend consuming 3 grams of leucine with every 1 gram of HMB, 3 times daily.

Lysine

Sources: Dietary sources of this essential amino acid include fish, chicken, beef, lamb, and other high quality, whole-protein sources (many vegetable proteins are lacking in lysine).

General Information: Lysine is an essential amino acid that your body uses to make carnitine, an amino acid that plays a role in transporting fatty acids into muscle cells, where they can be used as a source of energy.

Lysine is also of interest because it may interfere with viral replication; specifically, in herpes infections.[6] During a herpes infection, some researchers suggest taking 1,500 mg of lysine (along with a gram of Vitamin C). However, be sure to keep arginine intake low, because arginine often causes herpes infections to worsen.

There's also some evidence to suggest that a lysine deficiency might interfere with the ability to concentrate and synthesize protein, which mainly affects muscle and connective tissue.

Effectiveness: Personally, unless you've got a mean case of mouth sores or you are a vegetarian, supplemental lysine probably won't do you any good.

Dosage: For herpes infections, an extra 1,000-1,500 mg of lysine a day, taken in divided doses throughout the day with Vitamin C, has shown some promising results.

NON-ESSENTIAL AMINO ACIDS
Alanine

Sources: Alanine is found in peas, potatoes, beef, lamb, and most milk products.

General Information: Alanine, similar to glutamine, is involved in the inter-organ transfer of nitrogen and serves as a substrate to your body's energy source, ATP. One of the main functions of this non-essential amino acid is in the metabolism of tryptophan and pyroxidine (Vitamin B_6). If you experience low blood sugar (hypoglycemia), one cause may be intense exercise. When this happens, your body may use alanine as a source of glucose via gluconeogenesis to stabilize your blood sugar.[7] It does this by acting as a carrier to move amino groups out of tissues to prevent toxic ammonia buildup. The carbon skeleton of this carrier then is converted to glucose.

Effectiveness: I don't think alanine has any effects that are of particular interest to the performance athlete, and there's no real reason to take supplemental amounts.

Dosage: For general health, dosages between 200-600 mg a day are suggested, but also usually obtained through normal diet.

Glutamine

General Information: Glutamine is the most abundant amino acid in the human body. In fact, glutamine constitutes more than 60% of the total intra-muscular amino acid pool. Glutamine transfers nitrogen between organs, it can act as a fuel for the immune system, it's a precursor for the production of certain building blocks of DNA, and it regulates protein synthesis and protein degradation.[18]

As you can see, your body needs glutamine for numerous important functions. One of the main problems is that additional stress, like weight training or athletics, further increases its demand. After an intense workout, it takes your body several hours to rebuild its supply of glutamine. Supplementation may help your body recover and rebuild its stores.[8,9,10] When your body cannot recover, many times "overtraining syndrome" ensues, which typically involves low blood levels of glutamine for months or even years. On another side note, related with overtraining, glutamine levels tend to fall because of excess cortisol (the muscle-wasting hormone). The greater the exercise intensity, the higher cortisol levels go.[11] Cortisol, in addition to wreaking havoc on protein synthesis, growth hormone (GH), and numerous other functions, causes glutamine to be pulled out of muscle cells.

There may even be other possible benefits of glutamine supplementation, one being quicker recovery. The urinary excretion of 3-methylhistidine, a biochemical marker often used to measure the amount of muscle damage, is decreased with glutamine supplementation.[21] Glutamine may also increase circulating levels of GH. One study showed a four-fold increase in blood levels of GH an hour after taking only 2 grams of glutamine.

What do low amounts of glutamine mean to us athletes? Well, if you don't have enough in your body because you're chronically stressed out or overtrained, you'll have a hard time simply functioning, let alone putting on muscle or burning fat. Therefore, I certainly recommend consuming additional amounts.

Effectiveness: Will taking glutamine help you burn fat? Build muscle? Let's put it this way—adding glutamine to your diet may not result in any noticeable differences in the mirror right away, but over time, I think you will greatly benefit from glutamine supplementation. And, for those on low-carb or calorie-restricted diets, it is well worth it to help spare any catabolic effects that may happen while on these types of programs.

Dosage: Scientific studies have used varying amounts of glutamine, anywhere from 2 to 20 grams per day. For most athletes, 5 to 10 grams daily in addition to your diet seems to be standard protocol. However, it all depends on your body size and activity levels—the more you work out and the greater the intensity, the more you will probably need.

"Other functions of arginine include acceleration of wound healing, ensuring healthy thymus gland activity, reducing cholesterol…"

Taurine

Sources: Meat, poultry, eggs, dairy products, and fish are good sources of taurine. Legumes and nuts don't contain taurine, but they do contain methionine and cysteine, two amino acids that our bodies can make Taurine from.

General Information: Taurine isn't an essential amino acid, but it sure looks like it's an important bodybuilding supplement. There are indications that taurine acts as an "insulin mimicker." In fact, most studies seem to point at a "non-insulin" mechanism for taurine's effects. Researchers seem to believe taurine's effects may come from a direct action at the receptor level.[12,13]

Taurine is manufactured by your body, and it's also found in animal protein. Your body makes taurine from the amino acids methionine and cysteine, with assistance from Vitamin B_6. Most people, with the possible exception of vegetarians, get enough or make enough taurine. Roles for this amino acid include maintaining the solubility of cholesterol and normalizing the balance of other amino acids. It also seems to play a crucial role in heart function by controlling levels of potassium and calcium, which play a large role in controlling how your heart beats.

Effectiveness: All kinds of stress—including the stress imposed by weight lifting—deplete levels of taurine. Since it helps regulate blood sugar in much the same way as insulin, and apparently helps prevent muscle damage, I highly recommend a bit more taurine in your diet.

Dosage: Since active individuals do "use up" more of this amino acid than their sedentary counterparts, I recommend on the order of about 2 grams a day taken with carbohydrates (and creatine).

Arginine

Sources: Arginine is found naturally in peanuts, peanut butter, cashew nuts, pecan nuts, almonds, chocolate, and edible seeds of all types.

General Information: Back in the '80s, this amino acid gained a reputation as a potent GH releaser. That's true: In large doses, arginine will elicit greater GH production. Trouble is, no one has found a correlation between this and muscle gain or fat loss.

In the early '90s, researchers found out arginine could help control blood pressure, boost immune function, kill cancer cells, help control muscular activity, and regulate erections. It supposedly did this by contributing to the production of a chemical known as nitric oxide, or NO, a gas formed from arginine synthases.[14,15] NO has received much attention lately due to these effects, and I believe we will see much more information on this "conditionally essential" amino acid in the days to come. Along the same lines, arginine is intimately involved with the production of insulin. In fact, scientists often use an arginine-induced insulin response as standard protocol for insulin tolerance tests.

Other functions of arginine include acceleration of wound healing, ensuring healthy thymus gland activity, reducing cholesterol, and in treating the hardening of the arteries. Arginine may also promote insulin production and thereby assist in the transport of nutrients.

Deficiency: Individuals that are deficient in arginine display symptoms such as impaired insulin production, as well as impaired liver-lipid production.

Effectiveness: Arginine, like all amino acids, is crucial to building muscles, and though I'm not convinced of the GH-muscle link, I do think there's enough evidence with NO to prove that supplemental arginine will help in the quest to attain a lean, muscular physique.

Dosage: As far as eliciting an insulin/nitric oxide response, I recommend 3 to 5 grams following your workout. To enhance the sex life, guys should take between 4 and 8 grams of arginine, mixed with water, about 45 minutes before sex.

"As far as eliciting an insulin/nitric oxide response, add 3 to 5 grams of arginine following your workout."

Ornithine

Sources: Ornithine is found in milk products and meats, especially chicken.

General Information: Ornithine, along with arginine, was a "hot" amino acid in the '80s. At that time, some people made the claim that

these amino acids, taken together, could elicit GH release, and consequently lead to muscle growth and fat loss. However, that anecdotal data has never been validated to have any effect on muscular growth or fat loss.

Regardless, ornithine, like all amino acids, is important. Although ornithine isn't incorporated into protein, it does play an important metabolic role, as it enhances the transportation of other amino acids into cells. It also helps detoxify ammonia in the urea cycle, and there's some evidence to suggest it can help improve liver function.

Effectiveness: Overall, I don't think taking ornithine supplementation will help much.

Dosage: If you're looking for GH release, try 1 to 2 grams daily before bed.

Histidine

Sources: Histidine is found mainly in beef, poultry, cottage cheese, eggs, and cheese. Most vegetables and grains are devoid of histidine.

General Information: Histidine is an essential amino acid during childhood, but once you reach adulthood, your body can manufacture its own, and it then becomes a non-essential amino acid. Histidine is important in that it's vital to the maintenance of myelin sheaths—the tissue that surrounds nerve cells. In fact, histidine has been used to combat some forms of deafness, since of course, hearing is often nerve related.

Histidine, by the process of removing the COOH group by histidine decarboxylase, is converted into histamine, a powerful vasodilator that is involved in many allergic reactions. For these reasons, histidine has been used to treat certain circulatory and cardiac problems.

Effectiveness: It's clear that histidine is important for overall health, but I see no real need to add anything extra beyond that in your normal diet.

Dosage: Children require a dosage of about 33 mg per kilogram of bodyweight, but no recommendations have been established for adults.

Proline

Sources: Proline is found in meat, dairy products, and gelatin.

General Information: Your body does makes proline, but there might be some rare situations where additional supplementation is useful. The amino acid is one of the main components of collagen, the protein that binds and supports all other tissues. (You know, the stuff plastic surgeons love.) In fact, burn patients, compared to normal individuals, have decreased proline synthesis and a three-fold increase in proline oxidation. Therefore, some researchers have proposed that proline may increase tissue repair. Reportedly, the body uses proline to manufacture a chemical called hydroxyproline, which is incorporated into the structure of tendons and ligaments.[22]

Effectiveness: It stands to reason that proline might also help athletes who suffer from soft tissue sprains or "loose" joints. If you suffer from either of these problems, some experimentation with proline might be worth it.

Dosage: 500-1,000 mg a day, combined with Vitamin C, glucosamine, and chondroitin might be worth experimenting with.

Carnitine

Sources: It can be found in muscle and organ meats.

General Information: The human body manufactures carnitine, and supplemental amounts are found in muscle and organ meats. Plant proteins, however, don't contain carnitine. For some reason, it seems that men have a higher need for this amino acid than women, and large amounts are found in the epididymis of the testis.

Much of the evidence and physiological pathways suggest that carnitine might be a valid fat-burning supplement, but I've never heard of anybody who used it successfully to overcome a weight problem. In the body, carnitine transfers fatty acids across cell membranes to the mitochondria, where they can be used as energy. Given this effect, it seems that carnitine would be useful to help get leaner. Trouble is, data has not shown that increasing the amount of carnitine in your system increases the rate or the amount of fatty acids that can be converted into energy by the cell.

In order for your body to make its own carnitine effectively (out of its amino acid precursors, methionine and lysine), you have to take adequate amounts of Vitamin C, and optimally niacin and B$_6$ too. In fact, people who are deficient in carnitine are often actually deficient in Vitamin C. However, carnitine deficiencies are rare.

Effectiveness: Though I haven't seen much good data on carnitine, many people swear by it to reduce bodyfat. My thoughts are they might be deficient due to a vegetarian diet or poor eating habits. For enhanced cognitive function, you may also want to try the acetyl ester, Acetyl L-Carnitine, which is showing promise for cognitive enhancement.

Dosage: For fat burning, 1 to 3 grams in divided dosages throughout the day may have some effect in people with carnitine deficiencies.

Tyrosine

Sources: This amino acid is found in meat, dairy, and eggs, as well as in almonds and bananas.

General Information: Tyrosine is probably my favorite "non-essential" amino acid. Why? Well, tyrosine is an amino acid that plays a large role in your overall energy levels, as discussed above. Let me explain... remember how tryptophan, once crossing the blood-brain barrier, is converted to seratonin? Well, similarly when tyrosine enters your brain, it is "ganged up" on by Vitamins B_3, B_6, C, folic acid, and the minerals iron, copper, and zinc to transform it into two "alertness" chemicals called norepinephrine and dopamine. If you recall, norepinephrine stimulates the release of stored bodyfat and helps control the release of endocrine hormones, which regulate your metabolism and appetite, among other things. Dopamine, on the other hand, can affect the muscle movement and tissue repair, in addition to influencing your sex drive and immune system (both positively). It

also stimulates your pituitary to release GH. Overall, because of these conversions, tyrosine makes a great pre-workout energy formula, especially when combined with ephedrine and caffeine. Tyrosine also has been implicated in reducing the physiological and behavioral effects of stress—both conditions that are catabolic if not checked.

Deficiency: Tyrosine has many applications for bodybuilders and other athletes. Being deficient in this particular amino acid can be very detrimental, especially if you're a bodybuilder trying to put on muscle. Some of the deficiency symptoms include edema, weakness, liver damage, and loss of muscle and fat.

Effectiveness: As I stated above, tyrosine is one of my favorite non-essential amino acids. Its applications for bodybuilding and other sports are numerous.

Dosage: If you're looking for a pre-workout boost, I recommend 500-1,000 mg, 30 minutes prior to your workout. For enhanced fat loss, try taking 1 to 2 grams, 3 times a day.

Cysteine and Cystine

Sources: Found in poultry, eggs, wheat, and broccoli.

General Information: Metabolically, cysteine and cystine are pretty much interchangeable. Cystine is simply the stable form of cysteine, and your body changes one to the other as the need arises. Cysteine, along with another "sulfur-rich" amino acid methionine, is used by your body to make coenzyme A, heparin, biotin, lipoic acid, and glutathione. Cysteine also determines the flexibility and texture of skin, as the amino acid can prevent the collagen cross-linking, a side effect of overexposure to the sun and old age. The amino acid(s) also seem to offset some of the cellular damage caused by smoking or drinking.

One cautionary note: Diabetics or people who have problems controlling blood sugar should stay away from cysteine, as it can actually inactivate insulin.

Effectiveness: I don't think athletes need to take supplemental cysteine unless they want to experiment with its antioxidant properties. For those looking for an antioxidant, I recommend the acetylated variation known as NAC or N-Acetyl Cysteine.

> "...tyrosine is one of my favorite non-essential amino acids. Its applications for bodybuilding and other sports are numerous."

Dosage: In order to take advantage of its skin-protecting or cell-protecting qualities, try 1 gram 3 times a day, along with Vitamin B$_6$. Some research indicates that adequate levels of cystine or cysteine are necessary for proper utilization of Vitamin B$_6$. For those wishing to try NAC, a dose of 600 mg in 3 divided doses daily is definitely worth trying.

Glycine

Sources: Glycine is present in fish, meat, beans, and dairy products.

General Information: Although it's a non-essential amino acid, glycine is interesting in that it, along with arginine, seems to influence the natural production of creatine. Experiments with rats show that is also may play a part in the healing of damaged tissue, as it, again along with arginine, significantly improved nitrogen retention in traumatized and non-traumatized lab animals.

Other functions of this non-essential amino acid include the biosynthesis of nucleic acids, and the production of glutathione, an important naturally occurring antioxidant.

Effectiveness: Again, I think most bodybuilders get adequate amounts of this amino acid through a good, high-protein diet.

Dosage: None established for therapeutic purposes.

Asparagine and Aspartic Acid

Sources: Asparagine is found in food sources like dairy products, beef, poultry, and eggs.

General Information: Aspartic acid and asparagine play an important role in human metabolism. These amino acids help transform other amino acids into the ones your body needs at any particular time. They do this by donating an amino group. Once asparagine donates this amino group, it becomes known as aspartic acid. This process, known as "transamination," is important in the metabolic control of your brain and nervous system, urea cycle, and cellular function. It also helps cancel out the toxic effects of ammonia in your system (a byproduct of protein metabolism).

Effectiveness: Will aspartic acid help you in your quest to attain a lean, muscular physique? I doubt very much that taking supplemental amounts would help your endurance unless you were somehow deficient in the amino acid.

Dosage: None established for therapeutic purposes.

Citrulline

Sources: Not found in a lot of foods, although it was originally isolated from watermelon.

General Information: This non-essential amino acid, like aspartic acid, may help reduce fatigue by helping clear ammonia from your system, but this sure isn't conclusive. Since it's a precursor of both arginine (the arginine-citrulline cycle) and ornithine (the GH-releasing amino acids), it may, indirectly affect GH release and possibly nitric oxide and insulin.

Effectiveness: Most likely supplemental citrulline won't do a thing. However, the combination of arginine and citrulline may prove to be something of value.

Dosage: None established for therapeutic purposes.

Glutathione

General Information: Glutathione, although a non-essential amino acid, is essential as it is a

> "Weight training and general activity causes the production of pro-oxidants, so... glutathione can help your body heal itself."

naturally occurring antioxidant. Glutathione is one of your body's main defense mechanisms, taking care of toxins and repairing damage wherever it occurs. Glutathione, in conjunction with catalase and super-oxide dismutase (SOD), comprise your body's main "weaponry" against foreign invaders.

Glutathione is actually made up of three amino acids—cysteine, glutamic acid, and glycine. It scours your system for the pro-oxidants that suppress your immune system, cause cancer, and contribute to the aging process.[17] And like many processes that seem to dissipate as we age, glutathione production is no exception. In one experiment looking at different aged animals, glutathione levels were up to 34% lower in older animals. Other experiments have shown it to protect against the damage caused by cigarette smoking, kill liver tumor cells, and even detoxify heavy metals (cadmium, mercury, and aluminum) in the body.[16]

Effectiveness: Weight training and general activity causes the production of pro-oxidants, so potent antioxidants like glutathione can help your body heal itself. I take glutathione, and I highly recommend it in conjunction with other antioxidants like alpha-lipoic acid, super-oxide dismutase, and Vitamin E.

Dosage: As an antioxidant, 1 to 3 grams daily.

References Cited:

1 Feroci, G. and Fini, A., "Study of the antioxidant effect of several selenium and sulphur compounds." *J Trace Elem Med Biol.* 12.2 (1998) : 96-100.

2 Ballinger, A.B., Clark, M.L., "L-phenylalanine releases cholecystokinin (CCK) and is associated with reduced food intake in humans: Evidence for a physiological role of CCK in control of eating." *Metabolism.* 43.6 (1994) : 735-8.

3 Wurtman, R.J. and Wurtman, J.J., "Do carbohydrates affect food intake via neurotransmitter activity?" *Appetite.* 11.1 (1988) : 42-7.

4 Wagenmakers, A.J., "Muscle amino acid metabolism at rest and during exercise: role in human physiology and metabolism." *Exerc Sport Sci Rev.* 26 (1998) : 287-314.

5 MacLean, D.A. and Graham, T.E., "Branched-chain amino acid supplementation augments plasma ammonia responses during exercise in humans." *J Appl Physiol.* 74.6 (1993) : 2711-7.

6 Eaton, M.D., Scala, A.R., Birnie, H., "Lysine inhibition of cell protein and viral synthesis. Reversal by other amino acids." *Proc Soc Exp Biol Med.* 119.4 (1965) : 998-1004.

7 Wasserman, D.H., Williams, P.E., Lacy, D.B., Green, D.R., Cherrington, A.D., "Importance of intrahepatic mechanisms to gluconeogenesis from alanine during exercise and recovery." *Am J Physiol.* 254.4 (1988) : E518-25.

8 Rowbottom, D.G., et al., "The Emerging Role of Glutamine as an Indicator of Exercise Stress and Overtraining." *Sports Medicine* 21.2 (1996): 80-97.

9 Smith, R. J. "Glutamine: Conditionally Essential?"

10 Bowtell, J.L., Gelly, K., Jackman, M.L., Patel, A., Simeoni, M., Rennie, M.J., "Effect of oral glutamine on whole body carbohydrate storage during recovery from exhaustive exercise." *J Appl Physiol.* 86.6 (1999) : 1770-7.

11 Flynn, N.E. and Wu, G., "Enhanced metabolism of arginine and glutamine in enterocytes of cortisol-treated pigs." *Am J Physiol.* 272.3 Part 1 (1997) : G474-80.

12 Maturo, J., and Kulakowsk, E.C., "Insulin-like activity of taurine." *Adv Exp Med Biol.* 217 (1987) :217-26.

13 Lampson, W.G., Kramer, J.H., Schaffer, S.W., "Potentiation of the actions of insulin by taurine." *Can J Physiol Pharmacol.* 61.5 (1983) : 457-63.

14 Nishimura M., et al., "Cardiovascular Regulation by L-Arginine in the Brain of Rats: Role of the Brain Renin-Angiotensin System and Nitric Oxide." *Am. J. Hypertens.* 10.4 Part 1 (1997) : 389-396.

15 Guoyao, W.U. and Morris, M., "Arginine metabolism: nitric oxide and beyond." *J. Biochem.* 336 (1998) : 1-17.

16 Green, G.M., "Cigarette smoking: protection of alveolar macrophages by glutathione and cysteine." *Science* 162 (1968): 810-811.

17 Ross, D., "Glutathione, free radicals and chemotherapeutic agents. Mechanisms of free-radical induced toxicity and glutathione-dependent protection." *Pharmacol Ther.* 37.2 (1988) : 231-49.

18 Pasquale, M. *Amino Acids and Proteins for the Athlete* CRC Press, 1997. Pgs 127-130

19 Khoury, A.E., Fukagawa, N.K., Sanchez, M., Tsay, R.H., Gleason, R.E., Chapman, T.E., Young, V.R., "The 24-h pattern and rate of leucine oxidation, with particular reference to tracer estimates of leucine requirements in healthy adults." *Am J Clin Nutr.* 59.5 (1994) : 1012-20.

20 Mero, A., Pitkanen, H., Oja, S.S., Komi, P.V., Pontinen, P., Takala, T., "Leucine supplementation and serum amino acids, testosterone, cortisol and growth hormone in male power athletes during training." *J Sports Med Phys Fitness.* 37.2 (1997) : 137-45.

21 MacLennan, P.A., Smith, K., Weryk, B., Watt, P.W., Rennie, M.J., "Inhibition of protein breakdown by glutamine in perfused rat skeletal muscle." *FEBS Lett.* 237.1-2 (1988) : 133-6.

22 Manning, J.M. and Meister, A., "Conversion of proline to collagen hydroxyproline." *Biochemistry* 5.4 (1966) : 1154-65.

"It takes more than just a
good-looking body.
You've got to have the heart
and soul to go with it."

-Lee Haney

Chapter 12

The Basics—Vitamins and Minerals

We all know that vitamins and minerals are important to our health, but it is easy to forget exactly how and why. It's kind of like changing the oil in your car every three thousand miles. You are not really sure why it needs to be done, but you know that it is essential to the maintenance and performance of your car. In this chapter, I am going to give you a quick reference guide for all the vitamins and minerals so you can find out, at a glance, things like the Recommended Dietary Allowance (RDA), natural food sources, and special applications for active individuals like yourself. But first, let's talk about the overall importance of vitamins and minerals (micronutrients), the history and current status of vitamin and mineral consumption, and when and how you should be using vitamin and mineral supplements.

The History

The metabolic roles of vitamins and minerals vary, but they all contribute to the normal function, growth, and maintenance of your body.[1] Had these micronutrients not been discovered, we might be faced with the common diseases and conditions of history's past, like scurvy from lack of Vitamin C or anemia from lack of iron. Although nutrition experts and doctors have realized that vitamins and minerals play a crucial role in maintaining good health for more than a century, it became apparent during World War II that an official dietary recommendation of these nutrients was needed. In 1941, a group of 25 scientists formed the first Food and Nutrition Board, establishing dietary standards for evaluating the nutritional intakes of populations. This Board developed the first RDA. Now, you are probably thinking, that's really great historical information, but what does that mean for me in terms of meeting my daily needs for vitamins and minerals? Well, to answer that question, I have to dig a little deeper into these RDAs that were established.

To generate the RDAs, the Food and Nutrition Board of the National Academy of Sciences, determined the intake of a nutrient that met the needs of almost all (about 97%) healthy people of similar age and gender. These approximations only accounted for the amount of each nutrient needed to reduce the risk of deficiency diseases, such as scurvy and rickets. Although the RDAs were updated every 4 to 5 years, with the latest edition published in 1989, the recommendations have never considered optimal levels of nutrients to help prevent chronic disease, like heart disease and osteoporosis, nor have they taken into account the needs of highly active individuals. So, next time you consume your favorite "healthy" foods, which hype they contain 100% of this vitamin or that mineral, remember that you may still be cheating yourself out of the optimal levels of nutrients that you need as an active individual!

The Current Status of Vitamin and Mineral Consumption

As more and more of the population becomes nutrition savvy, we tend to rely more heavily on governmental recommendations as a guideline. After all, how could the Food and Nutrition Board, made up of highly qualified scientists, lead you astray? Now that you know the story behind the RDAs, you may be thinking the government has not done such a good job at making recommendations to ensure your health. Well, don't lose faith just yet. New research has made it clear that some of the 1989 RDAs do not maximize human benefit from food components and the new Food and Nutrition Board members have been making updated recommendations since 1997 that will continue to be released in stages through the year 2001. The framework

of these new recommendations will be renamed Dietary Reference Intakes (DRI). The DRI is intended to shift the emphasis from preventing deficiency to decreasing the risk of some diseases that are diet related. However, because the DRI is set for the general population, these levels will not necessarily be optimal for intensely exercising individuals. The DRI will encompass four categories. The first is Estimated Average Requirement (EAR), which specifies the intake that meets the estimated nutrient need of 50% of the individuals in a specific group. The second is RDA, which I described earlier. The third is Adequate Intake (AI), which specifies an amount when sufficient scientific evidence is not available. And the fourth is Tolerable Upper Intake Level (UL), which specifies the maximum intake by an individual that is unlikely to pose risks of adverse health effects in almost all healthy individuals in a specified group.

The following information in this chapter provides the most updated information available on the newest RDAs. The RDAs I have provided refer for the most part to men and women between the ages of 19 and 50. If you are interested in obtaining RDA information for another age category, you can go to www.nationalacademies.org or check your local medical libraries for books on Dietary Reference Intakes. Remember that new DRIs will be established throughout the year of 2001. Only about 65% of the vitamins and minerals have been updated through the end of 2000. For the most updated information, be sure to check the National Academies web site often.

The Newest Requirements

As I mentioned earlier, even with these new DRIs, the likelihood of meeting your optimal nutritional needs through whole and processed foods is questionable because of manufacturing and environmental factors, some of which you will read about later in this chapter.[12,13,14] Fortunately, dietary supplements have become widely available in the last few decades, including stand-alone multivitamin/mineral supplements and fortified nutrition shakes, bars, and other health-related products. These products can not only help ensure that you meet your daily requirements set by the government, but that you also support your extra needs prompted by exercise, stress, lack of sleep, and other tensions that your body is exposed to.

> "I recommend a good multivitamin/mineral supplement and some additional antioxidants as part of your basic nutritional program."

Based on the above information I have provided, it is no surprise that I recommend a good multivitamin/mineral supplement and some additional antioxidants as part of your basic daily nutritional program. Now, probably any quality vitamin/mineral supplement available on the market will meet the stan-dards set by the Food and Nutrition Board. However, you might want to consider using some blends specifically designed for exercising individuals like yourself. EAS' Multi-Blend, a multivitamin/mineral formula, combined with AAB, a potent antioxidant combination designed to support recovery from intense bouts of exercise and protection against free radicals, are two such products. Some of you might be wondering what you should take—a capsule or tablet? It really doesn't matter. Just be sure to look for quality supplements and follow the recommended use on the label. Now that we have covered all that, on to the details....

Vitamins

Fat-Soluble Vitamins

The fat-soluble vitamins include A, D, E, and K. These vitamins are lipid-like molecules that are absorbed along with dietary fat. Adequate absorption of the fat-soluble vitamins depends on efficient fat absorption. About 40 to 90% of all fat-soluble vitamins consumed are absorbed when they are taken in typical amounts. Once absorbed, these vitamins are delivered to target cells in your body, with any remainder being stored in your liver for future use.

Vitamin A (Beta-carotene, Retinol)

Retinol is the pure form of Vitamin A, and comes from animal products. Beta-carotene is a provitamin A (which converts to Vitamin A in your body) found in plants, and it converts

> "A recent study suggests that Vitamin A intake is associated with enhanced insulin-mediated glucose disposal."

to Vitamin A at about a rate of 50%.

Natural Sources: Asparagus, broccoli, cantaloupe, carrots, eggs, leaf lettuce, liver, milk, pumpkin, sweet potatoes, tomatoes, and watermelon.

RDA: 5000 IU (Retinol: 1 mcg = 1 RE = 3.3 IU, Beta-carotene: 6 mcg = 1 RE = 10 IU)

Function: Essential for night vision and proper function of the retina;[2] supports mucus-forming cells, which provide essential lubricants used throughout the body; promotes bone growth and maintenance; helps the body combat bacterial, parasitic, and viral infections; and it can also be used as a topical treatment for acne.

Deficiency Symptoms: Americans are at little risk for developing deficiency symptoms. Liver reserves for Vitamin A are up to five times greater than needed to provide for good health. Deficiency symptoms include, night blindness, lack of tear secretion, changes in eyes, dry or rough skin, weight loss, poor bone growth, diarrhea, acne, and fatigue.

Toxicity: Ten times the RDA or more for

Retinol Vitamin A, for an extended period of time, can lead to toxicity symptoms. One large dose at a time (100 times or more the RDA) can cause acute toxicity.

Fitness Applications: A recent study suggests that Vitamin A intake is associated with enhanced insulin-mediated glucose disposal.[3] Not only is Vitamin A a valuable antioxidant, but it also seems to be one of the simplest ways to increase your insulin sensitivity, so be sure to take in ample amounts of Vitamin A, or better yet, carotenoids. I suggest about 120 mg per day of beta-carotene or a carotenoid blend.

Did You Know? Worldwide, Vitamin A deficiency is the leading cause of non-accidental blindness.

Vitamin D (Calcitriol—the active form of Vitamin D)

Natural Sources: Vitamin D is synthesized by your skin when it is exposed to sun. In fact, the majority of our Vitamin D supply comes from sun exposure, so if you tend to spend most of your time inside or live in a very cloudy climate, you may need to supplement Vitamin D with foods or a good multivitamin/mineral. Foods containing Vitamin D include fatty fish, fortified milk, and fortified cereal.

Adequate Intake (AI): 5 mcg (micrograms)

Function: Regulates blood calcium by increasing the absorption of calcium from the small intestine and reducing calcium excretions by the kidneys, increases calcium deposition in the bones,[4] and prevents rickets.

Deficiency Symptoms: Elderly people and anyone else who spends most of the day inside and ingests little or no Vitamin D are at risk for deficiency. Deficiency symptoms include rickets, a childhood disease causing bent or bowed legs, malformation of joints or bones,[5] and late tooth development; and osteomalacia, an adult disease causing pain in the ribs, lower spine, pelvis, or legs, brittle bones, and muscle weakness.

Toxicity: Vitamin D can be a very toxic substance. An intake of just five times the RDA over an extended period of time can be harmful, especially for children. The main symptom of Vitamin D toxicity is over-absorption of calcium and calcium deposits in the kidneys, heart, and blood vessels. Excess Vitamin D intake can have similar effects as getting too little Vitamin D. Sun exposure causes no risk of Vitamin D toxicity.

Fitness Applications: There are really no specific uses related to fitness, but if you live in a cloudy climate you should take in a little more Vitamin D, about 600-700 IU per day. In sunny climates, you can take in about 400-500 IU per day unless you spend all of your time inside. In that case, I recommend sticking with 600-700 IU. Anyone who has low intakes and spends time inside, especially in the winter, may have low levels of Vitamin D and experience muscle weakness or imbalance problems.

Did You Know? You should spend five to ten minutes per day in the sun without sunblock protection. Sunblock products with a SPF of eight or above reduce Vitamin D synthesis in the skin.

Vitamin E (also called tocopherol)

Natural Sources: Almonds, asparagus, avocados, broccoli, canola oil, corn, corn oil, cottonseed oil, fortified cereals, hazelnuts, peanuts/peanut oil, safflower nuts/oil, soybean oil, spinach, sunflower seeds, walnuts, wheat germ, and wheat germ oil.

RDA: 15 mg or 22 IU natural Vitamin E, 33 IU synthetic Vitamin E (If Vitamin E is originates from food, 1 mg = 1.5 IU. If Vitamin E is of synthetic origin, 1 mg = 1 IU.)

Best Available Sources: The most active form of Vitamin E is d-alpha-tocopherol.

Function: Acts as anti-blood clotting agent; promotes normal red blood cell formation; promotes Vitamin-C recycling; reduces risk of fatal first myocardial infarction in men;[6] protects against prostate cancer; improves immunity,[7] especially in Vitamin-E deficient people; serves as an antioxidant for cancer, heart disease, and free radicals in the body.

Deficiency Symptoms: Lethargy, apathy, inability to concentrate, and nerve dysfunction.

Toxicity: Tolerable Upper Intake is 1,500 IU of the natural d- form.

Fitness Applications: When following a heavy training regimen, you might want to take 800–1,200 IU per day. According to a study published in the *International Journal of Sports Medicine*, Vitamin E may help prevent exercise associated muscle damage.[15] During maintenance training, take 200–400 IU per day.

Did You Know? Obtaining Vitamin E through food sources can be a hit-or-miss undertaking. The actual Vitamin E content of a food depends on harvesting, processing, storage, and cooking, because Vitamin E is highly susceptible to destruction by oxygen, light, metals, and deep fat frying.[16]

Vitamin K
(phylloquinones from plants and menaquinones from fish oils and meats)

Natural Sources: Alfalfa, asparagus, broccoli, Brussels sprouts, cabbage, cheddar cheese, green leafy vegetables, liver, seaweed, spinach, and turnip greens.

RDA: 80 mcg (micrograms)

Function: Essential for normal blood clotting, treats bleeding disorders due to Vitamin K deficiency, and promotes bone health.

Deficiency Symptoms: Abnormal blood clotting that can lead to nosebleeds, blood in urine, stomach bleeding, bleeding from capillaries or skin, causing spontaneous bruising, and prolonged clotting time.

Toxicity: Even though this is a fat-soluble vitamin, toxicity is unlikely because it is readily excreted from the body.

Fitness Applications: For athletes, I recommend 100–150 mcg per day, which you can easily get from eating about 3 oz of green leafy vegetables.

Did You Know? Vitamin K can be synthesized by bacteria in the human intestine. However, newborns lack the gastrointestinal bacteria that synthesize Vitamin K. To prevent deficiency in infants, physicians routinely provide Vitamin K by injection to newborns at birth.

Water-Soluble Vitamins

The rest of the vitamins are known as water-soluble. These include primarily Vitamin C, Biotin, and the B vitamins. Because they are water soluble, many of these vitamins are more easily excreted from the body than the fat-soluble vitamins. Moreover, some of the water-soluble vitamins are rather easily destroyed during cooking due to heat or pH changes. Typically about 50 to 90% of the water-soluble vitamins are absorbed. The nutritional status of most Americans for these vitamins is generally good.

Vitamin C (Ascorbic Acid)

Natural Sources: Broccoli, Brussels sprouts, cabbage, collards, grapefruit, green peppers, guava, kale, lemons, mangos, orange juice, oranges, papayas, peppers, potatoes, rose hips, spinach, strawberries, tangerines, tomatoes, and watercress.

RDA: Women: 75 mg, Men: 90 mg

Function: Promotes healthy capillaries, gums, and teeth; helps heal wounds, burn, and broken bones; prevents and treats scurvy; enhances immune function;[8] helps form collagen in connective tissue; increases calcium absorption; contributes to hemoglobin and red blood cell production in bone marrow; aids adrenal gland function; and reduces free-radical production.

Deficiency Symptoms: Scurvy, muscle weakness, swollen gums, loss of teeth, tiredness, depression, bleeding under skin, bleeding gums, easy bruising, swollen or painful joints, nosebleeds, frequent infections, slow wound healing, and anemia, which includes symptoms such as weakness, tiredness, and paleness.

Toxicity: Vitamin C is really not toxic, but excessive intake, such as 10,000 mg (10 g) or above, can cause unwanted side effects such as diarrhea, frequent urination, and possible skin rashes. Should you suffer from any of these side effects, cut back on your dosage.

"If you are a vegan, be sure to take Vitamin B_{12} supplements."

Fitness Applications: For antioxidant protection and because exercise makes your body excrete Vitamin C faster (you can sweat it out), I recommend 1-3 g per day.

Did You Know? Vitamin C is found in all living tissues and most animals are capable of synthesizing their own supply from glucose. Guinea pigs and humans are two of the very few organisms that are unable to synthesize their own supply of Vitamin C.

Vitamin B_{12} (Cyanocobalamin)

Natural Sources: Beef, beef liver, blue cheese, clams, dairy products, eggs, flounder, herring, liverwurst, mackerel, milk, oysters, sardines, snapper, and Swiss cheese.

RDA: 2.4 mcg (micrograms)

Function: Aids in folate metabolism, vital in maintaining the insulation for nerve cells, treats some types of nerve damage, treats anemia, prevents Vitamin B_{12} deficiency in vegan vegetarians and persons with absorption diseases, and treats Alzheimer's disease.

Deficiency Symptoms: Vegans are especially at risk for Vitamin B_{12} deficiency. Symptoms include enlarged red blood cell size, fatigue, weakness (especially in arms and legs), irreversible nerve damage, sore tongue, nausea, appetite loss, weight loss, numbness and tingling in hands and feet, difficulty maintaining balance, poor memory, and bruising.

Toxicity: There is a very low incidence of Vitamin B_{12} toxicity, even with amounts up to 1,000 mcg per day.

Fitness Applications: If you are a vegan, be sure to take Vitamin B_{12} supplements. Try 500 mcg per day.

Did You Know? All Vitamin B_{12} compounds are synthesized exclusively by bacteria, fungi, and algae. Animals such as cows and sheep obtain Vitamin B_{12} either from bacterial synthesis in the stomach or from ingested soil. The only reliable source for humans is animal foods. Plants do not contain Vitamin B_{12}.

Biotin (Vitamin H)

Natural Sources: Almonds, bananas, brewer's yeast, brown rice, bulgur wheat, butter, calf liver, cashew nuts, cheese, chicken, clams, eggs, green peas, lentils, liver, mackerel, meats, milk, mushrooms, oat bran, oatmeal, peanut butter, peanuts, salmon, soybeans, split peas, tuna, and walnuts.

Adequate Intake (AI): 30 mcg (micrograms)

Function: Aids in the formation of fatty acids; facilitates the metabolism of amino acids and carbohydrates; promotes normal health of sweat glands, nerve tissue, bone marrow, male sex glands, blood cells, skin, and hair; and minimizes symptoms of zinc deficiency.

Deficiency symptoms: Deficiency is very rare, but symptoms include fatigue, depression, nausea, loss of appetite, loss of muscular reflexes, smooth pale tongue, hair loss, increased blood-cholesterol levels, anemia, conjunctivitis, and liver enlargement.

Toxicity: Biotin is relatively non-toxic. Large doses have been given over an extended period of time without harmful side effects.

Fitness Applications: Biotin may increase insulin sensitivity.[9] Try 500 mcg per day for general health.

Did You Know? Egg yolks are one of the most nutrient-dense sources of biotin, but raw egg whites contain a protein called avidin, which inhibits biotin absorption. An occasional raw egg is of no concern, but in general, cook your eggs to destroy avidin (and salmonella).

Folate (Vitamin B$_9$, Folic Acid):

Natural Sources: Asparagus, avocados, bananas, beans, beets, brewer's yeast, Brussels sprouts, cabbage, calf liver, cantaloupe, citrus fruits/juices, endive, fortified grain products, chickpeas, green leafy vegetables, lentils, sprouts, and wheat germ.

RDA: 400 mcg (micrograms)

Function: Promotes normal red blood cell formation; maintains nervous system, intestinal tract, sex organs, white blood cells, and normal patterns of growth; regulates embryonic and fetal development of nerve cells and prevents neural-tube defects;[10] aids metabolism of amino acids and protein synthesis (RNA and DNA).

Deficiency Symptoms: Megaloblastic anemia, in which red blood cells are large and uneven in size; irritability; weakness; lack of energy; loss of appetite; paleness; and mild mental symptoms, such as forgetfulness and confusion. Deficiency in pregnant women can cause neural tube defects leading to spina bifida and anencephaly in infants.

Toxicity: Probably up around 10 mg per day.

"Some people take niacin in dosages of 500 to 1000 mg daily to help reduce cholesterol."

Consuming excessive amounts of folate can mask a Vitamin B_{12} deficiency.

Fitness Applications: Excessive amounts will not boost your performance, so I recommend about 1 mg per day.

Did You Know? Cooking vegetables causes loss of folate content.

Niacin (Vitamin B_3):

Natural Sources: Beef liver, brewer's yeast, chicken, fortified cereals and breads, halibut, peanut butter, peanuts, pork/ham, potatoes, salmon, soybeans, swordfish, tuna, and turkey.

RDA: Women: 14 mg, Men: 16 mg (Each 60 mg of dietary tryptophan contributes to the synthesis of approximately 1 mg of niacin. The number of milligrams of niacin supplied by dietary protein can be estimated by dividing protein intake by 6.)

Function: Prevents pellagra; acts as a coenzyme in over 200 metabolic reactions, including the production of ATP; reduces cholesterol and triglycerides in blood; dilates blood vessels if taken in doses larger than 75 mg; and treats vertigo and ringing in ears.

Deficiency Symptoms: Delirium; general fatigue/lethargy; loss of appetite; headaches; swollen, red tongue; skin lesions; indigestion; dermatitis/dark pigmentation; diarrhea; irritability; and dizziness.

Toxicity: Because niacin is water soluble, you would have to take in extremely exorbitant amounts to experience any toxicity.

Fitness Applications: Some people take niacin in dosages of 500 to 1,000 mg daily to help reduce cholesterol. Niacin is probably one of the first treatments prescribed for reducing blood cholesterol. These people experience the flushing and itching, but it is not toxic; it is just a side effect of the medication. Some physicians advise taking an aspirin to prevent these symptoms.

Did You Know? Niacin is very heat stable, and coffee and tea provide a little niacin to the diet.

Pantothenic Acid (Vitamin B_5):

Natural Sources: Avocados, bananas, blue cheese, broccoli, chicken, collard greens, eggs, lentils, liver, lobster, meats, milk, oranges, peanut butter, peanuts, peas, soybeans, sunflower seeds, wheat germ, and whole-grain products.

Adequate Intake (AI): 5-10 mg a day.

Function: Helps produce coenzyme A (CoA), which is essential for metabolism of carbohydrates, protein, and fat; aids the release of energy from foods; and helps synthesize numerous body materials.

Deficiency Symptoms: No proven symptoms exist for pantothenic acid. However, lack of one B vitamin usually means lack of other B nutrients. Pantothenic acid is usually given with other B vitamins if there are symptoms of any Vitamin-B deficiency, including excessive fatigue, sleep disturbances, loss of appetite, nausea, or dermatitis.

Toxicity: There is no known toxicity for pantothenic acid.

Fitness Applications: No special applications for this vitamin.

Did You Know? The Greek word "pantothen," meaning "from every side," reflects the ample supply of pantothenic acid in foods.

Pyridoxine (Vitamin B$_6$):

Natural Sources: Avocados, bananas, beef liver, chicken, fortified cereals, ground beef, ham, hazelnuts, lentils, potatoes, salmon, shrimp, soybeans, sunflower seeds, tuna, and wheat germ.

RDA: 1.3 mg

Function: Participates actively in many chemical reactions of proteins and amino acids; helps normal function of the brain; promotes normal red blood cell formation; helps in energy production; acts as a coenzyme in carbohydrate, protein, and fat metabolism; and treats some forms of anemia.

Deficiency Symptoms: Reduced protein synthesis, weakness, mental confusion, irritability, nervousness, insomnia, poor walking coordination, anemia, skin lesions, tongue discoloration, and muscle twitching.

Toxicity: Over 2 g per day for 2 months or more, or 200 mg per day over an extended period of time may cause toxicity. Toxicity symptoms include walking difficulties, and hand and foot numbness.

Fitness Applications: Athletes need more Vitamin B$_6$[11] because of their increased use of glycogen as a fuel, and their high protein intakes. Try 20-50 mg per day.

Did You Know? If we didn't have the biochemical action of Vitamin B$_6$, every amino acid would become "essential" and would have to be supplied by the diet.

Riboflavin (Vitamin B$_2$)

Natural Sources: Bananas, beef liver, milk, yogurt, cheese, eggs, enriched breads, fortified cereals, ham, mixed vegetables, pork, tuna, and wheat germ.

RDA: Women: 1.1 mg, Men: 1.3 mg

Function: Aids in the release of energy from food; maintains healthy mucous membranes lining respiratory, digestive, circulatory, and excretory tracts when used in conjunction with Vitamin A; preserves integrity of the nervous system, skin, and eyes; and activates Vitamin B$_6$.

Deficiency Symptoms: Cracks and sores in corners of mouth; inflammation of the tongue and lips; eyes that are overly sensitive to light and easily tired; itching and scaling of skin around nose, mouth, scrotum, forehead, ears, and scalp.

Toxicity: There is no known toxicity.

Fitness Applications: 50-100 mg per day for hard-training athletes.

Did You Know? The name riboflavin comes from its yellow color ("flavin" means yellow in Latin).

Thiamin (Vitamin B$_1$)

Natural Sources: Baked potato, beef kidney/liver, brewer's yeast, flour (rye and whole-grained), chickpeas, ham, kidney beans, navy beans, orange juice, oranges, oysters, peanuts, peas, raisins, brown rice, wheat germ, and whole-grain products

RDA: Women: 1.1 mg, Men: 1.2 mg

Function: Keeps mucous membranes healthy; maintains normal function of nervous system, muscles, and heart; prevents beriberi.

Deficiency Symptoms: Loss of appetite; fatigue; nausea; mental problems such as rolling of the eyeballs, depression, and memory loss; rapid heartbeat; gastrointestinal disorders; pain or tingling in the arms or legs; decreased reflex activity; fluid accumulation in the arms and legs; and heart enlargement.

Toxicity: Surplus dietary thiamin is rapidly lost in the urine via the kidneys, so there is no danger from excessive intake through supplements.

Fitness Applications: 50-100 mg per day. You will excrete whatever you don't need.

Did You Know? Psychological disturbances such as irritability, headache, depression, and weakness can be seen after only ten days on a thiamin-free diet. Therefore it is important to consume thiamin on a daily basis.

References Cited:

1 McKay, D. L. et al., "The effects of a multivitamin/mineral supplement on micronutrient status, antioxidant capacity and cytokine production in healthy older adults consuming a fortified diet." *J Am Coll Nutr* 19.5 2000 : 613-621

2 Berson, E. L. "Nutrition and retinal degenerations." *Int Ophthalmol Clin* 40.4 (2000) : 93-111.

3 Facchini, F. et al., "Relation Between Dietary Vitamin Intake and Resistance to Insulin-Mediated Glucose Disposal in Healthy Volunteers." *Am. J. Clin. Nutr.* 63.6 (1996) : 946-949.

4 Cymet, T. C. et al., " Osteoporosis." *J Am Osteopath Assoc* 100.10 (2000) : s9-S15.

5 Chapurlat, R. et al., "Therapeutic strategies for osteoporosis." *Ann Med Interne (Paris)* 151.6 (2000) : 471-476.

6 Gey, K. F., "Vitamins E plus C and interacting conutrients required for optimal helath. A critical and constructive review of epidemiology and supplementation data regarding cardiovascular disease and cancer." *Biofactors* 7.1-2 (1998) : 113-174.

7 Lee, C. Y. et al., "Vitamin E Supplementation Improves Cell-Mediated Immunity and Oxidative Stress of Asia men and Women." *J Nutr* 130.12 (2000) : 2932-2937.

8 McDermott J. H., "Antioxidant nutrients: current dietary recommendations and research update." *J Am Pharm Assoc (Wash)* 40.6 (2000) : 785-799.

9 Maebashi, M. et al., "Therapeutic Evaluation of the Effect of Biotin on Hyperglycemia in Patients With Non-Insulin Dependent Diabetes Mellitus." *J. Clin. Biochem. Nutr.* 14 (1993) : 211-218.

10 Hernandez-Diaz, S. et al., "Folic Acid Antagonists during Pregnancy and the Risk of Birth Defects." *N Engl J med* 343 (2000) :1608-1614.

11 Manore, M. M., "Effect of physical activity on thiamine, riboflavin, and vitamin B-6 requirements." *Am J Clin Nutr* 72.2 (2000) : 598S-606S.

12 Prochasda, L.J. et al., "Effects of Food Processing on the Thermodynamic and Nutritive Value of Foods: Literature and Database Survey." *Med Hypotheses* 54.2 (2000) : 254-62.

13 Shi J., Le Maguer M., "Lycopene in Tomatoes: Chemical and Physical Properties Affected by Food Processing." *Crit Rev Food Sci Nutr* 40.1 (2000) : 1-42.

14 Reddy M.B., Love M., "The Impact of Food Processing on the Nutritional Quality of Vitamins and Minerals." *Adv Exp Med Biol* 459 (1999) : 99-106.

15 Itoh H., et al., "Vitamin E Supplementation Attenuates Leakage of Enzymes Following 6 Successive Days of Running Training." *Int J Sports Med* 21.5 (2000) : 369-74.

16 Allwood M.C., Martin H.J., "The Photodegradation of Vitamins A and E Parenteral Nutrition Mixtures During Infusion." *Clin Nutr* 19.5 (2000) : 339-42.

Minerals

Minerals are categorized based on the amount you need per day. Generally speaking, if you require 100 mg or more per day of a certain mineral, it is considered a major mineral. The rest are considered trace minerals. Foods contain and supply us with many minerals, but our bodies vary in their capacity to absorb and use available minerals. Although minerals may be present in foods, they are not bioavailable unless your body can absorb them.

Minerals in the average American's diet come from both plant and animal sources. Overall, minerals from animal products are absorbed better because binders and fiber are not present to hinder absorption. A diet free of animal products is likely to be marginal in calcium and other minerals. Because bioavailability is in question, a multi-mineral supplement is always a good idea. Vegans should be especially aware of taking a good mineral supplement.

Sodium (Na)

Natural Sources: Table salt, white bread and rolls, processed meats, cheese, soups, spaghetti and tomato sauces.

RDA: 2,400 mg

Function: Helps regulate water balance in the body, plays a crucial role in maintaining normal blood pressure, aids in muscle contraction and nerve transmission, and regulates the body's acid-base balance.

Deficiency Symptoms: Muscle and stomach cramps, nausea, fatigue, mental apathy, muscle twitching and cramping, and appetite loss.

Toxicity: Some experts say that adults should limit their intake to 3,000 mg per day, but the verdict is still out on toxicity. Approximately 10 to 15% of adults are sodium sensitive and for these people, high sodium intakes can contribute to hypertension.

Fitness Applications: If you are going to be heavily exercising and sweating considerably, be sure to take in some extra sodium before or during exercise for proper electrolyte balance. According to the Gatorade Sport Science Institute, each liter of sweat can contain 1.8 grams of sodium or more, and a loss of just a few grams can affect nerve endings and muscle fibers, which may lead to cramping.

Did You Know? Table salt is 40% sodium and 60% chloride. The range of sodium intakes seen in adults of 3 to 6 grams per day, which translates to 7.5 to 15 grams of salt. A teaspoon of salt contains about 2 grams of sodium.

Phosphorus (P)

Natural Sources: Milk, cheese, yogurt, bakery products, meat, cereals, bran, eggs, nuts, fish, and soft drinks.

RDA: 700 mg

Function: Builds strong bones and teeth; promotes energy metabolism; promotes growth, maintenance, and repair of all body tissues; and buffers body fluids for acid-base balance.

Deficiency Symptoms: Deficiency is very unlikely since phosphorus is widely available and easily absorbed, but symptoms can include bone pain, loss of appetite, weakness, and easily broken bones.

Toxicity: Typical phosphorus intakes do not seem to be toxic. The Tolerable Upper Intake for phosphorus is 3-4 grams per day.

Fitness Applications: No special applications for athletes.

Did You Know? Phosphorus is the second most abundant element (after calcium) present in our bodies, and makes up about 1% of our total bodyweight.

Potassium (K)

Natural Sources: Asparagus, avocados, bananas, beans, cantaloupe, carrots, citrus fruit, juices, milk, molasses, nuts, peas, potatoes, raisins, salt substitutes, sardines, spinach, whole-grain cereal, coffee, and tea.

RDA: 3,500 mg

Best Source: Potassium chloride is the most common form used in supplements.

Function: Maintains water balance in body tissues and cells; promotes regular heartbeat; promotes normal muscle contraction; regulates transfer of nutrients to cells; preserves or restores normal function of nerve cells, heart cells, skeletal muscle cells, and kidneys.

Deficiency Symptoms: People who exercise heavily may need to replenish their potassium. Symptoms include loss of appetite, muscle cramps, confusion, constipation, and weakness. Eventually these symptoms can lead to low blood pressure and an irregular heartbeat, which can cause cardiac arrest and death.

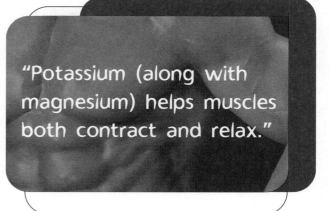

"Potassium (along with magnesium) helps muscles both contract and relax."

Toxicity: If the kidneys function normally, typical intakes of potassium are not toxic. When the kidneys function poorly, potassium can build up in the blood, inhibiting heart function.

Fitness Applications: Potassium (along with magnesium) helps muscles both contract and relax. When the body is low in potassium, muscles can cramp more easily and fatigue can occur quicker.

Did You Know? The intracellular fluids (fluids inside cells) contain 95% of the potassium in the body.

Calcium (Ca)

Natural Sources: Milk, cheese, leafy green vegetables, broccoli, sardines, canned salmon, fortified juice, breakfast cereals, and tofu.

RDA: 1,000 mg

Function: Calcium requires a slightly acidic pH and Vitamin D for efficient absorption. Calcium carbonate is the most common form of calcium used in supplements, and it has the highest concentration of calcium by weight (40%) compared to calcium citrate (21%) and calcium phosphate (8%). Calcium carbonate is a good form to take, but calcium citrate may be better due to its acidic properties and enhanced absorption. Remember that calcium citrate has a little less calcium concentration per weight so you will have to take in more total grams than the carbonate form.

Benefits: Builds bones and teeth, maintains bone density and strength,[1] helps prevent osteoporosis,[2] assists in blood clotting, important for transmission of nerve impulses to target cells, aids in muscle contraction, and helps regulate metabolism.

Deficiency Symptoms: Frequent fractures, muscle contractions, convulsive seizures, and muscle cramps.

Toxicity: 2,500 mg is the Tolerable Upper Intake. Toxicity symptoms can include headache, irritability, kidney failure, kidney stones, and decreased absorption of other minerals.

Fitness Applications: Most athletes need 1,000-1,500 mg per day.

Did You Know? To estimate your calcium intake, use the "300" rule. For a moderate

"To help ensure adequate intake of magnesium and support optimal hormone balance, including testosterone, try EAS' ZMA HP."

energy intake from typical daily foods, give yourself 300 mg. For every cup of milk or yogurt or 1.5 oz of cheese, add another 300 mg. From there, you can add any fortified foods or supplements you are taking.

Magnesium (Mg)

Natural Sources: Almonds, avocados, bananas, bluefish, carp, cod, collards, dairy products, flounder, halibut, herring, leafy green vegetables, shrimp, swordfish, wheat germ, whole-wheat bread, broccoli, beans, nuts, and seeds.

RDA: Women: 310-320 mg, Men: 400-420 mg

Function: Aids in nerve and muscle function,[3] including regulation of normal heart rhythm,[4] conducts nerve impulses; helps activate ATP; supports optimal hormone balance; contributes to potassium and calcium metabolism; aids in many enzyme reactions; acts as antacid in small doses; strengthens tooth enamel; and contributes to bone health.

Deficiency Symptoms: Muscle contractions or pain, convulsions, confusion, concentration difficulties, irregular heartbeat, irritability, nervousness, and skin problems.

Toxicity: The Tolerable Upper Intake for supplements above and beyond what food sources supply is 350 mg. Toxicity is of higher concern to those people with compromised kidney function because the kidneys primarily regulate blood magnesium. High blood magnesium can lead to weakness, nausea, and depression.

Fitness Applications: The average man consumes about 350 mg of magnesium per day,

50 mg below the RDA.[5] Vitamin D enhances magnesium absorption. To help ensure adequate intake of magnesium and support optimal hormone balance, including testosterone, try EAS' ZMA™ HP.

Did You Know? A link between magnesium deficiency and sudden heart attacks has been observed. Now, an intravenous dose is being investigated as part of the treatment during the early phases of a heart attack.

Chromium (Cr)

Natural Sources: Beef, brewer's yeast, calf liver, cheese, chicken, egg yolks, molasses, sweet potatoes, tomatoes, whole-grain products, mushrooms, and nuts.

RDA: 120 mcg (micrograms)

Function: Promotes glucose metabolism,[6] helps insulin regulate blood sugar, decreases insulin requirements and improves glucose tolerance of some people with Type II diabetes, and aids in protein synthesis.

Deficiency Symptoms: Impaired glucose tolerance, and elevated blood cholesterol and triglycerides.

Toxicity: Based on average intake levels of chromium, toxicity is unlikely. However, there may be some concern of long-term high intake. Because chromium is a metal, it may accumulate in the body with extended use. Some toxicity has been reported in people exposed to chromium in industrial settings. Liver damage and lung cancer may result from such high intakes.

Fitness Applications: Chromium supple-

mentation has been reported to improve glucose metabolism, improve blood lipid concentrations, and reduce bodyfat. However, current research clearly indicates that chromium provides no benefits to healthy individuals.[11,12,13] I do not recommend supplementing chromium as part of your diet or weight-loss efforts.

Did You Know? The amount of chromium in foods is closely tied to the local soil content of chromium. To ensure a sufficient chromium intake, regularly choose whole grains over refined grains.

Copper (Cu)

Natural Sources: Organ meats, avocados, legumes, lentils, liver, lobster, nuts, oats, oysters, peanuts, raisins, salmon, shell fish, soybeans, spinach, whole-grain breads, and cereals.

RDA: 2 mg

Function: Copper promotes normal red blood cell formation, acts as a catalyst in storage and release of iron to form hemoglobin for red blood cells. It assists in the production of several enzymes involved in respiration, assists in production of several enzymes involved in forming melanin, promotes normal insulin function, and helps maintain connective tissue and myelin (the insulation material around nerves).

Deficiency Symptoms: Anemia, which is low red blood cell count associated with reduced resistance to infection; faulty collagen formation; bone demineralization; and loss of hair or skin pigmentation.

Toxicity: Dietary copper is not toxic because

intakes are usually low and our bodies can regulate storage through excretion. At single supplemental dosages of 10-15 mg, copper tends to cause vomiting.

Fitness Applications: No special applications.

Did You Know? Use of large doses of antacids may bind enough copper in the intestine to cause a deficiency.

Iodine (I$_2$)

Natural Sources: Iodized salt, saltwater fish, seafood, molasses, and some plants grown near the sea.

RDA: 150 mcg

Function: Supports hormone synthesis in the thyroid gland and prevents goiter (an enlargement of the thyroid gland).

Deficiency Symptoms: Goiter, which is the insufficient function of the thyroid gland, and leads to a fall in metabolic rate and an increase in blood cholesterol. In children, a deficiency can cause depressed growth, delayed sexual development, mental retardation, and deafness.

Toxicity: Iodine intakes up to 2 mg per day appear to be safe. However, when very high amounts of iodine are consumed, thyroid hormone synthesis is inhibited (same as a deficiency). A "toxic goiter" results.

Fitness Applications: No special recommendations.

Did You Know? Some areas of Europe have yet to adopt the practice of fortifying salt with iodide. People in these areas still suffer from goiter. In fact, about 1 billion people worldwide are at risk of iodine deficiency, and approximately 20% of these people have goiter.

Iron (Fe)

Natural Sources: Meat, spinach, oysters, liver, peas, legumes, bakery products, bread, and crackers.

Iron that is part of hemoglobin and myoglobin molecules in animal flesh is called *heme iron*. Elemental iron found in plant foods is called *nonheme iron*.

RDA: Men: 10 mg, Women: 15 mg

Best Source: Ferrous sulfate to cure iron-deficiency anemia.

Function: Prevents and treats iron-deficiency anemia due to dietary iron deficiency or other causes,[7] stimulates bone-marrow production of hemoglobin (the red blood cell pigment that carries oxygen to body cells), forms part of several enzymes and proteins in the body, and supports immune function.

Deficiency Symptoms: Listlessness, heart palpitations upon exertion, inadequate temperature regulation, loss of appetite, fatigue, irritability, pale appearance to skin, brittle nails, decreased mental capacity, and learning deficit.

Toxicity: 150-200 mg per day for 4 to 6 months is usually the treatment for deficiency, so high amounts can be tolerated. However, they should not be continued for an extended period of time. Severe toxicity can lead to organ damage, especially in the liver and heart, diabetes, and bronze skin pigmentation.

Fitness Applications: Athletes should be especially aware of their iron intake, as they can lose a significant amount through perspiration, which can lead to impaired performance.[14,15] Female athletes may want to take in even more iron, 18-25 mg per day.[16]

Did You Know? A good source of iron is from cooking utensils. When acidic foods such as tomato sauce are cooked in iron cookware, some iron from the pan is taken up by the food. The replacement of iron cookware with stainless steel and aluminum in recent times has likely increased the risk for iron deficiency.

Manganese (Mn)

Natural Sources: Beans (dried), blue and blackberries, bran, buckwheat, carrots, chestnuts, hazelnuts, oatmeal, peanuts, peas, pecans, seaweed, spinach, tea, and whole grains.

RDA: 2-5 mg

Function: A co-factor for certain enzymes, it aids in carbohydrate metabolism and the formation of connective tissue and bones, promotes nerve function, and it's involved in antioxidant processes.

Deficiency Symptoms: Deficiency in adults is highly unlikely, and symptoms have not been observed in adult humans. Deficiency in children can lead to abnormal growth and development.

Toxicity: Toxicity is also highly unlikely, as average intakes fall within the RDA range.

Manganese toxicity has been seen in people who work in manganese mines, and includes severe psychiatric abnormalities, irritability, violence, hallucinations, and impaired control of muscles.

Fitness Applications: No special applications.

Did You Know? Consuming high amounts of calcium and phosphorus can inhibit manganese absorption.

Molybdenum (Mo)

Natural Sources: Milk, milk products, beans, whole grains, and nuts.

RDA: 75 mcg

Function: Necessary for the function of the enzyme xanthine dehydrogenase, which functions in the formation of uric acid and the mobilization of iron from liver stores.

Deficiency Symptoms: No deficiency symptoms have been observed in people consuming a normal diet, though deficiency signs have appeared in malnourished people. These symptoms include increased heart and respiration rates, night blindness, mental confusion, edema, and weakness.

Toxicity: Toxicity has not been established in humans, but lab animals consuming very high dosages of molybdenum have developed evidence of toxicity.

Fitness Applications: No special applications.

Did You Know? High intakes of molybdenum can inhibit copper absorption.

Selenium (Se)

Natural Sources: Bran, broccoli, brown rice, cabbage, chicken, garlic, kidney, liver, milk, mushrooms, nutritional yeast, oatmeal, onions, seafood, tuna, and whole-grain products

RDA: Men: 70 mcg, Women: 55 mcg

Benefits: Complements Vitamin E as an efficient antioxidant, plays a role in thyroid hormone metabolism, supports immune system function[8], reduces free radical production, and may protect against cancer.

Deficiency Symptoms: Symptoms include muscle pain and muscle wasting. Selenium deficiency has resulted in cardiomyopathy and myocardial deaths in humans.

Toxicity: Daily intakes as low as 1-3 mg can cause toxicity symptoms if taken for many months. These symptoms include hair loss, nausea, diarrhea, fatigue, and changes in fingernails and toenails.

Fitness Applications: Since selenium is an antioxidant, I recommend 150-250 mcg for hard-training athletes to fight free radicals caused by intense exercise.

Did You Know? Much of the selenium present in plant sources is determined by the content of selenium in the soil that they are grown. Northeast China, New Zealand, and Finland have especially low soil concentrations of selenium.

Zinc (Zn)

Natural Sources: Beef or other red meats, egg yolk, fish, herring, lamb, maple syrup, milk, molasses, oysters, pork, sesame seeds, soybeans, sunflower seeds, turkey, wheat bran, wheat germ, whole-grain products, and yeast.

RDA: 15 mg

Benefits: More than 300 enzymes require zinc as a co-factor for optimal activity. It supports synthesis and function of DNA; aids in wound healing, metabolism, and growth;[9] essential to normal immune function, ensures development of sexual organs and bone; and supports insulin function.

Deficiency Symptoms: Loss of taste and smell, slow growth in children,[10] rashes, multiple skin lesions, impaired appetite, hair loss, sterility, low sperm count, and delayed wound healing.

Toxicity: Supplements 5 to 20 times the RDA for extended periods of time can inhibit copper absorption and reduce HDL (good cholesterol). Intakes over 100 mg per day can also result in diarrhea, nausea, cramps, vomiting, and depressed immune function.

Fitness Applications: No special applications.

Did You Know? If you're taking both iron and zinc, make sure to take them at separate times as they interfere with each other's absorption.

References Cited:

1 Chapurlat, R., et al., "Therapeutic strategies for osteoporosis." *Ann Med Interne (Paris)* 151.6 (2000) : 471-476.

2 Wood, B., et al., "Osteoporosis." *J Am Ostoepath Assoc* 100.10 (2000) : S9-15.

3 Lukaski, H. C. "Magnesium, zinc, and chromium nutriture and physical activity." *Am J Clin Nutr* 72.2 (2000) : 585S-93S.

4 Seelig, M. G., "Interrelationship of magnesium and congestive heart failure." *Wien Med Wochenschr* 150.15-16 (2000) : 335-341.

5 Morgan, J. K., et al., "Magnesium and Calcium Dietary Intakes of the US Population." *J. Am. Coll. Nutr.* 4.2 (1985) :195-206.

6 Preuss, H. G., et al., "Chromium update: examining recent literature 1997-1998." *Curr opin Clin Nutr Metab Care* 1.6 (1998) : 509-512.

7 Hindmarsh, O. C. et al., "Effect of early maternal iron stores on placental weight and structure." *Lancet* 356.9231 (2000): 719-723.

8 Rayman, M. P., "The imporance of selenium to human health." *Lancet* 356.9225 (2000) : 233-241.

9 Semrad, C. E. "Zinc and intestinal function." *Curr Gastroenterol Rep* 1.5 (1999) : 398-403.

10 Sayeg Porto, M. A. et al., "Linear growth and zinc supplementation in children with short stature." *J Pediatr Endocrinol Metab* 13.8 (2000) : 1121-1128.

11 Lukaski, H.C., "Magnesium, Zinc, and Chromium Nutriture and Physical Activity." *Am J Clin Nutr* 72.2 (2000) : 585S – 93S.

12 Amato P., Morales A.J., Yen S.S., "Effects of Chromium Picolinate Supplementation on Insulin Sensitivity, Serum Lipids, and Body Composition in Healthy, Nonobese, Older Men and Women." *J Gerontol A Biol Sci Med Sci* 55.5 (2000) : M260-3.

13 Joseph L.J., et al., "Effect of Resistance Training With or Without Chromium Picolinate Supplementation on Glucose Metabolism in Older Men and Women." *Metabolism* 48.5 (1999) : 546-53.

14 Chatard J.C., et al., "Anaemia and Iron Deficiency in Althetes. Practical Recommedations For Treatment." *Sports Med* 27.4 (1999) : 229-40.

15 Waller M.F., Haymes E.M., "The Effects of Heat and Exercise on Sweat Iron Loss." *Med Sci Sports Exerc* 28.2 (1996) : 197-203.

16 Beard J., Tobin B., "Iron Status and Exercise." *Am J Clin Nutr* 72.2 (2000) : 594S-7S.

"You miss 100% of the shots you never take."

-Wayne Gretsky

Chapter

13

The Herbal Truth

The purpose of this chapter is to tell you about some of the latest, exciting trends in the herb industry and whether they "pass the test" for use as either a performance enhancer or some other application related to making you look and feel better.

As was mentioned in the last edition of the *Sports Supplement Review*, the vast majority of herbal medicines actually play a very small role in physique augmentation. Now don't get me wrong, science is discovering new herbal compounds at a rapid pace. However many of these herbal products are not intended to make you a better athlete, but are best suited to enhance a healthy lifestyle, combat stress or prevent, ***not cure,*** specific disease states. There are a few excellent herbs that athletes should consider using for improved performance, bodyfat loss, and even protein utilization, but at the same time, issues revolving around herbs are somewhat of a controversial nature. The reason for this is that if an herb delivers the same benefits of

a pharmaceutical compound, this could in essence undermine large pharmaceutical firms. The case for this is evident in the latest hearings dealing with Cholestin™, a dietary supplement used to decrease cholesterol levels, which caused major controversy in the pharmaceutical/herb business.

In the United States, research on herbal medicine lags behind pharmaceutical research, partly because herbs are natural products that can't easily be patented. Many manufacturers are reluctant to invest the amount of money it takes to perform clinical studies when they can't get exclusive rights to sell the product. In Europe, however, many herb manufacturers have chosen to invest money in studies. One reason they have been able to do this is that a proven herbal product can be authorized for use as medical treatment in Germany and other European nations, allowing the manufacturer to recoup its investment. In contrast, U.S. law prohibits the sale of herbs as remedies for specific medical conditions unless they have been approved by the Food and Drug Administration (FDA) as drugs. It is for these reasons that many of the most effective herbs have been researched and or discovered in countries outside of the United States.

A Simple Technique to "Weed" out Ineffective Herbs

One of the problems with herbs is the inconsistency with their potencies. Some manufacturers just dump in herbal powder (weeds?) and call it a day. They have no interest in making sure the plants are potent, just an interest in riding the next news story about the purported effects of a particular plant. Yet still there are others—true herb companies and manufacturers—who have worked painstakingly to create a set of **standardization** methods. The results are standardized extracts that serve to "guarantee" the potency of a particular herb. These standardized extracts are noted on supplement labeling as a percentage of the total weight of the compound. For example, on a label you might read that the product contains 300 mg of Ephedra standardized for 6% ephedrine (the active constituent in ephedra). This means the product yields 18 mg of ephedrine. This is the most critical aspect when choosing herbal products because if the end material or herbal extract does not contain a high enough concentration of the "active" compounds, you might as well just go ahead and burn up your money.

In most instances when researchers collect enough scientific data to support the effectiveness of different herbs, they also have identified the specific active compound(s). For example, dieters should know that the active ingredient in popular fat burners is *ephedrine alkaloids,* which can be extracted from the herb Ephedra, also known as Ma Huang. It is imperative that consumers shopping for herbs never make a purchase without first knowing which active component the herb is supposed to deliver. Because it is difficult for any athlete to keep track of data for the thousands of herbs on the market today, I have taken a few of the familiar herbs—some with bodybuilding effects, some without—and briefly describe their benefits and active compounds. We'll look at some of the more common herbs in the marketplace. And because often your favorite vitamin or sports supplement contains herbals, it is a good idea to familiarize yourself with a few key items. This way you'll at least feel comfortable when you see them.

Cyanotis

Latin Name: Cyanotis vaga

Parts Used: Leaf

Benefits: I wanted to start the section with an herbal compound that is very high on my list of hot new supplement trends, Cyanotis vaga. This herb contains an active component called beta-ecdysterone which, if taken in the right dosages, I believe will prove to be one of the most significant bodybuilding supplements ever in the years to come. Why? Well for starters there have been over 50 studies regarding one the active components of Cyanotis vaga—beta-ecdysterone. These studies all point to a marked increase in protein synthesis, work capacity, or an antioxidant effect. I have been using this stuff for about six weeks now and am extremely impressed with the results. This stuff is the real deal.

What to Look For: When purchasing a Cyanotis vaga product, look for a standardized herbal extract containing 96% ecdysterone.

Dosage: 30-40 mg three times per day (with high-protein meals).

Warning: Not recommended for persons with hypertension or anxiety.

References: See Chapter 9, "The Next Wave of Supplements."

Leuzeae

Latin Name: Rhaponticum Carthamoides
Parts Used: Leaf/root

Benefits: Like Cyanotis vaga noted above, there have been over 50 studies regarding beta-ecdysterone, which is one the active components of Leuzeae. Here again, these studies all point to a marked increase in protein synthesis, work capacity, or an antioxidant effect. Make no mistake, herbs standardized for about 96% beta-ecdysterones are my bet as the hottest new supplement this year.

What to Look For: When purchasing a Leuzeae product, look for a standardized herbal extract containing 96% ecdysterones.

Dosage: 30-40 mg three times per day (with high-protein meals).

Warning: Not recommended for persons with hypertension or anxiety.

References: See Chapter 9, "The Next Wave of Supplements."

Ginkgo

Latin Name: Ginkgo biloba

Parts Used: Leaf

Benefits: The ginkgo biloba tree is the oldest species of tree on the earth. It's been around for about 300 million years. Extracts of the leaves of the gingko biloba tree have been used by the Chinese for thousands of years to cure a variety of ailments. Today, ginkgo biloba is used to enhance brain functioning; users claim it improves mental alertness and increases energy. Does it really work? I don't know, but European physicians write over 1.2 million prescriptions for it every month.

"One of the problems with herbs is the inconsistancy with their potencies."

There have been close to 40 studies done on the herb since 1975, and it supposedly works by increasing blood flow throughout the brain and the body.[1] There's also evidence it may increase the production of ATP. Can it help bodybuilders? I suppose anything that improves concentration can help you get a better workout, but I've never heard of anyone putting on a significant amount of muscle because they use ginkgo biloba.

What to Look For: When purchasing a Ginkgo biloba product, look for a standardized herbal extract containing 24% flavone glycosides and 6% terpene lactones.

Dosage: Ginkgo biloba appears to be safe, inexpensive, and easily obtained in health-food stores. For improved mental abilities, I recommend 120-160 mg a day, taken in three divided doses.

Warnings: Due to ginkgo's ability to enhance mental function, it should not be used in conjunction with an MAO inhibitor or other anti-depressant medications. Also, it shouldn't be taken with anti-coagulants. It works similar to a blood thinner.

Turmeric

Latin Name: Curcuma aramatica, Curcuma domestica

Parts Used: Rhizome

Benefits: Turmeric is the major ingredient of curry powder, and it's also used in certain varieties of mustard. The herb is raised in India, China, and Indonesia, and its active ingredient, curcumin, is prescribed as an anti-inflammatory agent in the treatment of numerous diseases including jaundice, bruises, chest pain, menstrual difficulties, even flatulence.

I'm not sure it cures all of those things, but it's pretty clear that it does have use as an antioxidant, anti-inflammatory, anticarcinogenic, cardiovascular, hepatic, gastrointestinal, and antimicrobial agent.

The antioxidant effect of turmeric (or curcumin) is said to be comparable to that of Vitamins C and E (less effective than C, but more effective than B or even superoxide dismutase). As far as its anti-inflammatory effects, it's said to be comparable to cortisone. However, this last property might be problematic for bodybuilders. Turmeric supposedly stimulates the release of glucocorticoids; sensitizes cortisol receptor sites; and increases the half-life of cortisol. Although these things might help an acute injury heal, chronic use for a chronic injury could theoretically lead to protein catabolism.

On the other hand, turmeric seems to be an effective hepatoprotectant similar to silymarin. This liver-protecting characteristic is most likely due to turmeric's antioxidant properties.

What to Look For: Make sure your turmeric is standardized to 95% curcumin.

Dosage: You'd have to eat a lot of turmeric to enjoy its healing powers, so people generally use curcumin to treat illnesses. The general dosage for curcumin is 400-600 mg, three times a day. To ingest an equivalent dosage through turmeric alone, you'd have to take roughly 8,000-60,000 mg a day.

"The most common application for natural athletes is to use dandelion alone or in combination with glycerol..."

Warnings: Should not be taken by individuals with bile duct obstruction or gallstones.

Dandelion

Latin Name: Taraxicum officionale

Parts Used: Root

Benefits: Although it is known as dandelion in the U.S., this common plant is also known as wet-a-bed in other countries because of its diuretic action. Although dandelion is generally regarded as a liver tonic, it has also been used to treat fever, boils, heartburn, appendicitis, and various skin problems. Dandelion also contains the most Vitamin A of any known plant: 14,000 IU per 100 grams of raw greens.

Dandelion's beneficial effects on the liver have apparently been proven in laboratory studies. It supposedly increases the flow of bile, which could improve such conditions as bile duct inflammation, hepatitis, gallstones, and jaundice. Dandelion's high choline content might be responsible for these hepatoprotectant properties.

In other studies, dandelion has proven to be an extremely effective diuretic. However, because dandelion replaces the potassium normally lost through diuresis, it doesn't have many of the potential negative side effects of prescription drugs. The most common application for natural athletes is to use dandelion alone or in combination with glycerol before a photo shoot or competition.

What to Look For: A dandelion formula should contain a 4:1 extract of dandelion root.

DOSAGE: As powdered solid extract, 250-500 mg, three times daily.

Warnings: Should not be taken by people with kidney damage. Could cause dehydration if not enough water is consumed.

Synephrine

Latin Name: Citrus aurantium

Parts Used: Fruit

Benefits: Synephrine is the main "active" compound found in the fruit of a plant called citrus aurantium. The fruit is also known as zhi shi (in traditional Chinese medicine), and as green orange, sour orange, and bitter orange in other parts of the world. Synephrine is often found in diet and energy products as a substitute for or in addition to ephedra. Because synephrine is a stimulant, similar to caffeine and ephedrine, it is thought to have similar effects in terms of providing an energy boost, suppressing appetite, and increasing metabolic rate and caloric expenditure. In traditional Chinese medicine, zhi shi is used to help stimulate the Qi (energy force). Although synephrine and several other compounds found in zhi shi are structurally similar to ephedrine and are known to act as stimulants (via adrenergic activity), zhi shi does not appear to have the same impact on the central nervous system (CNS) as ephedra. In essence, zhi shi or products that contain its active component synephrine seem to be better tolerated by individuals who simply do not handle the more pronounced stimulatory effects of ephedrine.

What to Look For: Citrus aurantium should be standardized for 3-6% synephrine.

Dosage: Most formulas contain about 20 mg of synephrine which equates to about 340 mg of a 6% standardized citrus aurantium extract.

Warning: Since synephrine is a stimulant, its warning is the same as ephedrine

Goldenseal

Latin Name: Hydrastis canadensis

Parts Used: Root and rhizome

Benefits: Many herbs including goldenseal appear to be interchangeable as far as their alleged healing powers go because they all contain high amounts of their active ingredient, berberine. Berberine is an iso-quinolone alkaloid, and it's said to have a variety of beneficial effects, including: antibiotic activity, anti-infective activity (the ability to prevent bacteria from adhering to cells), immuno-enhancing effects, fever-lowering characteristics, and anti-cancer activity.[2]

These herbs are also used clinically to treat infectious diarrhea, trachoma (an infection of the eye), and liver disorders (cirrhosis). Other possible uses include treating gonorrhea and syphilis, as well as being useful in treating symptoms of the cold and the flu.

Unfortunately, there haven't been any real detailed studies done on berberine's effects.

What to Look For: Many companies standardize for hydrastine or alkaloids within

goldenseal. When more data becomes available we'll give you a better idea of what to look for in a goldenseal product.

Dosage: As powdered preparations vary widely in content, standardized preparations are recommended. Goldenseal appears to be the most widely available, so for treating ailments, 250-500 mg of powdered extract, three times a day is what's generally recommended.

Warning: Higher doses than that listed here might interfere with Vitamin B metabolism. Likewise, pregnant women are advised to avoid berberine-containing plants.

Milk Thistle

Latin Name: Silybum marianum

Parts Used: Seed

Benefits: Milk thistle is generally prescribed as a liver protectant. Since many oral pharmaceuticals and everything we ingest are eventually metabolized in the liver, tremendous strain is constantly placed on this organ. Studies also seem to supports its use as a hepatoprotectant in athletes who chronically overdose on acetaminophen.[3]

Although several research studies support its hepatoprotective properties, most experts believe it to be effective because it's a potent antioxidant.[4,5]

What to Look For: Milk thistle extract should be standardized to 80% silymarin

Dosage: A dosage of 150 mg three times daily is recommended.

> "Yohimbe, however, may also increase blood pressure, especially when combined with... caffeine or ephedra."

Echinacea

Latin Name: Echinacea angustifolia, pupurea, pallida

Parts Used: Roots, seed, above-ground parts

Benefits: Echinacea has long been used as a tonic for health and wellness. Often taken when symptoms of a cold or the flu come on, echinacea may help to ward off colds and flu.[6,7] Studies on echinacea vary, some show evidence of immunostimulatory effects, others do not. Those that do take echinacea either swear by it, or never use it again. For performance-enhancing purposes, echinacea receives a low grade from me. However, for those needing to ward off a cold or flu, I say it's well worth a try.

What to Look For: Echinacea is often sold in a blended mixture of different plant species due to the over harvesting of certain families. For best results, a blended mixture of goldenseal is preferred to enhance echinacea's effect.

Dosage: 300 mg daily for no longer than 2 weeks.

Warning: Should not be used by anyone with advanced immune deficiencies.

Stevia

Latin Name: Stevia rebaudiana (Bertoni)

Parts Used: Leaf

Benefits: Stevia is a natural sweetener over 200 times sweeter than table sugar. Its application to the athlete is pretty much limited to what the supplement companies use in their products.

Dosage: Dependent on your sweet tooth.

Warning: N/A

Yohimbe

Latin Name: Coryanthe yohimibe

Parts Used: Bark

Benefits: Yohimbe is a somewhat controversial herb these days. For years it was only used by men looking to enhance sexual function. Thereafter, research examined its effects on women and lo and behold, it assisted in body-fat loss. Of particular interest, this herb possesses the ability to antagonize the alpha-2 adrenoreceptor, which are in great abundance in the hips and buttocks of women. Therefore, yohimbe may have potent actions in assisting women drop bodyfat in these trouble areas.

Yohimbe, however, may also increase blood pressure, especially when combined with other stimulants such as caffeine or ephedra. I therefore recommend those that take yohimbe use caution when combining such compounds.

What to Look For: Yohimbe should be standardized for the active ingredient yohimbine, typically in the amount of 1%.

Dosage: Typically a dose of 2-5 mg of yohimbine is used.

Warning: Should not be used by those with kidney or liver disease. Should not be used by people with hypertension or heart disease. Contraindicated in chronic inflammation of sexual organs.

Gymnema

Latin: Gymnema Sylvestre

Parts Used: Leaves and the roots

Benefits: Gymnema sylvestre is a rather new herb in terms of performance enhancing. I see its main benefit to lie in the realm of bodyfat loss. This herb may help with the disposal of blood glucose. As we have talked about in numerous sections in this book, the topic of glucose disposal is of extreme importance to those athletes looking to enhance their physiques. gymnema is quite possibly one of the hot new upcoming supplements.

Recently, gymnema sylvestre has become known as a "sugar blocker" because of its effects. In fact, recent clinical trials conducted in India have shown that an extract of gymnema sylvestre is useful for controlling blood sugar. It is speculated that gymnema sylvestre acts one of two ways: The first is in the taste buds in the oral cavity where it may prevent the taste buds from perceiving the sweetness level of sugar-containing foods. When the taste of sugar is blunted, it appears that a

reduction in **short-term** caloric intake can take place.[17] The second is that the glucose-like molecules in gymnema sylvestre, gymnemic acid, fill different receptor locations in the absorptive external layers of the intestine, thereby preventing the intestine from absorbing the sugar molecules.[16]

With all that said, it looks that gymnema may make for a great addition to the program of those looking to inhibit "over-carb" consumption.

Dosage: 200-400 mg daily in divided doses.

> "...it seems that ashwagandha may also help to increase performance and strengthen the cardiovascular system."

Ginseng

Latin Name: Panax Ginseng, Panax Quinquefolius.

Parts Used: Root

Benefits: The root of the plant panax ginseng has been used for centuries in Asia for its many beneficial properties. Its adaptogenic traits have been shown in increases in the body's ability to handle stress. It has been shown to strengthen the cardiovascular system as evidenced, for example, by decreased heart rates in clinical subjects who ingested panax ginseng.

The active components of panax ginseng, called ginsenosides, have been shown to deliver remarkable beneficial effects for oxygen-depleted animals. In white rats, the survival rate at 7.6% oxygen was nearly doubled.[8,9]

Panax ginseng has also been used to enhance intellectual performance and to reduce mental exhaustion.

What to Look For: Panax ginseng should be standardized for 7% ginsenosides.

Dosage: 300 mg, two to three times daily.

Siberian Ginseng

Latin Name: Eleutherococcus senticosus

Parts Used: Root

Benefits: Although not as popular as Asian ginseng, eleutherococcus (known as Siberian ginseng) use dates back 2,000 years. Siberian ginseng is also referred to as ci wu jia in Chinese medicine (and by crafty marketers).

Siberian ginseng's purported effects—increased stamina and endurance—led to its use by Soviet Olympic athletes. Some research has suggested that Siberian ginseng improves the use of oxygen by the exercising muscle.[18] But still other studies have been inconclusive[19] or have shown Siberian ginseng to have no beneficial athletic effect.[20]

What to Look For: Look for products standardized for the eleutherosides. These complex polysaccharides are the active compo-

nents of the Siberian ginseng.

Dosage: 300 mg, two to three times daily.

Warning: Do not use Siberian ginseng if you have high blood pressure or if you are pregnant or nursing.

Ashwagandha (Indian Ginseng)

Latin Name: Withania somnifera

Parts Used: Root

Benefits: Ashwagandha has an extensive history of usage in Indian and Ayurvedic medicinal applications. It is used to increase tolerance to stress and to increase mental function.[9] Similar to panax ginseng, ashwagandha is an adaptogen and tonic for the immune system. Though few studies have been performed, it seems that ashwagandha may also help to increase performance and strengthen the cardiovascular system.

The active components of ashwagandha are called withanolides, and since these molecules resemble, in action and in chemical structure, the active compounds in panax ginseng (ginsenosides), ashwagandha is sometimes referred to as "Indian ginseng."

What to Look For: Look for the herb standardized to 1.5% withanolides.

Green Tea

Latin Name: Camellia sinesis

Parts Used: Leaf, stems

Benefits: This herb has been used for thousand of years as a health tonic and immunostimulant. In recent years its many benefits beyond this have just recently started to receive attention. For example, a recent study showed that green tea may help to inhibit the enzyme amylase, thereby slowing carbohydrate absorption.[10] This may not necessarily sound like a good thing, but trust me, it is. By slowing the absorption, you may also inhibit the insulin response. All of this equals to a much lower propensity to store excess calories as bodyfat.

In addition, a recent study showed that green tea increased resting energy expenditure by 4%.[11] For those of you looking to reduce bodyfat, green tea would make an excellent addition to your traditional thermogenic formula. My guess? Well, I believe green tea will soon be the staple for anyone looking to trim off those unwanted pounds.

What to Look For: A green tea extract should be standardized for 50% polyphenols, 35% catechins. Some products may also standardized for a specific catechin, epigallocatechin gallate or EGCG of around 10%.

Dosage: 200-400 mg, two to three times daily.

> "...to reduce bodyfat, green tea would make an excellent addition to your traditional thermogenic formula."

Saw Palmetto

Latin Name: Serenoa repens

Parts Used: Fruit

Benefits: Saw palmetto is commonly used in the treatment of BPH or benign prostatic hypertrophy.[12] As men age, this often becomes a problem with the enlargement of the prostate gland. Saw palmetto is thought to work by inhibiting the conversion of testosterone to DHT by blocking the enzyme 5-alpha reductase.

What to Look For: Look for a high concentration of fatty acids, around 85 to 95% fatty acids and/or sterols.

Ephedra

Latin Name: Ephedra sinica

Parts Used: Stems

Benefits: Ephedra is an ancient Chinese herb and has been known to exist for well over 5000 years. Ephedra sinica is the Latin plant name, where Ma Huang is the Chinese name given to the plant. Hence, ephedra sinica and Ma Huang are often used interchangeably. Of particular interest, ephedra is one of the most commonly ingested herbs today.

Ephedrine (the active compound in ephedra) increases caloric expenditure through a process called thermogenesis. The process of thermogenesis causes a dynamic conversion of stored fat or ingested calories into heat, which is a form of increased metabolism. This process is mediated by the hormones, epinephrine and norepinephrine, also called catecholamines, specifically. These chemical messengers promote fat oxidation and the liberation of free fatty acids from adipose storage sites.

Literally hundreds of studies have been performed using ephedrine, or a combination of caffeine and ephedrine analyzing variables like fat loss, energy expenditure, and performance. Since it has been well established that ephedrine works, products containing this compound have become increasingly popular. For a full review on ephedrine, check out Chapter 7 called "Standard Issue."

What to Look For: Ephedra should be standardized to 6-8 % ephedrine alkaloids

Dosage: 20 mg standardized herb, 2-3 times daily

Warning: Since ephedrine is not for everyone, the following warning may seem a little lengthy ,but caution should be considered before taking an ephedrine-containing product.

NOT FOR USE BY INDIVIDUALS UNDER THE AGE OF 18. DO NOT USE IF PREGNANT OR NURSING. CONSULT A PHYSICIAN OR LICENSED QUALIFIED HEALTH CARE PROFESSIONAL BEFORE USING THIS PRODUCT IF YOU HAVE, OR HAVE A FAMILY HISTORY OF, HEART DISEASE, THYROID DISEASE, DIABETES, HIGH BLOOD PRESSURE, RECURRENT HEADACHES, DEPRESSION OR OTHER PSYCHIATRIC CONDITION, GLAUCOMA, DIFFICULTY IN URINATING, PROSTATE ENLARGEMENT, OR SEIZURE DISORDER, IF YOU ARE USING A MONOAMINE OXIDASE INHIBITOR (MAOI) OR ANY OTHER DIETARY SUPPLEMENT, PRESCRIPTION DRUG OR OVER-THE-COUNTER DRUG CONTAINING EPHEDRINE, PSEUDOEPHEDRINE OR PHENYLPROPANOLAMINE (INGREDIENTS FOUND IN CERTAIN ALLERGY, ASTHMA, COUGH/COLD AND WEIGHT CONTROL PRODUCTS). EXCEEDING RECOMMENDED SERVING MAY CAUSE SERIOUS ADVERSE HEALTH EFFECTS INCLUDING HEART ATTACK AND STROKE. DISCONTINUE USE AND CALL A PHYSICIAN OR LICENSED QUALIFIED HEALTH CARE PROFESSIONAL IMMEDIATELY IF YOU EXPERIENCE RAPID HEARTBEAT, DIZZINESS, SEVERE HEADACHE, SHORTNESS OF BREATH OR OTHER SIMILAR SYMPTOMS. INDIVIDUALS WHO CONSUME CAFFEINE, OR OTHER STIMULANTS, WITH THIS PRODUCT MAY EXPERIENCE SERIOUS ADVERSE HEALTH EFFECTS. KEEP OUT OF REACH OF CHILDREN.

St. John's Wort

Latin Name: Hypericum perforatum

Parts Used: Herb, flowering tops

Benefits: By now, you've probably heard of this herb for its tremendous benefits at combating mild to moderate cases of depression. A number of recent, well-controlled studies indicate that extracts of this herb may significantly work. In fact, a recent meta-analysis of the literature on St. John's wort determined that is much more effective than a placebo, ,and provokes response rates that are similar to, or even better than, conventional antidepressants. Current research also leads us to believe that St. Johns wort is better tolerated than conventional antidepressants.[13] Similar to that of traditional antidepressants, St. John's wort's mechanism of action is thought to be through the inhibition of the reuptake of seratonin at the pre-synaptic cleft, the point at which seratonin normally can be recycled.

Due to these effects, St. John's wort may be an invaluable tool for athletes and bodybuilders suffering from overtraining syndrome. It may also help to focus on your workout instead of being wrapped up in your day-to-day operations.

What to Look For: St. John's wort should be standardized for 0.3% hypericum

Dosage: A dose of 300 mg standardized to 0.3%, three times daily should do the trick.

Warning: St. John's wort should not be taken by pregnant women. In addition, because the herb affects the nervous system, most experts recommend against combining it with antidepressant drugs, including MAOIs, SRRIs (Prozac, Zoloft, etc.), and tricyclics. In addition, this herb may reduce the effectiveness of birth control pills by 50%.

Periwinkle Plant

Latin Name: Catharanthus roseus

Parts Used: Plant

Benefits: A truly remarkable compound known as vinpocetine can be derived from the periwinkle plant. Over 50 clinical studies involving over 1,300 people worldwide using vinpocetine have shown the value of this safe product in enhancing memory, improving cognitive performance, mental acuity, and awareness. Vinpocetine has shown remarkable properties in enhancing the viability of red blood cells, improving cerebral blood circulation, promoting oxygen utilization, and optimizing energy transport in the brain.[14] Glucose is vital to the brain as the only energy source that the brain uses. Vinpocetine was shown to enhance the transport of glucose throughout the brain.

Vinpocetine has been shown to have a protective effect against hypoxia in reducing the devastating effects of low oxygen utilization in the brain under oxygen stress conditions.

What to Look For: Supplements that contain periwinkle plant will likely list vinpocetine as the active ingredient and will be simply listed as such. Vinpocetine is more technically referred to as "ethyl apovincaminate."

Dosage: A dose of 5 mg of vinpocetine three times daily should enhance workout performance and memory.

Warning: Due to vinpocetine's ability to enhance mental function, it should not be used in conjunction with an MAO inhibitor or other antidepressant medications.

Guarana

Latin Name: Paullinia cupana

Parts Used: Seeds

Benefits: Guarana is commonly found in most diet products on the market today because of its high caffeine content. Physiologically, it is important to understand that similar to ephedrine, caffeine also possesses the ability to increase the rate of fat burning. Caffeine exhibits its action in the body by mobilizing fatty acids to be used as energy by the body.[15] In addition, caffeine also inhibits the key compounds adenosine and possibly phosphodiesterase enzymes that would normally decrease the rate of fat burning.

What to Look For: Guarana should be standardized for 22% caffeine.

Dosage: Shoot for a 10:1 ratio of caffeine to ephedrine when trying to rid yourself of unwanted fat.

Warning: Since caffeine is a stimulant, its warning is the same as ephedrine.

References:

1 Fungfeld, E.W. A Natural and Broad Spectrum Nootropic Substance for Treatment of SDAT—the Gingko Biloba extract," *Progress in Clinical and Biological Research* 317 (1989) : 1562-1592.

2 Murray, M. T. *The Healing Power of Herbs, 2nd Ed.* Rocklin, CA: Prima Publishing (1992).

3 Muriel, P., et al. "Silymarin protects against paracetamol-induced lipid peroxidation and liver damage," *J Appl Toxicol* 12.6 (1992): 439-442.

4 Muzes, G., et al. "Effect of the bioflavonoid silymarin on the in vitro activity and expression of superoxide disumutase (SOD) enzyme," *Acta Physiol Hung* 78. 1 (1991): 3-9.

5 Letterton, P., et al. "...evidence that silymarin acts both as a inhibitor of metabolic activation and as a chain-breaking antioxidant." *Biochem Pharmacol* 39.12 (1990) : 2027-2034.

6 Lindenmuth GF, Lindenmuth EB. The efficacy of echinacea compound herbal tea preparation on the severity and duration of upper respiratory and flu symptoms: a randomized, double-blind placebo-controlled study. *J Altern Complement Med.* 2000 Aug;6(4):327-34.

7 Melchart D, Linde K, Fischer P, Kaesmayr J. Echinacea for preventing and treating the common cold. *Cochrane Database Syst Rev.* 2000;(2):CD000530. Review.

8 Ong YC, Yong EL; "Panax (Ginseng) – Panacea or Placebo? Molecular and Cellular Basis of Its Pharmacological Activity"; *Ann Acad Med Singapore* (2000) 29(1): 42 – 46.

9 Grandhi A, Mujumdar AM, Patwardhan B; "A Comparative Pharmacological Investigation of Ashwagandha and Ginseng"; *J Ethnopharmacol* (1994) 44(3): 131 – 135.

10 Zhang J, Kashket S. Inhibition of salivary amylase by black and green teas and their effects on the intraoral hydrolysis of starch. *Caries Res.* 1998;32(3):233-8.

11 Dulloo AG, Duret C, Rohrer D, Girardier L, Mensi N, Fathi M, Chantre P, Vandermander J. Efficacy of a green tea extract rich in catechin polyphenols and caffeine in increasing 24-h energy expenditure and fat oxidation in humans. *Am J Clin Nutr.* 1999 Dec;70(6):1040-5.

12 Plosker, G.L., and R.N. Brogden, "Serenoa repens (Permixon). A review of its pharmacology and therapeutic efficacy in benign prostatic hyperplasia," *Drugs Aging* (1996), 9(5):379–95

13 Woelk H. Comparison of St John's wort and imipramine for treating depression: randomised controlled trial. *BMJ.* 2000 Sep 2;321(7260):536-9.

14 Santos MS, Duarte AI, Moreira PI, Oliveira CR; "Synaptosomal Response to Oxidative Stress: Effect of Vinpocetine"; *Free Radic Res* (2000) 32(1): 57 – 66.

15 Arciero PJ, Bougopoulos CL, Nindl BC, Benowitz NL. Influence of age on the thermic response to caffeine in women. *Metabolism.* 2000 Jan;49(1):101-7.

16 Fushiki T, Kojima A, Imoto T, et al. An extract of Gymnema sylvestre leaves and purified gymnemic acid inhibits glucose-stimulated gastric inhibitory peptide secretion in rats. J Nutr 1992;122:2367–73.

17 Brala PM, Hagen RL, "Effects of sweetness perception and caloric value of a preload on short term intake". Physiol Behav 1983 Jan; 30(1):1-9

18 Asano K, Takahashi T, Miyashita M, et al. Effect of Eleutherococcus senticosus extract on human working capacity. Planta Medica 1986;37:175–7.

19 Kelly GS. Sports nutrition: A review of selected nutritional supplements for endurance athletes. Alt Med Rev 1997;2:282–95.

20 McNaughton L. A comparison of Chinese and Russian ginseng as ergogenic aids to improve various facets of physical fitness. Int Clin Nutr Rev 1989;9:32–5.

"I learned that if you want to make it bad enough, no matter how bad it is, you can make it."

-Gale Sayers

Chapter

14

Buyer Beware—Brand Awareness and Reviews

In the last issue of the *Sports Supplement Review*, Bill Phillips talked a lot about the growth of the performance nutrition industry, and the recent trends contributing to the momentum. As we embark on a new era, those same forces are still in play. Today more than ever, science is validating the positive benefits of supplementation as an adjunct to a well-defined exercise and nutrition plan. These effects have been well publicized in the mainstream media, which has convinced more and more weekend warriors—not just athletes and bodybuilders—that proper supplementation can contribute significantly to an active lifestyle.

But with all this information swirling around, and all the companies that have ponied-up to meet the ever-growing demand for supplements, the buyer should be—now more than ever—aware of those companies that are committed to great products and those committed only to great profits. I have had the opportunity of working "inside" some of the most well-known of these supplement companies, and I can say without reservation from my experiences there are a whole lot of good, ethical companies out there. On the other hand, there are many companies for which I do not have a lot of information. So what I'm doing in this book, and what I'm suggesting to you, is to try to analyze the products and advertising claims of every company from the perspective of an educated consumer. This approach has led me to the conclusion, which probably is pretty obvious, that there are big differences between the best and worst companies. In addition, there seems to be no relationship between the size of the company and the quality of its products and advertising. So be a careful consumer and learn as much as you can about the supplement you're buying.

How Sports Supplement Companies are Born

In the past, nearly all sports supplement companies that I am aware of were started one of two ways. The most typical entry into the business was when a fitness "hobbyist" or even a former competitive athlete with great passion for nutrition and exercise started his or her own company. For example, entrepreneurs passionate about sports performance started brands such as Champion, MHP, SportPharma, Labrada, Next Proteins, ErgoPharm, Weider Nutrition International, and, of course, EAS. When the sports supplement industry first became popular around 1985, many established vitamin- and health-related supplement companies created sub-brands to get into the market, creating the other type of company. Examples include Twinlab's Fuel Line, and, more recently, Country Life's Biochem brand. Today things have changed dramatically. We have large food companies entering the market through acquisitions such as Kraft, who bought Balance Bar in 2000 and Nestlé who bought PowerBar. What does this mean to you? Well, as a consumer, maybe a lot. I don't want to bore you with psychobabble, but each of these different entries into the market has a certain "chemistry" that makes it unique. These unique business types have pluses and minuses when it comes to satisfying the needs of advanced fitness enthusiasts and bodybuilders. So before we start our company/brand review, here is brief summary of "pluses" I look for in a sports nutrition company:

• The company must have adequate resources committed to bringing performance-based bodybuilding products to market. I do not mean they cannot market products that have no use to bodybuilders (like brewers' yeast or children's vitamins), but they should focus at least one dedicated product line

specifically to the advanced athlete. This is a sign that they have people on staff who have the experience in, and are passionate about, sports performance. Bottom line: They understand the needs of a bodybuilding enthusiast.

• The company advertises its products in a straightforward way that does not imply miracles or magic in just a few weeks. Bottom line: This is a sign the company is concerned about its advertising claims, so that they don't mislead consumers. This is also a sign of good business ethics, because any company in today's marketplace that thinks pushing the envelope and exaggerating claims is the way to persuade consumers isn't likely to be around for long. Look for clear-cut and reasonable advertising claims. If the theory behind the formula seems to make sense, the product is probably worth a try.

• The company sometimes may be slow to enter a new market category, but when they do, their product offerings feature dosages that are more efficacious or have greater substantiation, such as university studies. After several years of product development, I realize how important it is to be first to market a product. However, it takes time to find out if a substance is safe and maybe even more time to determine an efficacious dose. Bottom line: This is a sign that the company wants to put out **safe and effective** products that they are confident deliver results.

• The company funds research—from monitoring the current scientific literature applicable to dietary supplements to sponsoring double-blind, placebo-controlled university studies—to validate supplement combinations with **fair comparisons.** Bottom line: Figures usually do not lie, but clever supplement marketers can rig the testing protocols so that to the **untrained** eye they seem legitimate.

With all of this in mind, you can now start to form your own judgements about what makes a reputable supplement company or product. In this chapter, I will take you through a review of some of the most popular supplement companies and give you my opinions, but as you read along, you should begin forming your own judgements too. Also, remember we cannot review every company and every "hot supplement," therefore, some of your favorites may not be included.

Twinlab® Corporation

Established In: 1968

Background: If you are new to the weight-training game, you may not realize the impact Twinlab has had on this industry. Back in the late '80s, as far as I am aware, Twinlab was the only major sports supplement company that funded university research. Twinlab still maintains a scientific review program to review relevant scientific studies validating their product development efforts. This forward-thinking approach to science-based sports nutrition helped position the Twinlab "Fuel" line as the industry leader for product research and development, and it became a model for other successful companies in the industry.

Today the Twinlab brand and reputation continue to be very strong, especially when it comes to vitamins, minerals, and specialty health formulas. The Twinlab portfolio of supplements has expanded over the years to include the herbal brands Nature's Herbs® and Alvita Teas®; a multi-level marketing firm, Changes International®; and PR* Nutrition Bars. Problems with label claims should not be a concern with Twinlab products. They manufacture nearly everything they sell onsite, and they have a reputation for excellent quality control. I feel this aspect of their operation is among the best in the industry. Strong distributor relationships have also put the Twinlab brand in just about every health food store in the country. Twin also runs the body-building magazine *Muscular Development*, which still seems to have "staying power" with advertisers and fitness enthusiasts. I feel that part of the reason this magazine is still a good value for advertisers and athletes is that Twinlab has always been "up front" with its readers about the fact that the magazine is related to Twinlab and promotes their supplement line.

Flagship Products: Diet Fuel and Ripped Fuel, ephedra-based fat burners; Fuel Plex, their new meal-replacement product (MRP); and a host of high-quality herbal, vitamin, and mineral supplements.

Key Personnel: The Blechman family is the original owner of Twinlab, and the five Blechman brothers truly drive the business. They were there from the start and got them to where they are now. Each brother heads up a key area of the business; Steve Blechman is in charge of *Muscular Development* magazine and product development, Dean Blechman leads the sales force, and so on. Many bodybuilders have "bagged" on the Blechman's lack of focus toward the sport of bodybuilding. However, the truth is, the Blechman family has given generously to bodybuilding by setting the early pace for product development and product quality. I also think hardcore bodybuilders took offense to Twinlab's anti-steroid stance a few years ago when they positioned *Muscular Development* as an all-natural publication. As an ex-competitor **and** someone who would like to see more classic physiques win bodybuilding shows, I see both sides of the coin, and I think that athletes should give Steve Blechman a break on this one. He was never a competitive bodybuilder, so he probably did not realize that drug use has infected all types of high-level athletics, not just bodybuilding. Overall, Twinlab has been a big part of the growth and validation of the sports nutrition industry, and should never be counted out.

What to Watch: Watch for Twinlab's constant introduction of new products. This is almost unavoidable, since they have so many sub-brands that specialize in different areas of nutrition. Twin likes to take advantage of its strong distribution power and throw tons of products into the market. This sometimes can be a disadvantage, because it is difficult to support many new product initiatives all at once. Nonetheless, they have also enlisted one of my old colleagues from Weider Nutrition/American Bodybuilding, Jeff Pell, to help revitalize their "Fuel" line of sports products. I can vouch that Jeff knows the core

bodybuilder very well, and with the guidance and blessing from Steve Blechman, we should see more Twinlab bodybuilding supplements in the future.

Labrada Bodybuilding

Established In: 1996

Background: It should come as no surprise that bodybuilding legend Lee Labrada owns and operates a company that bears his name. As one of my personal role models back when I pursued competitive bodybuilding, it is nice to know that Lee is a very ethical businessman and happens to know quite a bit about producing quality supplements. Lee seems to take the same methodical approach to business as he did in his former days as a competitive bodybuilder by focusing on the vital products he feels makes his line complete. I believe Labrada Bodybuilding products are of good quality and are marketed in an ethical manner.

Flagship Products: Lean Body™ and Lean Body for *Her*™ line of MRPs and bars

Key Personnel: In a recent conversation with Lee, he told me that *all* of his employees are key people within the company, which is a testament to his humble attitude. Lee also seems to drive product development from his personal nutrition experience and consumer demand.

What to Watch: Lee tells me that his company will continue to focus on the bodybuilding and fitness market. Look for his Lean Body for *Her* products in drug stores nationwide during the coming year. Please refer to the product review chapter for further discussions.

Cytodyne Technologies

Established In: 1997

Background: Here is a company that burst onto the scene pretty much unnoticed until they launched Xenadrine, their thermogenic product. Cytodyne seems to be focused on bodybuilding products, and seems to be willing to dedicate significant resources to marketing them aggressively. In general, I have no reason to believe Cytodyne puts out anything but quality supplements, although some of their formulas and product claims have me a bit puzzled.

Flagship Products: Xenadrine™ and Methoxy Pro™

Key Personnel: It is my understanding that Bob Chinery, the brother of Scott Chinery, who brought you Cybergenics, is the "brains" behind Cytodyne.

What to Watch: Since Cytodyne makes some pretty amazing product claims, a careful consumer should ask for the actual scientific studies or verification for these claims if they're interested in Cytodyne's products.

MET-Rx®

Established In: 1992

Background: This company pioneered the MET-Rx Original Drink Mix, a MRP, which still seems to do well in most mass merchandise accounts. Early last year MET-Rx was purchased by the large specialty nutrition company, Rexall Sundown, and now, along with Worldwide Sport Nutrition, is a key component of their Active Nutrition Division. To complicate matters further, a few months after Rexall bought MET-Rx and Worldwide Sport Nutrition, Rexall was purchased by Royal Numico, a large Dutch nutrition company, which also owns GNC. Pretty confusing isn't it?

Flagship Products: MET-Rx® Original Drink Mix, Glycemet™, and Mass Action™

Key Personnel: With all the recent changes at MET-Rx, it's hard to tell who's in charge, but the founder, Dr. Scott Connelly, stayed on as Chief Technical Officer. Royal Numico is still putting together its management team, and where Connelly figures into this new team still remains to be seen. Scott is getting some help from the old Worldwide management, because they understand traditional sports nutrition a bit more than Rexall. I think it's still not clear who will be the key personnel for this brand.

What to Watch: Many speculate that because MET-Rx did not upgrade the Original MET-Rx formula, and chose not to market key products such as creatine and thermogenics until after 1998, that its brands fell out of favor with dyed-in-the-wool bodybuilders. While this may be true, MET-Rx did launch two new sub-brands over the last two years directed primarily at the bodybuilding market. These two sub-brands are Substrate Solutions and Anabolic Drive Series. They seemed to be well received by consumers, but as of late it appears that the Substrate Solutions prohormone line does not fit into Rexall's Active Nutrition future plans, while the Anabolic

Drive Series, which was a good line of products, has recently gone through an overhaul.

With back-to-back sports nutrition acquisitions, MET-Rx's parent company, Rexall, will have their hands full. But never fear, with Royal Numico as an anchor and all the resources at their disposal, MET-Rx should have enough staying power to continue being a player. It will be interesting to see who has the most impact on future MET-Rx product development.

Weider Nutrition International

Established In: Circa 1940

Background: This company was founded by the "Godfather of Bodybuilding" himself, Joe Weider. Besides being present at the birth of the industry, both Joe and Ben Weider have helped take bodybuilding and supplementation to the industry it is today. With Joe at the helm of the publishing business (*FLEX, Muscle & Fitness,* and *Shape*) and Ben steering the IFBB, you would think the name Weider would be the Nike of sports nutrition—but they're not. Weider Nutrition appears to be reorganizing and rebuilding. They still have top-notch manufacturing facilities and the goodwill of their bodybuilding publications (*FLEX* and *Muscle & Fitness*). Now it seems that they are getting back to their bodybuilding roots.

The Weider Nutrition Group has very capable quality-control personnel in their production facilities, making it nearly impossible to get a product that does not meet label claims. In addition, if you are an avid bodybuilder who competes in local or nationally recognized shows such as those organized by the NPC, you should know that Joe and Ben have made it possible for athletes to be able to pursue this sport as a hobby and as a career. In my opinion, this industry would still be in its infancy if it hadn't been for Joe, who had the guts to take weight training and supplementation out of its cult status and see it through to the booming industry we all enjoy today.

Flagship Products: As far as sports-related products go, Weider appears to be putting all of their eggs in the last remaining sports line, American Body Building. Known for popular products such as the Steel Bar, Blue Thunder, and Ripped Force, the current leader in the gym-based beverage business has been the marketing arm for Weider's best sports nutrition products. ABB's "Extreme" line, originally slated for drinks, has now been extended to the world of capsules, tablets, and powders. This is a good move for Weider, because ABB enjoys a good reputation for all of its supplements.

Key Personnel: This is tough to figure out, but the leader of the revered ABB distribution system, Brian Baranowski, is the most logical and capable choice. Brian and I worked together for years, and he does have the "passion" it takes to bring Weider back from the dead. Weider Nutrition also has a couple of bright "science guys," namely Alan Shugarman and Chris Lockwood, who should help future product development efforts.

Weider has always had some of the best sports nutrition minds in the business bar none. But for some reason it seems many of these great minds have either left for greener pastures or moved over to the Weider publishing arm. Another interesting fact about the leadership hierarchy at Weider is that contrary to popular belief, when you work for Weider Nutrition, you really are not associated with the sister company, Weider Publications. This puts whoever is in charge at a disadvantage, because there always seems to be a power struggle between the publishing business and the supplement business. At least that's how I felt when I was at Weider.

What to Watch: Watch for the folks in Salt Lake City to continue to focus all their sports nutrition efforts on ABB, as it is still hardcore and the only pure sports brand that they have left. You will also see the Weider folks continue to provide other non-sports nutritional supplements to the mass-market channels.

Biotest Laboratories, LLC.

Established In: 1997

Background: For those of you who have been around the serious side of bodybuilding for the last few years you know that when former *Muscle Media* Editor in Chief T.C. Louma left that post, he joined forces with Tim Patterson to form the online magazine Testosterone.net and the branded line of supplements called Biotest. It should also come as no suprise that the Testosterone.net web site is very reminiscent of *Muscle Media* circa 1996, since the voice and tone of the writers all have a distinct resemblance to T.C. Simply put, they combine real information you can use with a nice air of humor and personal satire. I personally think that some of the

satire on their site is extremely timely and funny, even though from time to time these guys poke fun at EAS for taking *Muscle Media* to a broader audience. We take this humor in "T-Dude" fashion ("T-Dude" is their mascot for a real bodybuilder) and laugh at it like anyone would with any level of self-confidence. Just the other day I had an hour-long conversation with Tim Patterson where we quickly exchanged notes on both of our companies and the rest of the industry, and I can assure you that there is mutual admiration between both parties. Tim wanted me to be very clear on several points: First of which is that the Biotest guys realize that EAS and *Muscle Media* paved the way for their business to continue speaking to the hardcore bodybuilder. Second, that in his opinion, the efficacy and integrity of EAS products made every serious consumer expect more from their supplement dollars. And third, in their opinion, no other company has done a better job of taking the entire sports supplement market to a larger audience than EAS. I expressed my gratitude for his many compliments and then told him that I felt that his company was doing a good job of marketing with integrity and putting out quality product formulations.

Flagship Products: Methoxy 7™, a liquid delivery for methoxyisoflavone; Tribex 500, a non-hormonal testosterone booster; and MD-6™, a potent fat burner.

Key Personnel: Tim Patterson and T.C. Louma both own and operate Biotest. When it comes to product development, Tim tells me he either consults with outside help or they develop them in-house.

What to Watch: Look for continued product introductions based on new compounds and or emerging market trends. No doubt that they will continue to publish on their Internet site hard-edge recommendations for nutrition and exercise plus their brand of industry satire by a host of very good writers.

Worldwide Sport Nutrition

Established In: 1995

Background: This is one of the pioneers of the low-carb/high-protein bars. Worldwide also has an increasingly sophisticated drink distribution system, which was put together by a good friend of mine, Chris Conrad. Recently, Worldwide Sport Nutrition was picked up during Rexall's acquisition frenzy in 1999 and 2000 (remember that Royal Numico now owns Rexall Sundown and GNC). Again, big dollars can play a huge factor in growing the distribution of a product line, but only if they focus on the task at hand.

Flagship Products: Pure Protein™ bars and shakes and Thermo Speed™ sports beverages

Key Personnel: As with all conglomerates, it's sometimes hard to tell who is running the ship. In this case, David McCabe, former President and Chief Executive Officer of Worldwide, said, "Our new partnership with Rexall Sundown and MET-Rx will give Worldwide the opportunity to capitalize on the product development strength and entrepreneurial spirit of these two industry leaders." This statement by itself doesn't tell us much about who is pulling the switches at

Worldwide, but bet that McCabe will be somewhere in the management mix. I, for one, am curious to see how it all pans out.

What to Watch: As we watch this business roll forward, it should be interesting to see how the new management approaches their thermogenic drink line, because at one point this was one area where they tried to remain on or near cutting edge.

Max Muscle

Established In: 1988

Background: Most bodybuilders are familiar with Max Muscle, the clothing company. In reality, this firm is also a growing sports nutrition retailer, fitness magazine publisher, and developer of its own supplement brand. The company was founded by Joe Wells, an ex-pro football player who also is CEO, and Sean Greene, an ex-competitive bodybuilder who is the firm's President. I have known both Wells and Greene for several years, and I am quite impressed that they have managed to succeed in four very competitive areas: publishing, clothing, retailing, and supplements. Both of these guys have a lot of practical experience when it comes to training and supplementation, which shows in the success of their business. In the early years, Max Muscle catered to the gym or hardcore athlete. Most recently, the owners have dedicated more attention to getting people from all walks of life into the exercise scene. Max Muscle seems to produce quality products and doesn't make bombastic claims to sell their products. Here again, their magazine, *Max Sports and Fitness*, has always been "up front" with its readers about the fact that it is related to their supplement line.

Flagship Products: SuperPro™, Max Lean™, and MaxPro™

Key Personnel: Joe Wells and Sean Greene primarily oversee all new product development and marketing efforts for Max Muscle. Since Max Muscle is also a retail outlet, it would make sense that other key personnel are the store owners and managers themselves.

What to Watch: Max Muscle will continue to be a popular clothing line, while their retail outlets will have to battle it out with the big boys from GNC, Sports Nutrition Depot, and Nutri-Sport. According to Sean Greene, Max Muscle has dedicated resources to develop additional in-store staff training and bring unique products to market. This will help them to build brand/store loyalty, and effectively compete with the sports nutrition warehouses that rely on selling brand names at low prices.

AST

Established In: 1995

Background: AST continues to be a player in the thermogenic market, but with the number of products and price competition that saturates this segment, it's hard to tell whether AST is a prominent player. I haven't seen many new products from AST lately, but it appears that AST provides good quality products and is generally known as a reputable company. However, in 1998 the FTC entered an agreement with AST (MET-Rx too) to put clearer warnings on prohormone pack-

aging and advertisements.

Flagship Products: Dymetadrine, Creatine ASC

Key Personnel: Paul Delia is the owner and founder of AST. Recently, Paul Cribbs, an exercise physiologist, was named as head of Director of Research. They also enlist the services of bodybuilder Skip La Cour, who acts as the company spokesperson and motivational author.

What to Watch: Typically AST has not been a market leader with product innovations, nor have they funded much university research. However, maybe the combination of Paul Cribbs and Paul Delia will allow AST to become more innovative with their product offerings.

Prolab®

Established In: 1992

Background: Natrol®, a company that has a broad line of supplements sold through mass-market retailers, recently acquired Prolab. However, Prolab continues to cater to the hardcore crowd. In fact, dedication to the hardcore audience while using real science from internal means or the public domain seems to be one of their strengths. I have always felt that Prolab produces quality products and uses an honest and straightforward approach to marketing them.

Flagship Products: Metabolic Thyrolean™, Glycogen™, and the new Cory Everson's Solutions Line

Key Personnel: Elliott Balbert, the President

and Chairman of Natrol, is now leading the Prolab charge and recently hired Rich Stanley from GNC as VP for all the Natrol companies. Stanley is a real professional, which should help to give the company clearer direction in the future. It would appear that Balbert and Stanley will strive for both companies to co-exist, yet keep them focused on their strengths.

What to Watch: Recently it seems that Prolab has partnered up with the former Ms. Olympia and TV fitness hostess Cory Everson to produce the new "Solutions Line." I haven't had a chance to fully review this product line, but I do know that these supplements are formulated for women. As far as Prolab goes, look for continued product introductions with the latest market trends and probably a much tighter focus on their hardcore roots.

Nature's Best

Established In: 1985

Background: Nature's Best seems to have strong local distribution, primarily focused on handling ready-to-drink gym beverages. They also have excellent ties overseas, especially in the Europe. Nature's Best has always had at least one product that could generate enough revenue to keep them in the game. They also seem to work with several high-profile Madison Avenue media agencies, which produce some very attractive advertisements to complement their products. I feel Nature's Best markets good products and uses a straightforward non-sensational approach to advertising them.

Flagship Products: Solid Protein Bar and IsoPure, an ion-exchange, whey-based line including a drink and powder.

Key Personnel: Hal Katz is the Owner/President of Nature's Best. I met him about 15 years ago, right after he purchased the company. I believe he continues to drive the marketing efforts and product launches. Because of the distribution model, other key personnel are the local distributors who continue to support Nature's Best product offerings.

What to Watch: Continue to look for a heavy push on the Solid Protein bars and IsoPure products. However, with more and more data surfacing that demonstrates the benefits of proteins like casein, you may see Katz go into defensive mode, since he primarily is banking on whey protein for his brand.

SportPharma

Established In: 1992

Background: This company made inroads with bodybuilders with an "insulin mimicker" product called Vanadyl pH™. Since the vanadyl sulfate market is not very hot, SportPharma has turned its efforts to other product categories, primarily nutrition bars. Even though SportPharma may not be on today's cutting edge of product development, in my experience they've always sold good products that meet label claims.

Flagship Products: Promax™ Bar, Thermadrene™

Key Personnel: Mike Walls founded this Concord, CA-based company. Walls, a former college track star and former employee of Champion Nutrition, took the product line and grew it into a good business. However, after taking a few lumps from the "less-than-spectacular" launch of Actisyn™, Mike has refocused his product offerings, and recently he has picked up sales and marketing experience from a few ex-MET-Rx employees.

What to Watch: Watch for SportPharma to continue to push the Promax bars into wider distribution like grocery and drug stores. I believe SportPharma will begin to see the bigger companies selling into the large mass-market chains as a threat and therefore make another run at the hardcore bodybuilding market in the coming years.

ErgoPharm

Established In: 1998

Background: ErgoPharm's founder and gifted chemist, Patrick Arnold, started the whole prohormone phenomenon. Their underground following and their prohormone product line has set the stage for them to evolve into a major player in the prohormone market if they can battle the FDA to keep their products on store shelves. ErgoPharm's product line continues to grow, but the most interesting products are the Cyclodiol products. ErgoPharm has pioneered water-soluble versions of 4-androstenediol (not to be confused with androstenedione) and 19-nor-4-androstenediol, and produces them as sublingual tablets and powders. I have known Patrick for years, and I have been impressed with the data to support these newer compounds and delivery forms. From what I have

seen, these proprietary Cyclodiol products seem to work much better at increasing anabolic hormone levels than the "dione" or tablet versions of prohormones, while also apparently avoiding downstream estrogen metabolites. My sense is that the FDA will attempt to ban these products on the argument that they fit all of the criteria to be classified as true steroids. At the forefront of prohormone development, ErgoPharm is always looking for the next effective bodybuilding supplement, but they will need to watch the government's reaction to these innovations.

Flagship Products: Cyclo-Diol and Cyclo-Nordiol, specific cyclodextrin-delivered 4-androstenediol and 19-nor-4-androstenediol products.

Key Personnel: Patrick Arnold is definitely the most recognized name of all the folks at ErgoPharm, although his brother and Dave Garrett are very active in the company's day-to-day operations. Patrick has been doing prohormone research for several years, and he actually provides much of the "high-quality" raw material for these products as a supplier for several companies. Recently though, Patrick and his colleagues have decided to try their hand at branded products, thus they launched ErgoPharm. There is no doubt the hardcore enthusiasts recognize the name Patrick Arnold, but ErgoPharm's goal is to come out of the shadows of the bodybuilding newsgroups and really make some noise in the supplement industry.

What to Watch: Because ErgoPharm is a relatively small company, watch for them to continue to push the product development envelope to make their mark. The relationships that were forged by their raw material business will only help these guys in the future. You can also bet that the ErgoPharm group will have their eye on the regulatory environment surrounding prohormones. If the regulatory status for these compounds allows them to continue being sold as sports supplements, I do believe that ErgoPharm is a very reliable source.

Champion Nutrition

Established In: 1980

Background: Long-time industry experience has given this company the scars of a true warrior. Champion's products have always been solid in design and quality. Champion is still revered by those who remember what they contributed to the industry. Although not "best sellers" in today's marketplace, Champion was responsible for bringing us Metabolol and Cytomax, two innovations in sports supplements.

Flagship Products: After selling off their Cytomax brand, and missing some key opportunities in the marketplace, Champion today is left with a relatively small product portfolio. Their big guns seem to be Heavyweight Gainer 900, Metabolol II, and Ultramet, which are all good products.

Key Personnel: Mike Zumpano continues to be the mastermind behind this Northern California company. He has worked with some of the greats (and is one of the greats) in the industry. I never count him out of the game. He is a pioneer, and just when you

think he is out of ideas, he'll strike.

What to Watch: Watch for Champion Nutrition to hang in there. Who knows what will transpire during a time when industry players are getting snatched up by big business? Is Champion a target for acquisition or will they rally in the final rounds and find their way back to the innovative position they once held? Only time will tell.

Next Proteins
(formerly Next Nutrition)

Established In: 1993

Background: Their targeted focus has been Next Proteins' strong suit. They have stuck with their "unique" whey protein position. And up until recently, Next was a powder-only company.

Flagship Products: Designer Protein Powder built the house—there's no doubt about that. Next has finally released the Designer Protein Bar, which has some industry experts wondering—what took so long?

Key Personnel: David Jenkins, ex-Olympic sprinter, is the brains behind the operation. He has good company helping him on the backside of the business. His right-hand man (actually, woman), Teri Lugo, keeps the company's internal and external operations running with precision.

What to Watch: Watch for Next to continue as a focused company with a small product portfolio. Jenkins has always had a knack for giving the sports enthusiasts what they demand. Setting themselves up to tackle other products in the industry (bars, cereals, and snacks) may prove to be just what the doctor ordered.

MHP (Maximum Human Performance)

Established In: 1998

Background: I recently spoke to former world-class competitive bodybuilder Gerard Dente, who owns and operates MHP. I found him to be both knowledgeable and friendly. MHP is the culmination of a 12-year friendship between Gerard and medical advisor Dr. Vincent Giampapa, a noted expert in natural hormone manipulation and anti-aging. MHP caters to both the anti-aging and fitness markets. Dente has a good understanding of what athletes want in a product, and he benefits from the ability to run these theories by Giampapa.

Flagship Products: Methoxy Meal™; TRAC™, a creatine-loading drink; and Secretagogue-One™, a GH-releaser.

Key Personnel: As I stated above, Gerard Dente owns and operates MHP. When it comes to product development, Gerard tells me he consults with Giampapa to make sure any formula ideas he may come up with are grounded in science.

What to Watch: Look for continued product introductions based on the latest market trends and probably a tighter focus on the bodybuilding market.

GEN (Genetic Evolutionary Nutrition)

Established In: 1995

Background: GEN also caters to the more hardcore crowd. One of their strengths is that they are fairly quick to market products with new compounds based on current nutrition theories. I believe GEN produces quality products and their marketing approach is straightforward.

Flagship Products: Thermonol XS™, Growth Factor X™, and MX7™

Key Personnel: GEN is owned and operated by Craig Tapscott, who has been around the supplement business for several years now. He seems to have his hand in most of the marketing, and I believe he also drives the formulations for the company.

What to Watch: GEN may be pushing product development toward their core bodybuilder market. This seems to be true since I've seen quite a few "edgy" GEN products hit the market recently.

Biochem® and Iron Tek®

Established In: 1997

Background: Biochem Sports and Fitness is sub-brand of Country Life Vitamins, which has been selling quality health supplements for over 30 years. According to Marketing Manager Brian Casutto, Biochem Sports and Fitness was created to meet the demands for sports nutrition that the parent company Country Life simply was not focused on. Recently, Country Life purchased the Iron Tek brand of supplements, thus giving them two brands in the fitness market.

Flagship Products: Iron Tek: Nor Tek™, Thermo Tek™, Biochem: Low Carb-1™ bars, and Ultimate Protein System™

Key Personnel: Ryan Drexler is the owner, and is actively involved in the business, while Marketing Manager Brian Casutto handles their branding efforts.

What to Watch: Look for continued product introductions from both brands, and possibly a more defined focus on fitness for Biochem and bodybuilders with Iron Tek. With Country Life as their parent company, I feel these two brands will put out quality products.

Optimum Nutrition

Established In: 1985

Background: Optimum Nutrition is the brand name started by the Costello brothers, who are the owners of the successful sports nutrition distributor of the same name. Optimum caters to both the fitness and the hardcore markets.

Flagship Products: Pro Complex™ and various whey proteins

Key Personnel: Optimum is owned and operated by the Mike and Tony Costello, who are both supplement industry veterans. They seem to have their hands in all facets of the business including sales, marketing, and operations.

What to Watch: Look for continued product introductions based on the latest market trends and probably a broader focus on the general fitness market.

EAS®
(Experimental and Applied Sciences)

Established In: 1992

Background: All right, I know what you're thinking. This ought to be good. Here comes the review for the company that employs the author of this book. Am I right? Well, before you turn the page, let me offer you something different than just a simple review of EAS. You see, I think a better approach would be to tell you why I wanted to be associated with EAS.

After 20 years in this business, my decision to come to EAS instead of pursuing some other opportunities allowed me to continue to do what I love and have a passion for, which is developing products for advanced bodybuilders and athletes. This position has also afforded me the opportunity to bring all of my experience both in and out of the realm of competitive bodybuilding, as well as all of my industry experience, and put together this edition of the *Sport Supplement Review*.

I have named several companies that are good and ethical, but what makes EAS stand out for me personally is overall integrity. I can't think of any other sports supplement company that gives back more to the consumer in the way of research and education than EAS does year after year. The fact that you are reading this book, which was researched and funded by EAS, is just one more example of their commitment to educating bodybuilders and athletes on the science and art of nutrition and exercise. This is truly what sets EAS apart from the other supplement companies.

For the record, over the past several years EAS has grown rapidly and today is one of the most successful sports nutrition firms in the industry. In addition, in terms of performance-based sports supplements sold in legitimate health food, gym, and specialty outlets, EAS has always enjoyed an excellent reputation for quality and efficacy.

EAS has funded and collaborated on over 35 university studies since 1993 and continues to do so. Another reason EAS is the number-one "enthusiasts'" sports brand is because of the commitment to quality and service. For example, EAS provides free technical-support service to anyone (including you!) who wants to learn more about bodybuilding and nutrition. This service is provided even if you don't buy EAS supplements, just call the EAS technical-support hotline, and they will do whatever they can to help you. The people who man this hotline are trained nutritionists and bodybuilders themselves who go through monthly in-house nutrition and training seminars to keep abreast of the latest scientific developments.

Flagship Products: Myoplex™ MRPs and Ready-to-Drink shakes, BetaGen™, BetaLean® HP, and SyntheVol™ HP

Key Personnel: From 1994 to August of 1999 Bill Phillips served as the company CEO. Under Bill's guidance, he turned EAS into the number-one brand of sports supplements by bringing several unique concepts to the market, including meal supplements, lean mass stimulators, creatine, and HMB. In addition, he inspired millions of people to transform their physiques through the creation of *Muscle Media*® magazine, the national best-selling book Body-*for*-LIFE, and the Body-*for*-LIFE 12-Week Challenge.

During 1999, EAS set out to find additional expertise to grow the company on several fronts, including strengthening its management team, enhancing product development, and expanding sales of its performance nutrition products to a broader consumer base. This goal was accomplished when North Castle Partners committed to a substantial equity investment in EAS. North Castle Partners is the largest private equity fund committed solely to investing in the healthy living sector. It was at that time David Lumley, a sports equipment industry veteran, became President and Chief Executive Officer.

In working with Dave Lumley, it's easy to see that when it comes to satisfying the needs of specialized consumers such as athletes, while also bringing products to a broader consumer base, he **"gets it."** He has quickly taken the necessary components of the larger corporations he has run, such as state-of-the-art raw material sourcing and efficient product development processes, and combined that with the spirit and experience of key EAS executives who worked with Bill Phillips.

Since I get asked quite often about projects that Bill Phillips is currently working on, let me tell you what I know. First of all, he has taken on a new role as Director of Value

Creation, with plans to focus on further growing the Body-*for*-LIFE and EAS communities through books, videos, new media, and other ancillary markets. Bill is also a member of the EAS Board of Directors.

What to Watch: As I stated above, Dave Lumley has created an excellent environment for EAS to cater to both the advanced bodybuilding/athletic market and broaden its product offerings to all active individuals. To accomplish this, Dave has implemented a two-division approach to research, education, and product development. These two separate divisions each have a specific objective, allowing them to focus on unique markets. For example, I work in the division that focuses solely on science-based performance supplements for elite athletes. In contrast, EAS also has another division that focuses on convenient, easy-to-use high-protein foods and ready-to-drink beverages for people who lead an active lifestyle and want to improve their nutrition plan. I believe this approach will allow EAS to satisfy two very different and demanding consumer markets, and set the pace for the entire sports supplement and fitness industry in the years to come.

Chapter

15

Rating the Industry's Hottest Supplements

As with nutrition companies, there are literally hundreds of nutritional products—far too many to review. In this section, I have taken a sample of items based on the questions I get from consumers just like you. As you go through this section, keep in mind that all these products cost you hard-earned cash... take the time to know what you're buying. Don't let overzealous marketing hype influence your purchasing decision. But also keep in mind that you usually get what you pay for when you buy from companies with well-established reputations. So don't go bargain hunting before you're armed with the facts.

ZMA Force +

Company: American Body Building

Information: ZMA (zinc monomethionine, magnesium aspartate, vitamin B6) is a very popular supplement these days. Purported to increase testosterone and help induce better sleep patterns, ZMA has become the "alternative" to prohormones. ZMA Force + obviously

isn't the only ZMA product on the market, but I thought I would talk about this one because it contains an interesting compound called theanine. Here's the deal, in addition to the right dose of ZMA, ABB's version hits you with an amino acid isolated from green tea (Thea sinensis) called L-Theanine that serves as a GABA precursor. GABA is a neurotransmitter that plays a pivotal role in relaxation but it doesn't just knock you out cold. Theanine works by crossing the blood-brain barrier where it can then be converted to GABA through a series of reactions. The GABA receptors are a common target for prescription sedatives like Valium. As you may have guessed mild sedatives have the ability to "take the edge" off a hectic day of work and or training. I don't know about you, but more relaxation in my life is always a plus and the added benefits to recovery are icing on the cake. The researchers at ABB have put a great amount of effort into bringing theanine to the bodybuilding market. As far as I know they are the first company to market this combination. Does it work? Well, I've had the opportunity to try ZMA Force + and I was really impressed. It made me calmer and I felt more focused state during the day and slept better at night (the ABB guys tell me you could use straight theanine during the day to eliminate stress). Anyway, according to the folks at SNAC systems (the developers of ZMA) it's best to take ZMA at night without any calcium-containing products (calcium will compete with the zinc for absorption). And with theanine booting-up your GABA supply I must say ZMA Force + is a great nighttime formula.

SyntheVol HP™

Company: EAS

Information: Creatine is definitely not news. So the race has been to develop the best creatine delivery mechanisms. To meet this challenge EAS has recently launched SyntheVol HP, a low-carb, insulin-stimulating creatine delivery product.

Since I happen to know the product pretty well (hey my job at EAS *is* product development) let me tell you the "thinking" that went into designing the product. First, as many bodybuilders know carbohydrates are used in the majority of creatine products on the market today as an "insulin amplifier" or driver. This technique definitely works, in fact it works very well, but when we designed SyntheVol HP we wanted to look at developing a product for athletes on a modified low-carb diet such as the Muscularity Diet. It is during these specific lower carbohydrate diets that athletes cannot afford to put on excess

bodyfat, so we challenged the entire product development team to design a product that could in essence "amplify insulin" to drive creatine into muscle cells without loading up on extra calories from carbs. If we could pull it off we knew would alleviate one the main drawbacks associated with most creatine products—*unacceptable quantities* of carbohydrates, usually in the form of sugar—leading you down the path to excess fat accumulation.

After looking at the available research we decided that a zero-carbohydrate product would be self defeating because if you raise insulin without offering up enough available carbs to your system, you may start using valuable amino acids from protein to make glucose. We decided instead to use a modified blend of carbohydrates consisting of vitargo, maltose and dextrose. Vitargo is a high-molecular-weight carbohydrate isolated from potato starch that in research has shown to have the unique ability to rapidly replenish glycogen stores in your muscle cells.[3] In addition to vitargo, we have added dextrose and maltose, which are needed to "kick start" the insulin pathways needed for nutrient transport to facilitate creatine delivery.

Once the insulin mechanism has been set in motion with the modified carbohydrate blend, we sought to maximize the anabolic environment via insulin and nitric oxide production. To accomplish this, we started looking at research regarding insulin secretagogues (initiates the secretion of) and realized the amino acid arginine has a very solid scientific history as insulin "amplifier." One interesting note is that you should take amino acid secretagogues such as arginine without a lot of other whole proteins in your system. The reason is that amino acids that elicit specific physiological processes need to cross the blood-brain barrier to be effective and in the presence of a big protein meal this simply cannot be achieved.

By digging a little deeper we also found another mechanism by which arginine may induce amplified concentrations of insulin, which is through production of nitric oxide (NO). You've probably heard a thing or two about nitric oxide recently, but may be confused as to how it can benefit athletes. Well, nitric oxide is a gas that is formed from the amino acid arginine by a family of enzymes, called NO synthases (NOS). In theory—because researchers simply can't say for sure—nitric oxide has the potential to increase muscle growth by increasing muscle protein synthesis, blood flow, nutrient delivery, and possibly nitrogen balance. There also seems to be a link between nitric oxide, NOS activity, and their presence in insulin-producing cells.

To make SyntheVol HP an effective post-exercise supplement, we also added glutamine peptides. By now, you should be well aware of the positive effects associated with glutamine use. So it's no secret that glutamine is a conditionally essential amino acid that serves a variety of purposes in the muscle building-process, namely protein synthesis, cell volume, and overall immunity. However, you may not know that the source of glutamine in SyntheVol™ HP is hydrolyzed wheat gluten, which has been shown to possess

another "side" benefit that is perfect for our post-exercise recovery phase, ***insulin amplification!***

To round out the formula, SyntheVol™ HP contains a potent blend of glucose/insulin mediators and potentiators, namely d-pinitol and the amino acid taurine, which are both explained in detail in Chapter 9, "The Next Wave of Bodybuilding Supplementation."

I know that was a lot to digest, but I want you to see firsthand how EAS approaches product development and, of course, that SyntheVol HP contains a literal kitchen sink of all the latest gadgets designed to help trigger creatine uptake without the need to gorge on sugar. It's the creatine product I use, and considering everything it contains, I think it's a great value.

Xenadrine™ RFA-1

Company: Cytodyne Technologies

Information: Advertised as the number one diet supplement in America, Xenadrine is definitely a supplement I get asked a lot about. The company's recent advertisements claim the Xenadrine product is "clinically proven to increase fat loss 1700% more than exercise and diet alone." I haven't had the opportunity to review this study in detail but 1700% seems pretty unrealistic to me. Anyway, in this study the control group evidently complied with the same exercise and diet program as the Xenadrine group, but did not get the added benefits of any thermogenic product. It makes sense that the Xenadrine group would burn more fat than the control group, but the advertising claims and study results might be more meaningful to consumers if Xenadrine was compared to other thermogenic formulas head-to-head.

Xenadrine does appear to be an effective thermogenic product. After all it does contains the major "players": Ma Huang (standardized for ephedrine), guarana (standardized for caffeine), citrus aurantium (standardized for synephrine) and white willow bark (containing 15% salicin, the same chemical in aspirin) and a smattering of other ingredients the company refers to as "thermo synergists." Based on the ingredient list on the Xenadrine label it should be an effective thermogenic, but at the same time there's nothing in the ingredient list that would appear to make Xenadrine more effective than all the other fat burners on the market. What is puzzling to me is that while this thermogenic product is probably better than average, their advertising makes claims for results far better than the average fat burner, and that suggests they should have some controlled human studies to substantiate those claims. I haven't tried to find any studies supporting the claims for Xenadrine, but as a careful consumer you should never hesitate to ask a company about the support for advertising or label claims made for its products.

Would I say that Xenadrine is a good product? Yes. Should you expect to get similar results to their marketing claims? Well, results will vary from individual to individual, but if I were buying I'd want to know more about average results for all the persons participating in a controlled study.

Phosphagain 2®

Company: EAS

Information: In 1994, EAS introduced the world to a supplement known as Phosphagain. The was the first weight gainer that was dubbed a "lean mass stimulator." Since then, EAS has modified the original paradigm-shifting formula into what is known as Phosphagain 2.

Phosphagain 2, like its predecessor contains a healthy amount of creatine per serving (8 grams) and contains 25 grams of protein. In addition to an effective amount of creatine and protein, Phosphagain 2 contains 13 grams of carbs with only 5 grams of sugar.

Although Phosphagain 2 was a pioneering formula, you don't hear much about it any more. Why? Well, as the price of creatine has come down substantially many price-sensitive consumers have simply looked for cheaper sources of creatine and protein. Many people are just adding more creatine to their favorite MRP or protein powder. There's more to Phosphagain 2 than simply adding creatine to a protein powder—but for a lot of consumers that's as far as they've looked. Also, there's a lot more competition now than just a few short years ago when Phosphagain 2 was introduced, as you will see in this chapter, where several similar products are reviewed— products with creatine plus protein—but these new formulas don't tell you the whole story. Read on, there's still lots of benefit to be gained from the original Phosphagain 2.

Methoxy-Pro™

Company: Cytodyne Technologies

Information: Methoxy-Pro contains, as the name suggests, 5-methyl-7-methoxyisoflavone. This is currently the hot industry isoflavone for bodybuilders who want to minimize protein breakdown. "Methoxy" was designed to increase lean mass in animals and humans while steering clear of the hormonal pitfalls associated with steroids. Anecdotal evidence has suggested that this flavone can be powerfully anabolic, and may be capable of producing several pounds of lean mass in just a few weeks. See more detail on this subject in Chapter 9.

In addition, Methoxy's tagteam partner is this protein concoction, 7-isopropoxyisofalvone or ipriflavone. You may recognize this ingredient from its use in natural supplements designed to help maintain bone density or even prevent osteoporosis. From my perspective, and without scientific studies suggesting otherwise, ipriflavone seems to increase lean mass by enhancing BONE mass not muscle mass.

When I went to the Cytodyne web site to get a bit more information, I found the following question at the beginning of the Methoxy-Pro information page. "With a literal flood of new protein powders hitting the market every year, why does Methoxy-Pro stand alone as perhaps the greatest breakthrough in the history of bodybuilding supplements?" Well, after reading about the product, I have to ask a different question: why doesn't the product information clearly say that CREATINE is in the formula? Now, I'll

admit that the evidence for some of these isoflavones looks promising, but Cytodyne decided to enhance their Methoxy-Pro formula with creatine, which we know helps build lean muscle mass, without making clear to consumers that creatine is a key ingredient. It's not clear why Cytodyne chose to list creatine by its chemical name N-methyl-N-guanylglycine, but it's likely that not many consumers, even knowledgeable weight trainers, will recognize the chemical name. This is one of those cases where a consumer has to go the extra mile to fully understand what ingredients are in the product, when Cytodyne could just as easily have used the common name "creatine" to identify a key ingredient in their product. Seems like Cytodyne could have made things a lot easier for its consumers, so what gives? I don't know their reasoning but they do the same thing in their advertisements; they don't tell consumers that creatine is a key ingredient in Methoxy-Pro. Unless you really know your chemistry, you wouldn't know that creatine and whey protein appear to be the active strength-enhancing ingredients in this product, unless there's a lot of good science supporting the effectiveness of the flavones in Methoxy-Pro.

Diet Fuel®

Company: Twinlab

Information: Twinlab cut its teeth on the thermogenic market long before many of the other companies even existed (including EAS). Diet Fuel is one of several potent, solid thermogenic formulas offered by Twinlab. Nothing fancy here—just the usual suspects:

guarana extract (for caffeine) and Ma Huang extract in a 10:1 ratio. In addition, Diet Fuel contains 500 mg of Citrimax® (which due to recent research I'm not too crazy about)[1] and 200 mcg of chromium. As straightforward as this supplement seems, it has been extremely popular because it definitely works. But because Twinlab keeps a watchful eye on all their advertisements and product literature, you won't see sensational claims—don't be fooled, lack of hype does not mean lack of effectiveness.

SuperPro

Company: Max Muscle

Information: SuperPro is a blend of three proteins—calcium caseinate, egg white, and soy protein isolate—designed to deliver a unique array of amino acids. Touted as a dieter's protein, SuperPro is a thick, satisfying shake with very few carbs. Nothing completely novel here, but I like the way Max Muscle uses caseinate protein to ultimately enhance absorption. I've had the chance to taste SuperPro and found it to be like a very thick MRP, which could be good for dieters as it fills you up. I think SuperPro is a good-tasting protein for a reasonable price. The one problem is that as of this writing, SuperPro is hard to find. You can only get SuperPro through Max Muscle retail outlets and select gyms.

CycloDiol SR**

Company: ErgoPharm

Information: This is a very interesting product in the ever-growing sports nutrition market. Through the use of a special bio-adhesive,

CycloDiol SR is a prohormone product that delivers 4-androstenediol (available in norandrostenediol too) in a sustained-release fashion by adhering to the inside of your lip (yeah, I know, sounds bad but read on). In addition, the prohormone has been treated with HPB cyclodextrin to enhance solubility and delivery.

According to Patrick Arnold, the "father" of prohormones and maker of CycloDiol SR, this product is far easier to use than lozenges, because you're actually able to carry on a conversation with these things in your mouth. Water-soluble, sustained-release prohormone products—sounds like a recipe for growth.

CAUTION: Contains prohormones. See warning at end of this section.

Cell-Tech™

Company: Muscletech®

Information: Cell-Tech is a creatine transport product that has been around for quite some time. The Cell Tech formula contains 75 grams of dextrose, 10 grams of creatine, 200 mg of alpha-lipoic acid plus chromium picolinate, potassium, phosphates, taurine, ascorbic acid, and magnesium to further potentiate creatine uptake. If you're trying to restrict your calories or are on a low-carb diet, then Cell-Tech is probably not for you. But, if you are following one of the Periodized Bodybuilding and Nutrition programs that calls for higher carbohydrate intake outlined in this book, then this product may be useful to you.

Ecdysten™

Company: Thermo-Life International

Information: This is the first "real-deal" ecdysterone product that I've used. In fact, Ron Kramer and his crew at Thermo-Life International renewed my interest in this powerful compound with the quality of their raw materials. I had an independent laboratory analyze Ecdysten and found it to be about 96% pure ecdysterone, which is right on the money! Ron tells me this powerful substrate is extracted from the herb *Rhaponticum carthamoides,* otherwise known as leuzeae, and is imported directly from Russia, which is also where most of the scientific data originated.

This non-hormonal dietary supplement does not seem to trigger androgenic traits, but does seem to exhibit anabolic characteristics. The reported increases in nitrogen retention and increase in protein synthesis have the whole bodybuilding community talking about—and taking—this compound.

In addition to 12 mg of purified ecdysterone, this product also contains 5 mg of bioperine for added bioavailabity. If you're looking for a potent ecdysterone supplement, Ecdysten is a great choice.

Myoplex

Company: EAS

Information: Myoplex is a reliable meal replacement and has been the flagship product for EAS for several years now. As someone who had to compete with the Myoplex line of meal supplement powders, I can say that they are **by far** the most popular meal-replacement powders on the market. It is also no "secret" that if you want to compete in this category, you have to beat the Myoplex flavor, taste, and mouth-feel, which many think is the "gold standard" for meal replacements. Since I personally use about four to six packets per day (*I use double servings after training*), I really appreciate all the flavor options offered in the Myoplex line. It's a lot easier to stay regimented with Myoplex because they offer so many flavor choices beyond the normal chocolate, vanilla, and strawberry, including the Tropical pack flavors (orange, banana, peach, pina colada) and the Chocolate Lovers pack (chocolate peanut butter, chocolate mocha, chocolate mint, rich dark chocolate).

Myoplex is a simple and convenient way to get the extra protein and nutrients athletes need to build and maintain lean mass. No wild claims and no ridiculous advertising hype, just a great-tasting nutritional **foundation** product. Myoplex has 42 grams of high-quality proteins, which includes ion-exchanged whey protein, milk-protein isolates and slower digesting casein. According to new research, this just may be the best protein combination for athletes available today.[2] Myoplex also includes cell-volumizing amino acids, L-glutamine and taurine, as well as an abundance of vitamins and minerals. Each serving of Myoplex also contains 24 grams of carbohydrates and only 2 grams of fat per serving! It's definitely the type of product that can make following the Foundation Diet in Chapter 4 much easier to adhere to.

For those with calorie concerns, Myoplex comes in a lower calorie version called Myoplex Lite, which utilizes soy protein and phosphates for maintaining a healthy metabolic rate while on a lower calorie regimen. For those on a mass or hardgainer program, EAS also offers Myoplex Mass, which contains 33 grams of high quality protein and a greater amount of carbohydrates—75 grams, which is an ideal post exercise-recovery meal. If you are serious about your training, you'll need a solid foundation for your nutrition program, which is precisely what the Myoplex line of meal supplements is designed to do.

Promax

Company: SportPharma

Information: In my opinion, Promax is one of the best-tasting protein bars on the market. This product has been around for quite some time and is available almost everywhere. The Promax bar contains 20 grams of protein and 35-39 grams of carbohydrates, with 20-33 grams of sugar. As you can see, if you're trying to restrict your calories or are on a low-carb diet, the Promax bar is not for you. I mention this bar because there are those who are trying to gain size that have been hooked into this whole low-carb diet concept. But, when you're trying to grow and when you're training hard, you need carbs. Now, I'm not advocating drowning yourself with sugar to gain mass, but what I am suggesting is that there are products out there—that are NOT low carb—that can help support your quest for gains (more on this in Chapter 3, "Rock Solid Nutritional Strategies").

BetaLean® HP

Company: EAS

Information: I mentioned the effectiveness of Ma Huang and caffeine as thermogenics earlier. These ingredients have now been combined with other powerful ingredients to create the "next level" of thermogenic products. BetaLean HP is one such product.

Using the standard thermogenic foundation of ephedra and caffeine, BetaLean adds tyrosine, naringin, coleus forskolin, and green tea to enhance the overall thermogenic effect. In addition, to improve insulin sensitivity, a common thread associated with excess bodyfat, BetaLean HP also contains alpha-lipoic acid. I won't bore you with all the scientific stuff here, because many of the added ingredients in BetaLean HP are explained in detail in Chapter 9, "The Next Wave of Bodybuilding Supplementation"— just look for "Glycemic Response Modifiers, Thermogenic Amplifiers, and Glucose Disposal Agents."

Having a well-packed formula with all the latest ingredients is important, but what really "makes" this product in my opinion is the Precision Release Matrix. This technology allowed EAS to "dial-in" how they wanted the formula to behave. And in this case, the release matrix delivers an initial burst of about 80% of the active ingredients followed by a 2-hour trickle of the remaining 20%. The end result is a nice, smooth, and effective fat-burning product. No wild claims here. According to the scientific data on caffeine and ephedra, an athlete who follows a prudent nutrition and training plan (see Chapter 3, "Rock Solid Nutritional Strategies") should be able to accelerate fat burning between 30-50% compared to athletes who train without a thermogenic.

Using a potent thermogenic like BetaLean requires some extra caution. All the popular "fat burners" that contain ephedra or a combination of ephedra and caffeine are stimulants that must be used properly, and in fact, are not for everyone. In my view, it is important to consult with your physician before using this or similar products that contain stimulants. Most of these products contain extensive warnings about proper use but the basic cautions are these:

EPHEDRA AND CAFFEINE WARNING: NOT FOR USE BY INDIVIDUALS UNDER THE AGE OF 18. DO NOT USE IF PREGNANT OR NURSING. CONSULT A PHYSICIAN OR LICENSED QUALIFIED HEALTH CARE PROFESSIONAL BEFORE USING THIS PRODUCT IF YOU HAVE, OR HAVE A FAMILY HISTORY OF, HEART DISEASE, THYROID DISEASE, DIABETES, HIGH BLOOD PRESSURE, RECURRENT HEADACHES, DEPRESSION OR OTHER PSYCHIATRIC CONDITION, GLAUCOMA, DIFFICULTY IN URINATING, PROSTATE ENLARGEMENT, OR SEIZURE DISORDER, IF YOU ARE USING A MONOAMINE OXIDASE INHIBITOR (MAOI) OR ANY OTHER DIETARY SUPPLEMENT, PRESCRIPTION DRUG OR OVER-THE-COUNTER DRUG CONTAINING EPHEDRINE, PSEUDOEPHEDRINE OR PHENYL-PROPANOLAMINE (INGREDIENTS FOUND IN CERTAIN ALLERGY, ASTHMA, COUGH/COLD AND WEIGHT CONTROL PRODUCTS). EXCEEDING RECOMMENDED SERVING MAY CAUSE SERIOUS ADVERSE HEALTH EFFECTS INCLUDING HEART ATTACK AND STROKE. DISCONTINUE USE AND CALL A PHYSICIAN OR LICENSED QUALIFIED HEALTH CARE PROFESSIONAL IMMEDIATELY IF YOU EXPERIENCE RAPID HEARTBEAT, DIZZINESS, SEVERE HEADACHE, SHORTNESS OF BREATH OR OTHER SIMILAR SYMPTOMS. INDIVIDUALS WHO CONSUME CAFFEINE, OR OTHER STIMULANTS, WITH THIS PRODUCT MAY EXPERIENCE SERIOUS ADVERSE HEALTH EFFECTS. KEEP OUT OF REACH OF CHILDREN.

CytoPlex

Company: Cytodyne Technology

Information: There is a lot of interest in Cytodyne's products and product claims. And, it's a simple fact in this business that if you've got "hot" products, consumers want to know how they work and why.

Cytoplex claims to be the first meal replacement to include a revolutionary compound called Glucostatin-RFS, which is marketed as a unique blend of powerful substrates "clinically proven" to control appetite and stimulate rapid and dramatic weight-loss results, **even without dieting**. Well, when a product is advertised as "clinically proven," that's supposed to mean there's basically scientific agreement supporting how the product works or its results. An independent lab analyzed Cytoplex, at our request, and it appears that the "revolutionary" ingredient "Glucostatin-RFS" is nothing more than plain old chitosan (a fiber from shellfish commonly referred to as a fat trapper). In addition to this shellfish byproduct, Glucostatin-RFS contains other fibers in a blend stated as: maltodextrin, brown rice complex, oat fiber, and Glucostatin RFS (guar gum, glucomannon [hemi cellulose, cellulose, pectin substance, lignin], chitosan).

If you don't watch a lot of late-night TV, then I should tell you that chitosan is indeed a "fat trapper," and yes, it will retard the inevitable weight gain of those consumers who throw their diet into the wind. The real kicker is when the Cytoplex advertisements state that the "precision" formula is powered by an advanced blend of revolutionary substrates **individually** proven in published clinical studies to dramatically increase the rate of weight loss (even without dieting or exercise). The more basic issue is this: any bodybuilder or athlete worth his gym membership will tell you that fat or carb blockers are not revolutionary; this doesn't mean they don't work for some people, but the bottom line about effective long-term weight loss is still proper nutrition and moderate exercise. If you're serious about losing weight safely, go out and get yourself a high-quality meal supplement that tastes good **to you**, use the meal replacement as part of a good nutritional foundation, and start exercising. Include a high-quality thermogenic in your program if you want to accelerate weight loss, but understand there is nothing revolutionary about the right ways to lose weight and body fat. I may sound like a broken record, but none of these product combinations works well unless you train and eat wisely. So don't forget to read Chapter 3, "Rock Solid Nutritional Strategies."

Speed Stack

Company: American Body Building

Information: This ready-to-drink product is another thermogenic product that is definitely not for the TIMID—and if you think I've sounded like a broken record before, here I go again, thermogenics aren't for everyone, consult your physician before using them, and use only as directed! From ABB, the makers of the most popular bodybuilding drinks in gyms and health clubs, comes with yet another pre-

workout fat burner that's the next generation from Ripped Force in overall thermogenic muscle. What's the difference between this fat burner and Ripped Force? For one, it contains fewer carbs and calories than Ripped Force and, two, it contains 24 mg of ephedrine, instead of the 20 mg in Ripped Force. Speed Stack also contains 200 mg of caffeine and 11 mg of standardized synephrine, which will definitely ring your bell. I have used Speed Stack to train and based on my experience the product seems well designed and as a bonus it tastes pretty good.

All these advanced thermogenics are potent and should be used with care. Getting tired of hearing me say that? But it is true! These are products best suited to experienced athletes who have a fundamental understanding of how thermogenics work and how they can be used effectively and safely. Use only as directed, consult your physician, they aren't for everyone—enough said.

Horny Goat Weed

Company: Pinnacle

Information: Need some weed? This is the sophomoric question that is posed alongside the equally juvenile tagline, "Do the weed and you'll succeed," for Pinnacle's Horny Goat Weed. In my opinion, indirect references to street drugs, no matter how innocent or cute, have no place in the marketing of dietary supplements—and I think the FDA has stated a similar position. But my opinions aside, because I don't sell the products I just review them, this concoction of exotic herbs is supposed to increase sex drive and performance.

Sounds interesting right? Let's take a look at what's going on here.

Epimedium grandiflorum, also known as Horny Goat Weed, is an herb that has been marketed as an elixir of sorts for the male libido. From what I can see, it appears that epimedium grandiflorum and its active component may indeed have immune-enhancing effects, but as for your libido I just don't know. Another component of HGW is 250 mg of Maca Pure (Lepidium meyenii), which according to a recent study[3] can increase sexual behavior in animals. However, this study clearly stated that the amount needed to produce statistically significant results was over 45 mg per kg/bodyweight, which is 4,000 mg for a 200-lb person. HGW also contains macuna pruriens, a phytonutrient that contains L-dopa, which is a good GH releaser and may enhance your mood if taken in high enough quantities. Unfortunately HGW contains only 33.3 mg of macuna pruriens standardized for 15% L-dopa, which equates to a very small 5 mg amount. Next, HGW contains polypodium vulgare, which is another source of ecdysterone (see Chapter 9 for more info). Data on ecdysterone specifically state that this compound has **no effect** whatsoever on male hormone levels at all, and because the product only contains 25 mg of an 8% standardized extract, which equates to a paltry 2 mg, it probably won't increase protein synthesis either. I appreciate the proposed benefits (hey, don't we all work hard to attract the opposite sex?), but from what I can tell from the science, HGW doesn't appear to be an "over-the-top" libido enhancer, and doesn't seem to have much to do with building a bet-ter physique. It's probably safe to say that as every person is different, and you may or may not experience the results as advertised. Next product please...

3-Andro Extreme**

Company: AST Research

Information: This product is no slouch when it comes to products on the edge. It's really a "shotgun marriage" of purported hormone boosters and a potent thermogenic cocktail. 3-Andro extreme has 100 mg each of 4-androstenediol and 19-norandrodione to trigger production of testosterone and nortestosterone respectively, plus 100 mg of 5-androstenediol. I'm not sure why 5-andro made the list because there's not much science connecting it with muscle metabolism. But there are no superfluous ingredients when it comes to the thermogenic component of this product. 200 mg of caffeine is coupled with a hearty dose of ephedrine—32 mg—along with phenylalanine and tyrosine for a nice boost in dopaminergic neurotransmission. Remember all those warnings about potent thermogenics? Well read them again, carefully! Seriously, just like the car commercials on television, this is a product that in my opinion should only be used by professionals, meaning experienced strength-training athletes who really understand all the ingredients and how they may work synergistically, and then only with care. It is an extremely potent product that should be approached with caution and after consulting with your physician. If all the ingredients work synergistically, this is a product that could flip all the switches in your brain to "on" and send you off on a high-energy rocket ship ride to the Red Planet.

Proof of the products "edgy" nature is the sheer amount of ephedrine it contains—32 mg, which is 60% higher than the upper limit of ephedrine allowed by the folks at GNC, and really puts the FDA on edge. As such, don't expect to see 3-Andro Extreme at your local General Nutrition Center anytime soon.

CAUTION: Contains prohormones. See warning at end of this section.

BetaStatin-WPI2

Company: BetaStatin

Information: A relatively new meal-replacement powder on the market, BetaStatin-WPI-2 seems to be a decent formula, but the product claims... come on guys! Maker of the highest Biological Value (BV) meal replacement ever!? Where's the support for that? This is an example of a product that appears to have some decent attributes—whey-protein isolate, glutamine peptides, creatine monohydrate—but the good attributes are overpowered by sensational marketing claims (which apparently aren't supported with science—either clinical studies or current scientific literature). Products such as this that include lots of good ingredients can stand on their own, without claims that go way beyond sales puffery. Makes me wonder about the people behind it.

Secretagogue One

Company: MHP

Information: This was one of the first of the so-called growth-hormone-releasing peptide formulas. Each 12.5-gram effervescent packet contains a proprietary blend of amino acids, anterior pituitary peptides, and a smidgen of naturally occurring L-dopa. Apparently Secretagogue One transports active peptides to your pituitary gland in order to stimulate the release of growth hormone.

I think the jury is still out on natural hGH products, but if you want to give this category a try, MHP appears to have all the elements of a theoretically effective formula. The plethora of hGH-stimulating products that have surfaced in the last four years have a lot of industry people scratching their heads. Personally, I'd like to see more human clinical studies, and I think the marketers of these growth hormone products should provide more support for their claims—but that's me. However, it is likely that these products work for some athletes—otherwise they already would have gone the way of the dinosaur. And speaking of "scratch," if you feel you want to give this product a go, it'll cost you— about $2.00 to $2.50 per day.

Another two-cents about warnings. Any growth hormone product should be used carefully, and only after consulting a qualified physician who can help you understand whether or not growth hormone may be beneficial for you. The body's hormonal balance is delicate, and like advanced thermogenics, growth hormone products should be used only by experienced strength-training athletes, and even for these GUYS (sorry, no girls allowed with these products), consulting a qualified physician is an essential first step in using these products safely.

Ultimate Orange

Company: Next Proteins

Information: This one's a thermogenic classic. Ultimate Orange has been around for almost a decade and was the brainchild of David Jenkins, owner of Next Proteins and the late Dan Duchaine, steroid guru. The bottom line is, this formula is powerful—that's right, go back and read the warnings!

Designed for use prior to and during workouts, this powdered beverage contains ephedrine, caffeine, sida cordifolia (another source of ephedrine), coleus forskolin, green tea, guarana, cayenne pepper—a literal kitchen sink of thermogenic compounds. In addition, the Ultimate drinks (there's Ultimate Punch too) have 7 grams of protein from whey-protein concentrate (with glutamine peptides) and 17 grams of energy-sustaining carbohydrates.

Truly a hardcore product, Ultimate Orange is ONLY for experienced bodybuilders and strength training athletes who know what they're doing—and even they need to read the label and use advanced thermogenic products as directed.

Male Fuel

Company: Twinlab

Information: Here's another product that doesn't really have direct associations with bodybuilding or training. It does however have a few gadgets that have a definite biological effect.

A serving of Male Fuel is loaded with 800 mg of yohimbe and 2,800 mg of L-arginine HCl to help with penile blood flow. (Did you know arginine is intimately involved in nitric oxide production—can you say Viagra®?) In addition, it has ginkgo and tyrosine to make sure the right neurotransmitters are firing for proper sexual arousal. Male Fuel is also home to a host of other herbs and nutrients assembled together to make sure all the "plumbing" is operating normally. Like Horny Goat Weed, results will vary, and as the name suggests—ladies this one isn't for you.

Super Heavyweight Gainer

Company: Champion

Information: This is a high-calorie weight gainer. Now you may be thinking that this is an old-school approach to bodybuilding—and you're right. But if you look at the nutrition requirements set forth in the Hardgainer Diet (see Chapter 6), particularly the post-training caloric requirements, this is a product that can work well in that regimen.

With 60 grams of protein and 108 grams of carbs, this may be the ticket for post-workout glycogen resynthesis while delivering a nice shot of high-quality protein.

Ultra Pure Protein Shake

Company: Worldwide Sport Nutrition

Information: As of this writing, EAS has introduced several new ready-to-drink products under the AdvantEdge and Myoplex brand names, but with that said, I'm objective enough to tell you that I really like Worldwide's Ultra Pure Protein Shake. Ultra

Pure delivers 35 grams of protein from milk-protein isolates and caseinate and only 4 grams of carbs in a ready-to-drink format—and it tastes good considering the low-carb formulation. This is a good way to grab an extra dose of post-workout protein when you're leaving the gym.

Lean Body™ Bars

Company: Labrada Bodybuilding Nutrition

Information: Lean Body Bars fill a market niche somewhere between a traditional high-carb food bar and a low-carb protein bar. Really Labrada's bars are more like an MRP bar—with 30 grams of protein and around 17 grams of carbs, they're also loaded with vitamins and minerals. Although not considered low-carb bars by most standards, Lean Body Bars are relatively low in sugar. These bars are great for a post-workout meal or on-the-go snack, and I think they taste great.

Thermo-Tek

Company: Iron-Tek

Information: This is a very potent thermogenic product. If you look at the formula closely you'll notice similarities to the popular Xenadrine RFA-1. Like Xenadrine RFA-1, Thermo-Tek contains a Ma Huang and guarana combo, with synephrine riding along to enhance the thermogenic boost. In addition to these nearly identical ingredients, the folks at Iron-Tek threw in a few other gadgets, primarily 800 mcg of chromium and 200 mg of Hydroxycitric acid, which have been added for blood sugar control. Again I'm not

a fan of HCA in a thermogenic because of the most recent scientific data.[1]

Iron-Tek hasn't been around long, but their formula for Thermo-Tek appears to be solid, and they don't make sensational or unbelievable product claims. Country Life is the parent company of Iron-Tek and they're known for running a tight ship—so I would expect products from Iron-Tek to be effective and consistent with label claims. But, again, Thermo-Tek is an advanced thermogenic and subject to the same warnings that I've mentioned before.

MX7

Company: GEN

Information: GEN has been heavily involved in the flavone movement. Their introduction of Chrysin in 1997 established GEN as a company whose products are targeted at hardcore bodybuilders. Continuing in this marketing direction, GEN has launched MX7, which is their trade name for the largely popular 5-Methyl-7-Methoxyisoflavone, also known as Methoxy.

Like I said earlier about Methoxy-Pro, "methoxy" is currently the hot isoflavone for bodybuilders and serious strength-training athletes who strive to minimize protein breakdown that follows intense workouts. Methoxy was originally created and designed to increase lean mass in animals and humans. Anecdotal evidence has suggested that this flavone can be powerfully anabolic, and may be capable of producing noticeable effects in just a few weeks. I go into more detail on this in Chapter 9.

GEN has been known to put out solid products, and seems to always be on the cutting edge. MX7 contains 150 mg of methoxy per serving, and does not contain creatine. While there's a lot of market hype about the benefits of methoxy, and some pretty outrageous product claims, GEN seems to be reasonable in its marketing approach and product claims. As with all these advanced products, results will vary dramatically among individuals, and most of what you hear in the gym will be anecdotal and probably inflated in terms of the results people are getting from the various methoxy products. As more science becomes available, we'll be able to better evaluate the benefits of methoxy, but for now we're hearing about lots of good results.

Myoplex™ Ready-to-Drink Shakes

Company: EAS

Information: EAS is the first sports nutrition company to enter the ready-to-drink market using packaging called *Tetra® Prisma*, which appears to have some advantages over competitive products in metal containers. Since I am not a packaging or processing expert, I asked EAS' Director of RTD Product Development, Lorenzo Nicastro, to tell me the advantages of delivering products in a *Tetra® Prisma*. Here's the scoop: Products in a *Tetra® Prisma* package are first pasteurized and then aseptically processed and packaged. This means that the beverage and *Tetra® Prisma* package are separately heat treated (at temperatures sufficient to pasteurize the product and basically sterilize the packaging material), and then brought together in a sterile

environment for filling and sealing. Beverages packaged in metal containers are usually subjected to a longer heat-pasteurizing process, called retorting, where the temperature and duration of the heat processing is dependent on both the product and the package size, shape, and density, because the product is packaged before it goes through the retort process. The benefit to aseptic packaging, as with the *Tetra® Prisma*, is that it results in a cleaner taste. The retort process can impart to the beverage a metallic flavor, which results from the higher temperatures and generally longer duration of heat processing. Bottom line is that aseptically packaged beverages taste better.

Myoplex™ Ready-To-Drink have a calorie ratio of 40-40-20. Of the 200 calories, 40% of the calories come from protein, 40% from carbohydrate, and the remaining 20% from fat. The RTD Shakes contain 20 grams of quality protein from whey-protein isolate and soy-protein isolate. In addition, these are naturally sweetened drinks, with 20 grams of total carbohydrate.

Myoplex™ Pro Ready-To-Drink will contain about 45 grams of protein (whey, milk-protein isolate, and caseinate), 25 carbs, 5 grams of fat, and 24 vitamins/minerals. This product will be almost an exact copy nutritionally as the Myoplex packet products.

Myoplex™ Low Carb Ready-To-Drink will contain about 20 grams of quality protein (whey, milk-protein isolate, and caseinate), only 3 carbs, 4 grams of fat, and 24 vitamins/minerals. This product will be an ultra-convenient way for athletes to stay on any of the

Muscularity Diets mentioned in this book.

If you are looking for convenient, balanced, and great-tasting products to help you optimize your nutrition program; the family of Myoplex™ Ready-To-Drink Shakes will be a great addition to your supplement arsenal.

N-Large-2

Company: Prolab

Information: N-Large-2 is another mass-gaining formula designed to pack size on the hardgainer. This formula delivers a heap of calories, coming from 52 grams of protein and 89 grams of carbohydrates. It mixes pretty easily in a shaker cup and the taste isn't bad. This product could work its way into the diet of a hardgainer or as a post-workout recovery drink—but watch those calories. Eating too much of a product like N-Large-2 could make you large in all the wrong places.

ATP Advantage Serum Creatine™

Company: Muscle Marketing USA

Information: The samples of this product that I've had analyzed at an independent laboratory don't come close to meeting label claims. I'll be the first to admit it's always possible to find one or two samples of a product that doesn't meet label claims, but with the careful attention that most reputable suppliers give to quality control, even these occasional screw-ups are becoming increasingly rare. Muscle Marketing claims to have invented the world's only stabilized liquid creatine. In the case of ATP Advantage Serum Creatine, the lab analysis we had performed on two sep-

arate product lots found that the product contained less than one microgram of creatine, but the label claimed 2.5 grams. This is less than 1% of the amount of creatine claimed on the label. The lab analysis also found only traces of ginseng, royal jelly, and Vitamin B_{12}, when compared to the label claims.

In my opinion, the bottom line is this: The regulatory environment in this industry is tightening up, but at some level the industry has to police itself. We know our competitors analyze our products, just as we analyze theirs. Most of the time the products from all the major players, and many of the smaller companies, are right on label claim or very close. There will always be exceptions, but what separates the reputable companies from the others is attention to quality control and the fact that quality problems are addressed when their discovered. That's why you won't see reputable companies and their products having continuing problems with products not being close to label claims.

Muscle Milk

Company: CytoSport

Information: After "breaking away" from Champion Nutrition, Greg Picket set out to do something different. He purchased Cytomax, one of the strongest products from Champion, and with that he was off and running.

Muscle Milk is a new product from CytoSport designed to deliver, "metabolically favorable ingredients to stimulate growth and recovery in a similar manner to mother's milk…" so says their web site. If you read the ingredient panel, you'll be overwhelmed by the degree of proprietary ingredients and scientific jargon. This can be a convenient smokescreen when a company doesn't want you to know the ingredients in their products by common names, but sometimes it's also a sign of highly proprietary research and product development. In this case, we don't know what to think. Things like Evopro, Leanlipides, Betapol are all trademarks for a host of things including proteins and fats. And speaking of fats, Muscle Milk has 18 grams of the stuff. Now, I'm not saying that fat is completely bad, especially when it comes from unsaturated sources, but be careful. Those fat calories can add up quickly. So check your diet plan, and make sure a product like this will fit into your caloric requirements before you choose to believe the magic.

Methoxy 7™

Company: Biotest Laboratories, LLC.

Information: This was the first Methoxy-isoflavone product that I ever took seriously (for more in depth info on Methoxyisoflavone see chapter 9). In fact we bought several bottles here at EAS right about the same time we got some high potency ecdysterone materials so we could see what kind of results we could achieve by combining the two. I really liked the Biotest Methoxy-7 product for a couple of reasons. The first is potency—each 2-teaspoon serving contains 400 milligrams of 5-methyl-7-methoxyisoflavone so if you take it just once per day you're still getting a lot more bang for your buck than most of the other Methoxy products on the market. Second is the delivery system, which utilizes pure, USP-grade choles-

terol that acts as an "escort system" to help make the flavone more bioavailable. As for the cholesterol in this product remember that a sufficient quantity is required for hormone production. As far as methoxy products go this one seems to be a good choice.

Summary

I hope you found this chapter to be thought provoking, educational, and entertaining. I know that after two decades as a supplement consumer, some of the things that I discovered while playing "inspector" opened my eyes to many interesting bits of information about different branded supplements. This is the kind of stuff that typically isn't right on the surface, and I've tried to share some of my experience in this chapter. By reading this chapter, in combination with the rest of this issue of the *Sports Supplement Review*, I hope you'll become a more informed consumer—or at least a more careful consumer—when it comes to purchasing supplements. Don't be afraid to be skeptical of sensational product claims, and don't be afraid to ask questions. If you don't understand what's in a supplement—call the supplier, you're the consumer, you have a right to know. If you can't get satisfactory answers, spend your hard-earned money somewhere else. There's not a product in the market today that doesn't have a reasonably close substitute. I can say this because I am a reformed "supplement sucker," and I fully realize that when your number-one goal is a better body, it's easy to go for the hype and the sensational claim, and it's easy to be misled. To believe in something is not a crime, however, not taking the time to inform yourself can certainly make you an easier victim. The bottom line is awareness—reading supplement ads and labels carefully and asking experienced bodybuilders and athletes and others who have been around the strength-training scene for a while. Get their feedback, and take advantage of their experience, but remember they have their biases, and they aren't necessarily experts. As I said above, don't hesitate to call the company whose products you're interested in buying; ask your questions and expect to receive helpful answers. If you really get into it, take some time and read the studies that are cited to support product claims. Usually, these are too technical for most of us, but you'll be surprised how much of the information you will understand. There's a wealth of information available, and don't forget the Internet. If you don't want to go to all that trouble, a couple of good rules of thumb are these: First, trust the companies who have been around for awhile, and whose products have worked for you in the past. And, finally my favorite rule of thumb, which comes from years of experience: If a product or product claim sounds too good to be true, buy something else!

** WARNING Finally, for those athletes who are considering adding prohormones to your supplement program, please do not do so "blindly." These compounds, when designed properly, are very powerful, and can potentially alter your own hormonal environment. This **may not be appropriate** for many athletes, especially women. It appears that the best candidates for prohormones are aging males over 50 or those with hormones such as testosterone that have consistently hovered in the low ranges due to health-related problems or stress. In my view, the best approach to using these compounds is an educated one. This means that you will need to do a little "homework" on the biological effects of any compound you want to use, and bring this information to your physician. Only after you do this can you have an intelligent conversation with any medical professional concerning your personal needs, and if these products are right for you (not your training partner or friends). Your physician should then set up a full blood chemistry exam and analyze your current hormonal status. Once your physician looks at your hormonal status from a medical point of view, he or she can make a proper determination as to what products may benefit you. Remember that this is your endocrine system, and it is very delicate. The endocrine system you have has many built-in "feedback" systems that, if overloaded, may cause untoward health risks. I am sure you can get the most current prohormone data for your physician from the National Library of Medicine at www.nlm.nih.gov/. If your physician is unfamiliar with these compounds, you can always ask him or her to seek advice from colleagues. Just remember that the blood chemistry work should be the basis from which your doctor makes his or her recommendations.

References Cited

1 Luc JC van Loon, Johannes JM van Rooijen, Bas Niesen, Hans Verhagen, Wim HM Saris, and Anton JM Wagenmakers, "Effects of acute (-)-hydroxycitrate supplementation on substrate metabolism at rest and during exercise in humans." *American Journal of Clinical Nutrition*, 72.6 (2000) : 1445-1450.

Chapter

16

Altered States

Taking Your Training to the NEXT Level!

When my colleagues and I discussed the contents of this book, we were deadlocked on whether or not it should contain training advice. It wasn't long after we outlined the Periodized Bodybuilding Nutrition System that we realized training advice was a must. I firmly believe intelligent training programs look to exploit synergies within specific nutrition goals. Even so, there is a lot of conflicting training information out there. In fact, I would venture to say the Information Age has spawned the "Misinformation Age," making it tougher for athletes to get the real inside scoop on maximum training methods.

The Science of Workout Design

The training goal for any bodybuilder or athlete should be to thoroughly attack every muscle fiber type for maximum muscle size, vascularity, and fullness. Because of this, many bodybuilders think that an in-depth overview of muscle physiology is necessary to design an effective training program. After all, research has shown that muscle fiber types have different characteristics affected by varying training systems. While all of the above is true, this chapter will make it simple to understand how your muscles adapt to different systems of training, which in itself will save you years of frustration. I promised you in the beginning of this book I would cover all the questions I asked myself when I was desperately searching for the right formula. Fortunately for you, this chapter will help "clear the air" on the science of training in a format that is neither too rigid to apply or so haphazard it fails altogether. This chapter contains three parts, which coincide with our Periodized Bodybuilding Nutrition Systems outlined in the previous chapters.

I can say this because I have the benefit of writing this chapter with Russian Master Trainer Pavel Tsatsouline. I have read many books by coaches, trainers, and athletes who have all experienced renowned success, and I can say that Pavel is easily one of the most brilliant. As you might expect from a Russian specialist, Pavel has a complete and sometimes "over the top" understanding of training as it relates to different athletic events and muscle fiber types. But he has a keen understanding of how to design training programs within a specific nutrition phase. In just a few meetings, Pavel has opened up my eyes to exciting new ways to simplify and maximize my own training. And this may be the first time many of you have the chance to grasp the concept known as periodization or cycling, and actually be able to use it with great success. Now I know why various law enforcement agencies hire Pavel Tsatsouline to train their elite SWAT teams, and readers of hardcore iron publications like *MILO* or *Powerlifting USA* go nuts over Pavel's articles and books!

Training on the Foundation Diet

Pavel Tsatsouline is here to help me develop the training to "mirror" the diet protocols for each of the diets contained in this book. Let's begin with a discussion about the most effective training methods to practice while following this Foundation Diet.

Vince Andrich: Pavel, I know that you have reviewed each of the nutrition modules outlined in the previous chapters. What I'd like to do is start by discussing the most effective training methods for athletes who are on the Bodybuilding Foundation Diet. What shall we start with?

Pavel Tsatsouline: Let us divide the Bodybuilding Foundation Training Cycle into two 4-week long phases, or "mesocycles," if you prefer exotic Russian terminology, which utilize a different set of exercises and a different split. Russian studies have shown that the body adapts to a complex set of weight-training exercises in about four to six weeks. That gives us two different programs to work with. The only exercise that hangs on for the entire two-month stretch is the breathing 20-rep squat. The reason is simple: You can milk this painful goodie for gains a lot longer than any other drill! Since Paul Anderson made his historic power trip to the USSR, we have been impartial to squats.

VA: High-rep breathing squats for mass, now that takes me back quite a few years. I like it already. Could you explain your training model for building mass?

PT: Vince, I say "Long live Arnold!" and recommend a high volume of loading. Don't get me wrong. If you are trying to peak your strength, intensity is a good thing when taken in moderation. However, the rest of the time, high volume rules! Russian scientists uncompromisingly state that lasting muscle growth in elite athletes can only be achieved through a high volume of loading! Hey, if bodybuilding was as easy as just doing one set of an exercise, don't you think there would have been a lot more muscular studs walking around?

VA : I completely agree. We don't hear much about "muscle quality" any more, which was supposedly the hallmark of an athlete with years of combined volume and high-intensity training. Then again, it seems that the patent excuse has been that athletes who could do the higher volume routines were taking illegal substances to get them through it. I think most high-level athletes and authors like Jeff Everson will agree that the super-low volume approach is one that was developed more for mass-market appeal than for world-class results. In retrospect to my own training, I have realized that when I am eating enough protein, carbs, and fats, and sleeping properly, you can do much more volume than the one-set-to-failure proponents would like you to believe. Again, cycling periods of high-volume training in and out of your total training is the best approach. By the way, how do you define "high volume?"

PT : There are a couple of ways of measuring volume. Many Russian coaches like to add up the tonnage, or the total amount of weight lifted per workout. For example, 200 lbs x 10 reps x 5 sets = 10,000 lbs. Russian experts recommend that experienced athletes elevate 30 to 50 tons, or up to 100,000 lbs, per workout in the hypertrophy phase, while handling weights in the 60 to 80% one-rep-maximum (1RM) range.

This simplified approach works wonders for you lifters and hardgainers, who focus on a handful of basics that can work your entire body. But when you try to apply the tonnage method to a bodybuilder's split routine with isolation exercises, it becomes evident that 10,000 lbs will barely warm up your quads, but may put your triceps in a hospital. For a bodybuilder, it is more appropriate to express volume in total reps per muscle group. Russian coaches who prefer this volume calcu-

lation method specify that the reps fit in a given "intensity zone" or percentage of 1RM. If you are not a lifter, you will do just fine by simply adding up all your reps minus the warm-ups.

VA : So what rep total would you prescribe?

PT : Eastern European scientists recommend a very wide range, between 30 and 150 quality repetitions per muscle group. That gives you a lot of room to exercise your bodybuilding instinct. Bodybuilding is science as much as art.

VA : I'll go with that. And how about intensity?

PT : Vince, shall I presume that you refer to the closeness to muscle failure rather than the Russian definition of intensity as the percentage of 1RM?

VA : Yes.

PT : There are at least three reasons not to train to failure. First, extreme stress spikes the hormone cortisol, which is highly catabolic. Second, the gains achieved with intense training, be it training to failure, maxing out, or employing forced reps or negatives, are very short lived and easily reversed. And third, training to failure derails your strength gains, thanks to something neuroscientists refer to as the "Hebbian mechanisms." So go ahead and lift to your rep max on your top sets, but never start a rep that you might not complete in less than perfect form! And one more thing: Please lay off the melodrama in the gym! Impress people with your physique or with your strength, not with your emotional display of effort.

VA : I'll second that notion and add that weight training should be a lifelong endeavor that should not be mentally parallel to a car accident. I mean how can anyone possibly want to go to the gym, barely warm up, and then attempt to set a personal record in each lift such as is proposed by the "Heavy Duty" disciples? Your methodical training approach is right on the money in my book. Now what is the rep range for our Bodybuilding Foundation program?

PT : Eight and up. High repetitions are efficient for achieving a high volume of loading and great for stimulating the body's anabolic hormones.

VA : What about rest periods between sets?

PT : Professor Matveyev advises one to three minutes, because this time frame does not provide for complete muscle recovery and forces the accumulation of pumped fatigue and growth-hormone-producing lactate.

VA : A rest period of one to three minutes is a very wide range. So are you saying that bodybuilders on this program should pace their rest periods between sets according to their levels of fatigue, and not necessarily the clock?

PT : Exactly. You do not need to aim for complete recovery between sets in the Bodybuilding Foundation phase, but you do not want your workout to deteriorate into an aerobic class with pink Barbie & Ken dumbbells. Makes sense?

VA : Yes, it reminds me of advice I got from the original Iron Guru Vince Gironda years

ago. He simplified tempo between sets to mean pacing, which is all related to fatigue and pushing those limits.

PT: The bodybuilder will have a clearer understanding of our program and shall develop an instinctive sense for rest intervals and other load variables if he or she understands what stimulates muscle growth. Allow me to explain the energetic theory of muscle hypertrophy.

VA : Go ahead, let it rip.

PT : I'll use an analogy to explain it. Recall the old adage that a muscle needs to be "torn down" to be rebuilt bigger and stronger. Imagine that water in a pool represents this muscle. The more you can drain it during your workout the better. The in-pipe stands for the rebuilding processes that are constantly taking place in our cells. The drainage pipe would represent your sets and reps that degrade your muscle's proteins. The heavier the weight, the thicker this pipe. The time this pipe is open corresponds to the time under tension, or simply your sets multiplied by your reps.

VA : Aha, this is the basis for a high volume of loading.

PT : You bet. The obvious way to outrun the in-pipe and deplete the muscle "pool" most thoroughly is to get the biggest out-pipe (the heaviest weight) and to keep it open for as long as possible (many sets and reps). Obviously, a compromise is unavoidable. If you use a lot of weight, you will be unable to do many reps and sets. On the other hand, if the weight is light enough to enable you to knock off a zillion reps, you are using such a thin out-pipe that the pool keeps getting refilled at the same time it is depleted!

VA : That explains why there are so many successful bodybuilding routines; you can drain the pool with many combinations of weights, sets, and reps as long as you avoid the heavy and light extremes!

PT : Just do not forget to compress the breaks between your sets. The in-pipe keeps dripping in, so you will achieve the best results if you do all your sets and reps in the shortest time possible!

VA : One of Gironda's favorite lines was "More work in less time—equals quality muscle size."

PT : Beautiful, the energetic theory of hypertrophy in a nutshell. Old timers may not have known their physiology, but they surely had their act together. By the way, note that the Iron Guru's statement implies not training to failure. Terminating your sets a rep before you bite the dust keeps you relatively fresh, and enables you to maximize your tonnage with heavy weights.

VA : Now I have read your books and articles on stretching, and was impressed with your rationale. Can you elaborate?

PT : I encourage bodybuilders to stretch the worked muscles after each set.

Recently a number of bodybuilding magazines have reported on "breakthrough" American and Australian studies that show that proper stretching between the sets can up one's strength and mass. Old hat, my friends! Soviet Professor Arkady Vorobyev

made that discovery a quarter of a century ago. This weightlifting champion turned scientist studied the effect of stretching between sets on your muscles, and concluded that Loaded Passive Stretching (LPS) will fill your muscles with power! LPS is not your garden variety stretching. You are supposed to stretch the target muscle to the point of tolerable pain, and hold the stretch for 10 to 20 seconds after each set of a bodybuilding exercise. For example, after a set of benches, take a couple of light dumbbells and let them stretch your pecs in the fly position. Do not make an effort to either contract or relax your target muscles like you would for conventional or PNF stretches. For those unfamiliar with PNF stretches in simple terms, it involves the target muscle group being stretched to its maximum range of movement (ROM) at which point it is contracted strongly for at least six to eight seconds.

VA : How about cardio work?

PT : Fat loss is not your priority in the Foundation Diet, and aerobics would just distract your muscles from growing. Besides, high-volume weight training burns fat by sheer numbers and through natural stimulation of fat-mobilizing growth hormone.

VA : This type of laser-like focus makes perfect sense to me. All right, how about a sneak peak at the total program for athletes on the Bodybuilding Foundation Diet?

PT : I thought you'd never ask! Here it is. Follow my program or build your own based on the following principles:

The Bodybuilding Foundation Program

- Eight weeks long, two cycles of four weeks
- Follow one complex of exercises for four weeks, then switch to another
- Stay with the 20-rep breathing squats for the entire 8-week period
- Train with high volume; 30 to 150 reps per muscle group per workout
- Do not train to failure and stay away from high-intensity techniques such as forced reps or negatives
- Keep your repetitions in the eight-plus range
- Rest for up to one to three minutes between your sets
- Cycle your weights and reps
- Stretch for 10 to 20 seconds after each set with the LPS technique described previously
- Do minimal or no cardiovascular training

Split for Weeks One to Four

Split your body parts into two workouts, and alternate them:

Workout 1: legs, back, calves

Workout 2: chest, shoulders, arms, abs

There are many ways to arrange work and rest on this flexible classic split. For example, if your recovery ability seems above average, you could do six consecutive training sessions with Sunday as your off day:

Monday: Workout 1
Tuesday: Workout 2
Wednesday: Workout 1
Thursday: Workout 2
Friday: Workout 1
Saturday: Workout 2
Sunday: Off

A neat feature of this split is that if you skip a day or two, you can just easily fall back into the rotation:

Monday: Workout 1
Tuesday: Workout 2
Wednesday: Missed
Thursday: Workout 1
Friday: Workout 2
Saturday: Workout 1
Sunday: Off

Bodybuilders who need more recovery time could train two days on and one day off or perform each workout twice a week:

Monday: Workout 1
Tuesday: Workout 2
Wednesday: Off
Thursday: Workout 1
Friday: Workout 2
Saturday: Off
Sunday: Off

Older bodybuilders who don't recover as fast or anyone who prefers to train less frequently for some social or professional reason may want to hit the weights one day on and one day off or even work each body part three times every two weeks, as advised by Russian lifter and scientist Igor Sukhotsky:

Monday: Workout 1
Tuesday: Off
Wednesday: Workout 2

Thursday: Off
Friday: Workout 1
Saturday: Off
Sunday: Off
Monday: Workout 2
Tuesday: Off
Wednesday: Workout 1
Thursday: Off
Friday: Workout 2
Saturday: Off
Sunday: Off

Here are the recommended training programs:

WORKOUT 1: LEGS, BACK, CALVES

1. Breathing squats
2. One-arm dumbbell snatches
3. Calf raises in the leg-press machine
4. One-arm dumbbell rows

1. Breathing squats

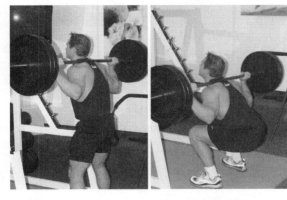

High-rep squats work magic on your legs and for overall mass, and the bodybuilding world owes the author of "Super Squats," Dr. Strossen, a big favor for reincarnating this classic program. To make gains with this simple, but not to be confused with easy, drill, all

you need is the most basic powerlifting style cycle. Breathing squats are actually just regular squats, although because of the high number of repetitions with the large muscles of the quadriceps, you will be breathing like mad!

Before you start the cycle, estimate your projected 20-rep max in the end of 8 weeks. Most bodybuilders should have no trouble knocking off 20 with their old 5RM after an intense 2 months' focus on the breathing squat. Start charting your squat cycle by figuring out how many squat workouts you are going to do in two months. If you decided to train each body part twice a week, you will have to survive 16 squat workouts. Round that number out to 15 to give yourself some slack for a skipped session.

Plan to add five pounds to your work set every session: 5 lbs x 15 workouts = 75 lbs.

Subtract this amount from your target weight, and you shall have your starting weight. Say, your best 5RM today is with 225 lbs. Your starting weight would be: 225 lbs – 75 lbs = 150 lbs. That is your target 20RM. Kick off your Foundation Phase with 20 reps at 150 lbs (150x20).

Do just one set of 20 reps. You are encouraged to follow up every set of your squats and snatches with a set of light pull-overs to open up your rib cage.

2. One-arm dumbbell snatches

The one-arm snatch was a key exercise in the Soviet Special Forces PT regimen, and is featured in my Russian Kettlebell Challenge video. American old timers like D. Willoughby

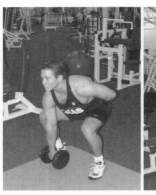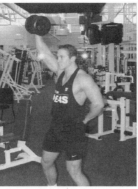

used to say that if you choose to do only exercise for your back, make it the one-arm dumbbell snatch or swing.

Stand in the ready-to-jump half-squat position with a dumbbell in one hand, and your arm hanging straight. With a powerful hip thrust, throw the weight overhead. Pause for a second, then let the weight nearly drop in front of you. Before the dumbbell hits the ground, swing it back up. Make sure your lifting falls in sync with your breathing. Keep your back reasonably straight, but do not lean back on the top; project your force straight up. Be forewarned: In addition to forging a rugged back and hamstrings, one-arm snatches may make you throw up your lung!

Here is how to set up your one-arm snatch cycle:

Start with a light dumbbell. A 30-lb dumbbell is enough for an intermediate male bodybuilder, half that will do for a lady. Of course, these are just rough guidelines. Use your judgment. Do a set of 12 reps, switch your arms, and immediately do another 12.

Stretch your back and hamstrings, and rest for one to three minutes. Take the next dumbbell off the rack and do another 12. Then another with five more pounds. Although Russian scientists frown upon pyramiding weight for pure strength training, anything goes during the mass quest. Keep working up until you feel that adding more weight would make you fight for survival or cheat.

Your first session may look like this: **30 lbs x 12 reps, 35 lbs x 12 reps, 40 lbs x 12 reps, 45 lbs x 12 reps, or 15 lbs x 12 reps, 20 lbs x 12 reps, 25 lbs x 12 reps**. This is plenty for starters, and you'll be convinced the morning after.

Next time do an unloading 60% tonnage workout. Follow the same sets and weights as before but do only eight reps: **30x8, 35x8, 40x8, 40x8, 40x8 or 15x8, 20x8, 25x8**. According to the Father of Periodization, Professor Matveyev, continuous variation of volume and intensity reduces the possibility of overtraining and amplifies the gains. The 60% rule is a standard for the light workout among Russian coaches.

Workout 3 will have you work up to a tough but not impossible set of 12 reps, again in 3 to 4 sets: **30x12, 35x12, 40x12, 45x12**.

Workout 4 uses the same principle with 8 reps: **30x8, 35x8, 40x8, 45x8**. Even if you could do 50x8, and I am sure you can, call it a day at the top weight of your previous session.

Keep repeating this pattern for two weeks. Work up to a near-maximal set of 12 in 3 to 4 sets, then do an unloading workout with the same sets and weights, but only 8 reps per set. This heavy-light format will keep your mind and muscles fresh, and will deliver greater gains than pushing pedal to the metal every workout.

For the final two weeks, increase the volume by adding back-off sets after reaching the top weight. You used to do 35x12, 40x12, 45x12, 50x12. Now you will suffer more with: **35x12, 40x12, 45x12, 50x12, 45x12, 40x12, 35x12**. Work down on your light days as well: **35x8, 40x8, 45x8, 50x8, 45x8, 40x8, 35x8**. You might ask if would not be better to gradually build up the volume for the duration of four weeks? The answer is no. Russian experts insist that a discreet jump in training load is superior to a slow buildup, at least in experienced athletes. A load spike just shocks your muscles into adaptation!

3. Calf raises in the leg-press machine

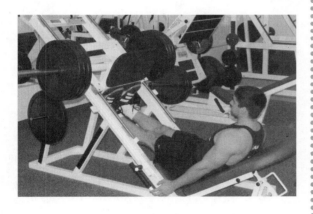

The hip sled is our choice piece of equipment for calf training, because your "diamonds" can handle a lot more weight than your back.

Use the same 100-60% loading format as with your snatches, but triple the reps: for sets of 12 do 36 and for sets of 8 do 24. Because of a shorter range of motion, your calves need more reps to get the same time under tension.

Do not forget to add back-off sets halfway into the phase. Reduce the rest periods on the down side of the pyramid almost to the point of doing a drop set. Top experts like Sorokin and Vorobyev, who would hear nothing of drop sets for weightlifters, readily endorse this technique for bodybuilding.

4. One-arm dumbbell rows

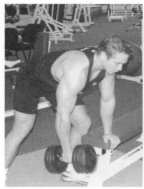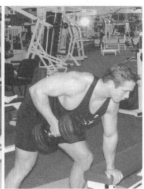

You may substitute this drill with a chest-supported two-arm row on a machine, but do not do anything that would stress your lower back. After squats and snatches, your back will be toast!

Exercises for smaller muscle groups or fewer muscles such as one-arm rows always gain a lot slower than your legs and lower back. This is why we need to resort to more sophisticated programming: 100-60-80. That means adding a day of 10 reps to the format you have used for snatches. An interesting wrinkle borrowed from strength coach extraordinaire Bill Starr is to finish your medium day—10 reps in our case—with the weight you are planning to use for your top weight on your next heavy day. For example:

Workout 1: 30 lbs x12 reps, 35 lbs x12 reps, 40 lbs x12 reps

Workout 2: 30x8, 35x8, 40x8

Workout 3: 30x10, 40x10, 45x10

Workout 4: 30x12, 40x12, 45x12
Workout 5: 30x8, 40x8, 45x8
Workout 6: 30x10, 40x10, 50x10

If you doubt that you will be able to better your PR (personal record) on your next heavy day, stay with the same weight:

Workout 6: 30x10, 40x10, 45x10, rather than 50x10

As with the previous drills, add back-off sets after two weeks, for example 30x12, 40x12, 50x12, 40x12, and 30x12. Take as little rest between your back-off sets as possible as long you can make your reps in good form. Enjoy that pump!

WORKOUT 2: CHEST, SHOULDERS, ARMS, ABS

1. Dumbbell military presses
2. Incline alternate dumbbell curls
3. Dumbbell bench presses
4. Seated top half barbell curls
5. Floor dumbbell triceps extensions
5. Weighted crunches

The 12-8-10-rep strategy, with back-off drop sets thrown in after 2 weeks, will serve you well on all of the exercises in this workout. Here is a sample cycle:

Workout 1: 30 lbs x 12 reps, 35 lbs x 12 reps, 40 lbs x 12 reps
Workout 2: 30x8, 35x8, 40x8
Workout 3: 30x10, 40x10, 45x10
Workout 4: 30x12, 40x12, 45x12
Workout 5: 30x8, 40x8, 45x8
Workout 6: 30x10, 40x10, 50x10
Workout 7: 30x12, 40x12, 50x12, 40x12, 30x12

Workout 8: 30x8, 40x8, 50x8, 40x8, 30x8
Workout 9: 35x10, 45x10, 55x10, 45x10, 32x10
Workout 10: 35x12, 45x12, 55x12, 45x12, 35x12
Workout 11: 35x8, 45x8, 55x8, 45x8, 35x8
Workout 12: 40x10, 50x10, 60x10, 50x10, 40x10

1. Dumbbell military presses

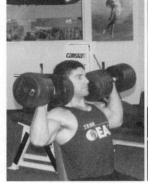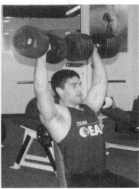

To work your delts effectively, keep your shoulders pressed down with your lats, an old trick of legendary Steve Reeves. Also let the dumbbells travel outward rather than straight up. If your back is giving you trouble, you are probably not keeping your abs and glutes tight enough. Flexing these muscles during overhead presses is an old weightlifter trick; use it!

2. Incline alternate dumbbell curls

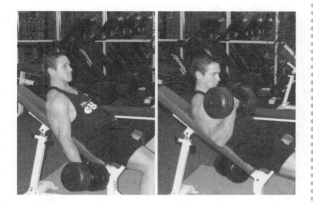

Sit on an incline bench steep enough to stretch your guns, but not enough to tear them. Squeeze your dumbbells for greater power and safety. Supinate or rotate your palm toward the ceiling as you are coming up.

3. Dumbbell bench presses

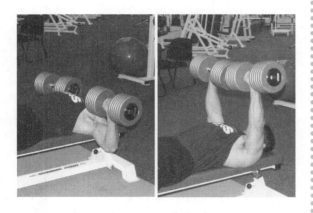

Let the dumbbells drift out into a semi-fly position to load your chest rather than your triceps.

Do not put your feet up on the bench! This supposed back safety measure will make you dangerously unstable, and reduce the pec stress by sinking your rib cage. Do not relax at the lowest point of the press as you could mess up your shoulders.

4. Seated top half barbell curls

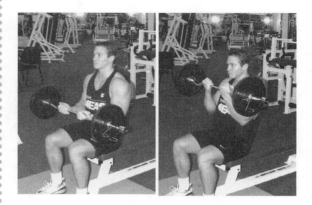

This old-time drill will put meat on your biceps in a hurry! Sit on a bench with your knees close together, and perform barbell curls with a straight or EZ curl bar. Your legs will chop the possible range of motion in half, which will enable you to use much heavier weights for superior gains.

5. Floor dumbbell triceps extensions

Lie on the floor and have your partner hand you over two dumbbells. With your elbows pointing to the ceiling and your forearms and the dumbbells parallel, lower them to the floor behind your head, and then muscle them back up. Squeeze your triceps hard on the top, and do not relax them on the bottom.

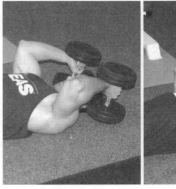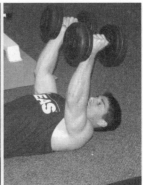

6. Weighted crunches

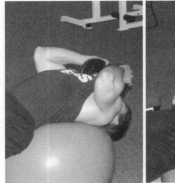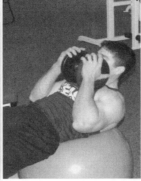

This one is pretty obvious, isn't it? Do not be afraid to use some serious weight. Your abs are muscles too.

Split for Weeks Five to Eight

You should have made great gains for the first two weeks on the Foundation Program. Now it is time to break things up to enjoy continued progress. A different workout arrangement always spurs new growth. This time split your body parts into a three-way split that allows maximum tonnage to be lifted:

Workout 1: legs, shoulders, abs and calves
Workout 2: chest and back
Workout 3: arms

The 12-8-10-rep strategy with back-off drop sets added after 2 weeks will serve you well on all of the exercises in this workout except for the breathing squat. Here is your new workout:

WORKOUT 1: LEGS, SHOULDERS, ABS AND CALVES

1. Breathing squats
2. Shrugs

3. Lateral raises
4. Calf raises in the leg-press machine, one leg at a time
5. Kneeling cable crunches

1. Breathing squats

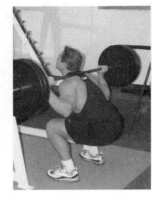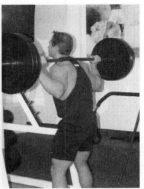

The squat is here to stay! By now you should be handling some respectable weight. Stick to the basic linear cycle.

2. Shrugs

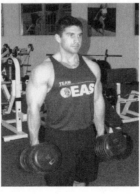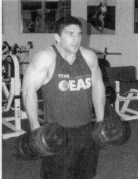

Shrug with a barbell or dumbbells, and do not relax on the bottom of the movement. It is OK to use straps.

3. Lateral raises

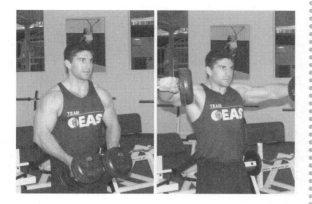

Do not shrug your shoulders up! Zero in on your delts with minimal joint stress. Instead of focusing on lifting the dumbbells, think of reaching your arms out as wide as possible as if pushing the walls apart. This little-known martial arts technique will make all the difference between strained and built shoulders.

4. Calf raises in the leg-press machine, one leg at a time

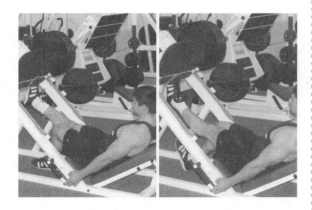

Thanks to something called "a bilateral strength deficit," you will be able to overload your calves more intensely when you work them individually. Upgrade the 100-60 program to 100-60-80, and use repetitions of 24, 16, and 20.

5. Kneeling cable crunches

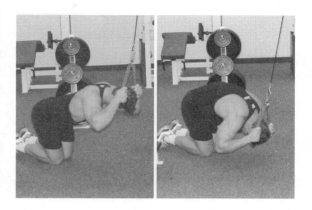

You can choose another ab drill. Personally, I am biased against crunches.

WORKOUT 2: CHEST AND BACK

1. Wide-grip bench presses
2. Decline flyes
3. Lat pull-downs
4. Nautilus pull-overs
5. Slightly bent-over rows

1. Wide-grip bench presses

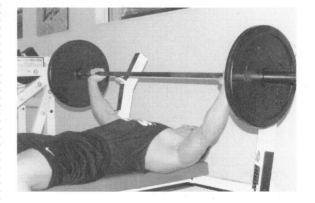

Use the maximum legal grip for powerlifting—your index fingers should be touching the outside of the rings on the bar.

Experiment with your hand position to minimize the stress on your wrists. Keep your chest high and your shoulders down. Press your feet into the floor. And remember that the barbell is not a basketball; do not bounce!

2. Decline flyes

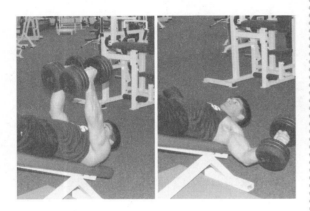

Keep your elbows slightly bent to protect them. Force your chest out for a good stretch and solid biomechanics.

3. Lat pull-downs

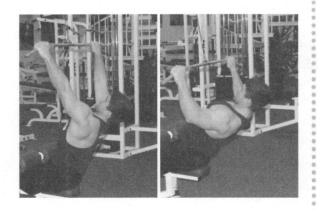

Pull the bar toward your breastbone, and arch your back in the contracted position. Visualize touching your elbows together behind your back. You will do a better job of overloading your lats if you use a palms-for-

ward thumbless grip. Weighted pull-ups are a better choice if you can do them. The Gravitron® machine is all right if you cannot.

4. Pullovers

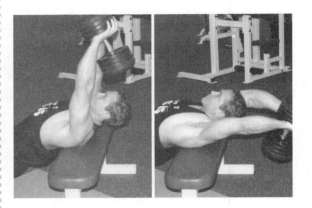

This is a rare machine that delivers. You can do dumbbell pullovers if this machine is not available. Do not let your elbows flare out, and keep your arms and forearms parallel to spare your shoulder joints. Think of pulling with your armpits rather than your arms.

5. Slightly bent-over row

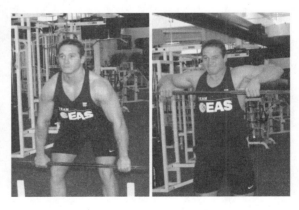

This hybrid of the bent-over and the upright row is awesome for your lateral and posterior deltoids. "Push the walls apart" with your elbows rather than curl them, and shrug the barbell or dumbbells. Do not strive for a great range of motion. If your shoulders start shrugging up, you are no longer doing a great deltoid exercise—just a poor trap movement.

WORKOUT 3: ARMS

1. Triceps pushdowns
2. Barbell curls
3. EZ bar French presses
4. Reverse barbell curls

1. Triceps pushdowns

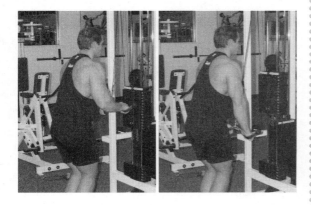

For ideal biomechanics, keep the pressure on the meaty base of your palm, straight below your little finger. Do not let your shoulders shrug up, and keep your lats contracted.

2. Barbell curls

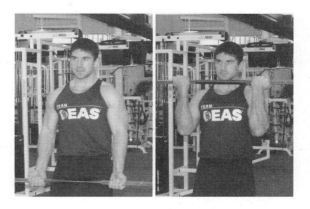

Keep your abs tight to protect your lower back, and grip the barbell wider than your shoulders if you are using a straight bar. It is easier on your joints.

3. EZ bar French presses

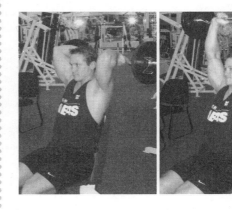

Use the narrow grip on the EZ bar. Put up the weight overhead, and then slowly lower it behind your head. Be careful not to relax in the stretched position as it may be too much for your triceps tendons. Muscle the barbell back up without an excessive elbow flare.

4. Reverse barbell curls

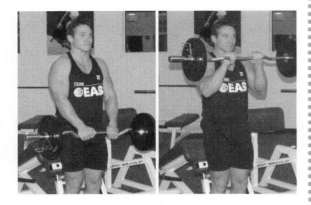

Watch your thumbs, and do not forget to squeeze the bar.

The Muscularity Training Phase

Vince Andrich: For many of our readers, training for muscularity is one of the most difficult areas to understand. That's because it takes an overall knowledge of how the body responds to stresses from training in conjunction to somewhat rigorous nutritional changes. In this section, our resident training expert Pavel Tsatsouline and I discuss the most effective training methods for athletes who are following the dietary recommendations in the Muscularity Diet.

PT: First of all, I want to let our readers know that even though the dietary modifications on the Muscularity Diet (which I believe are very solid) cut your calories back a bit, you still may end up gaining a bit of lean mass during the program. This is achievable because we are going to employ very radical training techniques in this phase.

VA: Well I'm sure our readers who have heard this before are saying "show me what you got!" But really, how long is the training program on the Muscularity Phase, and why is it so effective?

PT: The Muscularity Training Phase is six weeks long and employs a variety of exercises that hit your muscles from all angles. This is a standard bodybuilding practice during the cutting-up period of training, however, what makes the Muscularity Phase unique is the use of four to seven reps.

VA: OK, since I've already heard your rationale behind using sets in the four-to-seven-rep range (and happen to think it's brilliant), why don't you tell our readers.

PT: Our radical choice has two reasons behind it. First, doing a lot of reps in combination with the moderate-carb Muscularity Diet would deplete your glycogen stores. As a result, your muscles would look flat and your recovery would be severely compromised. Medium-rep power bodybuilding, although it drains your mind, does not impose unreasonable demands on your muscle energetics. Therefore it belongs in the Muscularity Training Phase. Second, low-rep heavier training forces greater tension on your muscle. One of the aspects of traffic-stopping definition is muscle tone. *And tone is nothing more than resting tension in a relaxed muscle.* The only way to improve your tone is through high-tension training. This is one of the reasons why we have made the revolutionary choice of training every exercise, even lat raises and ab drills, with heavy weights and reps in the four-to-seven range. Besides, power bodybuilding with heavier weights and greater rest periods increases your muscle density—the third reason for our madness. While higher repetitions and volume encourage the growth of many things in the muscle—mitochondria, capillaries, and sarcoplasm—only heavy training promotes noticeable hypertrophy of the myofibrils or the contractile proteins. The end result is a dense and rugged look that all bodybuilders seek and so few ever achieve. Powerlifting champions Arnold Schwarzenegger and Franco Columbo did not come to rule the Olympia by accident. Like everyone else, they did the high-rep work to fill out their guns, but they never forgot that only heavy training overcomes the soft pumped-up look. Our Muscularity Phase workout is YOUR ticket to the hard look.

VA: You have some other interesting observations that athletes should be in tune with before they embark on this training phase. Can you elaborate?

PT: Certainly, as I stated when we first spoke, one of the key concepts regarding power bodybuilding with heavier weights is that you must maintain a noticeable amount of volume; around 50 reps per body part. Many athletes here in the States never read about this in popular bodybuilding media. This is the major flaw in most high-tension programs, because according to the energetic theory of muscle hypertrophy, high tonnage combined with heavy weights delivers the goods.

Another problem with programs that advocate heavier weights is that they do not take into consideration the added stress of training to absolute muscle failure. Training with heavy weights combined with "absolute failure" should be avoided until the last week of the cycle, especially in a low-calorie/low-carbohydrate environment. Our program also employs rest periods of around three to five minutes, which is a better recovery model for the diet at hand. What I do recommend for added "intensity" in this phase is compensatory acceleration training on compound exercises like squats and benches. This is where you lower your weights under control, and then lift them explosively. This "dynamic effort method," excellent for recruiting your fast-twitch fibers, belongs in the Muscularity Training Phase. Besides, Russian research in the mid '70s showed that varying your weight-training tempo over a period of time delivered greater gains than lifting with any one cadence. You have mostly employed the moderate cadence in the Bodybuilding Foundation Phase. Now it's time to try something new!

VA: I am not sure that all of our readers are familiar with compensatory acceleration training techniques (called CAT for short). From my experience, a good analogy for this method of training is that of a sprinter trying to better his or her time in the 100 meters. To accomplish a better time, the sprinter must attempt to "condense" his or her start-to-finish time in the event. In other words, no amount of submaximal 100-meter runs will train his or her musculoskeletal system to deliver a better overall time. In weight training, this simply means that each rep is an all-out attempt to condense the time the load goes from point A to B, which in itself is like training each rep, not each set, to failure.

PT: Precisely. In addition to CAT techniques, the Muscularity Training Phase is the time to double your stretching efforts between sets. In the Bodybuilding Foundation Phase you stretched once, right after each set.

The Russian study I have referred to earlier has concluded that adding another stretching set, a minute before the next set, will amplify the gains even more. Squeezing in another set into the short rest periods of the last phase was tough. Not any more because in this phase you will lift, then immediately stretch, then rest enough to stretch once more about a minute before you lift again. It sounds complicated, but it is simply one stretch set after the lifting set and one stretch set one minute before the next lifting set.

As a part of the total Muscularity package, you are also encouraged to add brief high-intensity interval cardiovascular training to your program. These interval cardio sessions need only to last about 15-20 minutes and are meant to ramp up you metabolic rate and not have you laboriously trying to burn calories by merely trying to outpace the hours on the clock. Be careful not to overdo it though; you do not want to lose your hard-earned muscle!

VA: Basically, we're engineering one hell of a fat-burning and muscle-building machine—so what does the Muscularity Training Phase look like on paper?

PT: Here's a review of our previous notes, plus details on splits and exercises:

The Muscularity Training Phase

• Six weeks long

• Train in the four-to-seven-rep range
• Do around 50 total reps per body part
• Rest for three to five minutes between your sets
• Use compound and isolation exercises but stick to low reps even for your abs and calves
• Add another set of Loaded Passive Stretching (LPS) between the sets
• Feel free to use compensatory acceleration in compound exercises
• Do high-intensity interval training to facilitate fat loss

Workout 1: chest, biceps
Workout 2: legs, calves
Workout 3: abs, forearms
Workout 4: shoulders, triceps
Workout 5: back

Please note that because you are about to use a greater number of exercises per muscle group than in the Foundation Phase, you need to split your workout in the following manner. Here is an example:

Monday: Workout 1
Tuesday: Workout 2
Wednesday: Workout 3
Thursday: Workout 4
Friday: Workout 5
Saturday: Off
Sunday: Off

WORKOUT 1: CHEST, BICEPS

1. Moderate-grip bench presses
2. One-and-a-half wide-grip bench presses
3. Arm-wrestler's curls
4. Table curls

1. Moderate-grip bench presses

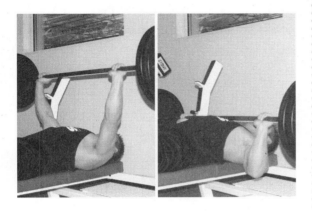

Nothing fancy, just your good old basic bench press. And don't forget to keep your feet off the bench! The reliable 5x5 format from the arsenal of Arnold's hero Reg Park is what the doctor ordered. Start by doing five explosive reps with a weight you think you could handle for seven repetitions or so. Rest for whole five minutes. Extra recovery between the sets is a critical component of the Muscularity Training Phase, because it allows you to generate more tension and therefore more strength and cuts. So for this phase, time your rest periods!

Loading Parameters

Do five sets with the same weight. This exercise will take you 25 minutes, but trust me it is worth it.

Next week add five to ten pounds and repeat the sequence. Do not get bummed out if you do not get all the fives. Just do as many reps as you can in good form, with no forced reps, **and** stay with the weight until you make it. For instance, one week you will do 225x5, 225x5, 225x4, 225x4, and 225x3, then 225x5, 225x5, 225x5, 225x5, and 225x4.

Conquer the two plates on the third week: 225x5, 225x5, 225x5, 225x5, and 225x5.

The fourth week you can jump to 230 lbs.

The above cycle will reward you with chiseled pecs and attention-getting bench power!

2. One-and-a-half wide-grip bench presses

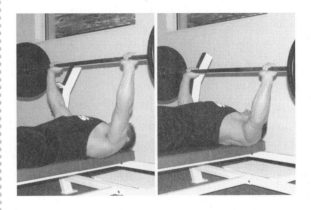

This secret powerlifting exercise is second-to-none in building up the pecs and developing unstoppable power off your chest. Take the bar right outside the power rings, and lower it slowly to your chest. Pause for at least a second while staying tight, then slowly squeeze the barbell off your chest and lift if halfway up with precise technique. Lower the bar back to your pecs, and after another pause, explode it to lockout.

Loading Parameters

Do four sets of four reps with four minutes of rest in between. Start light, and work up to your best set of four. For example, 135x4, 185x4, 195x4, and 200x4.

3. Arm-wrestler's curls

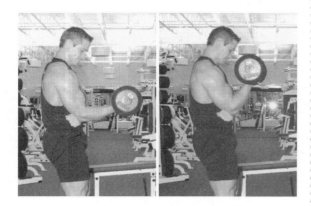

The arm-wrestling curl is a dynamite exercise that will make your guns grow in front of your eyes. It is performed with a dumbbell, one arm at a time. Place your non-working forearm under the elbow of your working arm, between the elbow and your rib cage. Swing a heavy dumbbell to the top of the curl, and then perform partial curls. Lower the weight no further than what arm benders call "the elbow lock" or to the spot slightly above parallel where you will feel very strong. Do not be afraid to use a quick cadence. Make sure to keep your abs super tight to protect your lower back. Help yourself with your other arm to lower the weight when you are done.

Loading Parameters

Start light, with a dumbbell you could full curl five times or so, and work up the rack in sets of seven: 35x7, 40x7, 45x7, 50x7, and 55x7, then work back down in the same fashion: 50x7, 45x7, 40x7, and 35x7.

Alternate your arms naturally. You should not rest much between your sets of the arm-wrestling curl. Use your gut feeling.

For the first three weeks, train with sevens, switch to fives for weeks four and five, and come back to sevens for the sixth week of the phase.

Stretching is important for every exercise of the Muscularity Phase, but for the AW curl it is critical! Just hold the dumbbell you have curled with a palm-up grip, and let it stretch out your arm.

4. Table curls

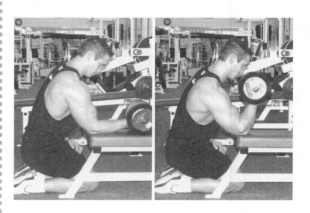

The table curl just may have been invented in one of those Harley Davidson biker bars in which cops are afraid to show their faces. Arm wrestlers use a table; a bodybuilder will find a padded bench handier. Set a dumbbell across a bench, and sit or kneel on the floor facing it. Place your elbow on the padded surface and grip the dumbbell with the usual curl grip. Inhale, tighten your lat, and squeeze the dumbbell off the bench. That is the hard, result-producing part. Once you have reached the point where your forearm is vertical, head back to the bench. Totally relax before the next rep to get the max effect from the tough start.

WORKOUT 2: LEGS AND CALVES

1. Front squats
2. Romanian deadlifts
3. Plate drags
4. Negative accentuated calf raises in a leg-press machine

1. Front squats

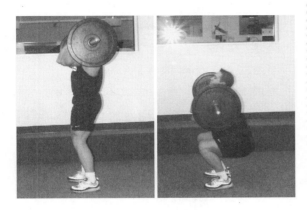

Front squats, especially if your technique and joints allow you to go rock bottom, are awesome for cutting up your thighs and developing the much sought-after tear-drop vastus medialis.

Loading Parameters

Follow the 5x5 program, just like the bench press.

2. Romanian deadlifts

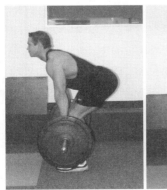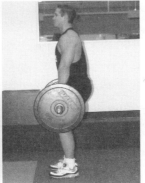

By now scientists have settled the dispute: Yes, Romanian deadlifts work your hamstrings much more intensely than leg curls! Besides, nothing will define your glutes better than this Eastern European import. Deadlift a relatively light barbell, then stick your butt out while keeping a tight arch in your back. Keep your weight on your heels. Let the barbell descend along your shins, which should be vertical, until you feel that you are about to lose your arch, slightly below the knee for most bodybuilders. Then squeeze your glutes and lift the weight back to the lockout in a crisp motion. Do all your reps without setting the bar down.

Loading Parameters

Again, 5x5 is the program of choice. If you wish, you may alternate front squats (FSQ's) and Romanian Deadlifts (RDL's), but not in a superset fashion. FSQ-2min-RDL-2min, and so on.

3. Plate drags

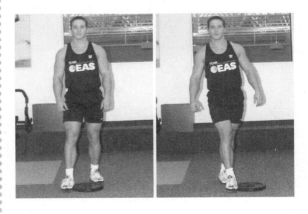

This weird drill from the arsenal of Eastern European track and field athletes cannot be beat for defining your inner and outer thighs! Stand in front of a barbell plate, and push it from side to side with the inside and then the outside of your foot. Keep the muscles around your knee tight. Feel free to hold on to the power rack for balance. Because the drill is missing the eccentric component, it does not build muscle, but just tones and strengthens it; just what the doctor ordered for your hip adductors and abductors!

Loading Parameters

Work up from a light to heavy weight in sets of seven, with a moderate amount of rest between the sets. Pile small plates on top of the big one.

For the first three weeks train with sevens, switch to fives for weeks four and five, and come back to sevens for the sixth week of the phase.

4. Negative accentuated calf raises in a leg-press machine

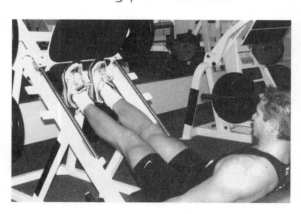

Lift the weight with two feet, and lower it slowly on one. This intense technique will jar your calves into new growth, and carve a few more striations.

Loading Parameters

Do 6 reps per foot, which is 12 per set.

Work up to a heavy set and then work back down.

Switch to sets of four per foot or eight per set after three weeks.

WORKOUT 3: ABS AND FOREARMS

1. Janda sit-ups
2. One-arm deadlift lockouts
3. EZ bar wrist curls
4. EZ bar reverse wrist curls
*Follow the 5x5 format for all these exercises

1. Janda sit-ups

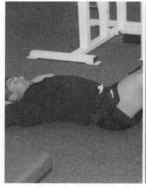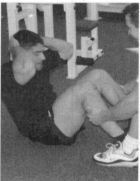

This exercise, devised by Eastern European back rehab expert Vladimir Janda, just might be the most effective abdominal exercise in the world!

Assume the standard bent-knee sit-up/crunch position with your knees at a 90-degree angle. Have your partner place his or her hands underneath your calves, just the opposite of regular sit-ups. Your partner should give you about 15 lbs of steady pressure, as if trying to drag you across the floor.

Make sure that your partner only pulls back and does not help you keep your feet down in any manner; that is your job!

Inhale, squeeze your glutes tight, and slowly sit up all the way while pulling against your partner. Relax, flex your glutes again, and head back down. You will go nowhere if you relax your glutes. Do not be surprised if you can only do negatives; Janda sit-ups are very tough. I once challenged the studly audience at the Arnold Classic, where I gave an abdominal training seminar, to try to do five Janda sit-ups. A full-of-muscle volunteer barely finished two!

Loading Parameters

Do negatives if you cannot get up. Feel those abs like never before!

2. One-arm deadlift lockouts

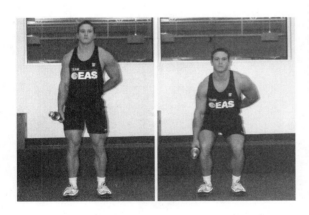

Powerlifting legend Ed Coan does these to strengthen his grip, but one-arm deadlifts are just as effective for tightening up those obliques. Lift a long bar from like a suitcase knee level in a power rack, without bending sideways. Pause, park, and repeat on both sides.

3. EZ bar wrist curls

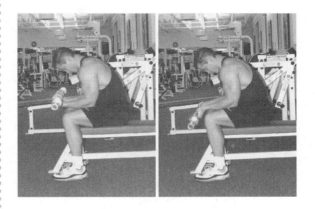

Place your forearms on the bench or your thighs, and go for it!

4. EZ bar reverse wrist curls

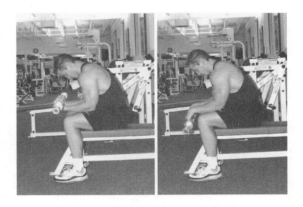

Alternate—don't superset—these with the regular wrist curls. Don't forget to watch those thumbs.

WORKOUT 4: SHOULDERS, TRICEPS

1. Military presses
2. One-arm lateral raises
3. Overhead barbell triceps extensions
4. Reverse-grip bench presses
*Follow the 5x5 format for all these exercises

1. Military presses

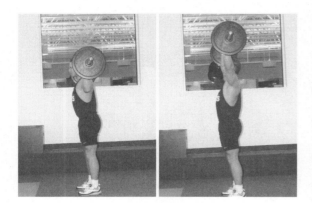

Clean the barbell or take it off the rack. Be certain to keep your abs and lower body tight.

2. One-arm lateral raises

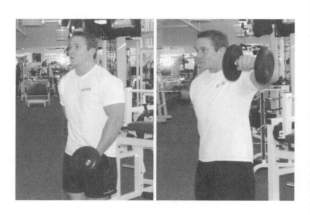

This is one of the favorite deltoid moves of legendary bench presser Pat Casey. Keep your shoulder down and feel free to hold on to the power rack for balance.

3. Overhead barbell triceps extensions

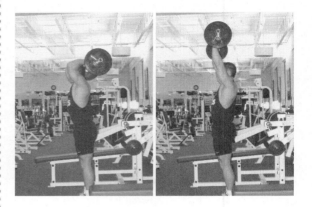

This is a favorite exercise of another world bench press record holder, Mike McDonald of Duluth, Minnesota. Military press the barbell overhead with a close grip, then lower the bar to the top of your head while flaring your elbows comfortably.

4. Reverse-grip bench presses

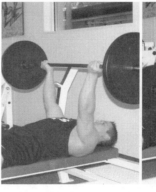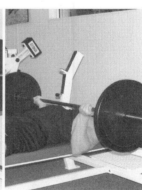

Bench with a curl grip, and you will be amazed how your lateral triceps head, the most visible part of the horseshoe, will stand out in bold relief! Research shows that you must train your triceps heavy if you want to hit all three heads!

WORKOUT 5: BACK

1. Pull-ups
2. Explosive shrugs
3. Back hyperextensions

*Follow the 5x5 format for all these exercises

1. Pull-ups

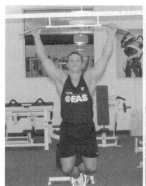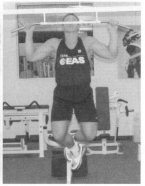

Grip the bar with a thumbless grip to emphasize your lats rather than your biceps. Follow the 5x5 format with extra weight, or do pull-downs if you cannot pull your weight yet.

2. Explosive shrugs

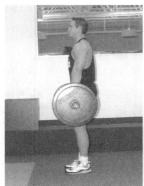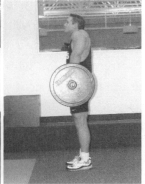

Give the bar a kick with your hips, but do not pull with your arms.

3. Back hyperextensions

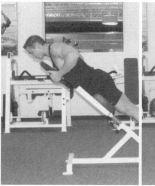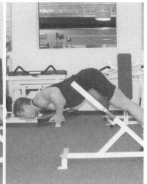

This is a favorite exercise of Russian weightlifters. Do not forget to hold a plate on your chest.

Muscularity Training Phase—Notes

Since low-rep, high-tension training combined with isolation drills like curls is a total surprise to your body, expect new growth in spite of reduced caloric intake. You will be so impressed with the results from this program that you will be tempted to repeat the cycle. If you decide to do this training phase again, go for it, just re-arrange the exercises. If not, proceed to the Maximum Muscularity Phase.

The Maximum Muscularity Training Phase

So far we have pretty much gone against the grain on nearly every key topic mainstream bodybuilding publications and authors have promoted over the years. I know from my perspective, Pavel's insights have brought much-needed clarity to the "big picture" of diet and exercise. The next section is probably the most critical, because we attempt to optimize one of the most widely used means for getting lean—the high-protein, low-carbohydrate diet.

Vince Andrich: Pavel, many athletes have struggled when faced with the many variables associated with achieving maximum muscularity. What are your initial thoughts on this topic—especially in conjunction with a reduced carbohydrate intake?

Pavel Tsatsouline: Well, as you know many athletes are using a high-protein, low-carbohydrate diet to get leaner. This is a good strategy if indeed there is method to your madness. I would like to say that your Maximum Muscularity Diet recommendations incorporate two very key elements, which are carbohydrate timing and the overall length of each phase. These two points are critical and should eliminate many of the problems that athletes may encounter when following this type of diet. Having these two factors in line allows me to fully exploit the diet with thermonuclear training tools, which cannot be maintained longer than your four-week plan.

VA: What is the European outlook on maintaining peak condition?

PT: Russian scientists warn that attempting to maintain peak condition may be detrimental to your future progress! This phenomenon was observed by Soviet scientists who realized high-caliber athletes who use intense training and diet interventions enjoy quick but fleeting gains. Doggedly attempting to maintain the peak condition just dooms the bodybuilder to failure, something powerlifters learned the hard way three decades ago. This is another reason why most of the time, volume rules over intensity.

VA: Things obviously change when an athlete is engaged in a low-carbohydrate diet phase, right?

PT: Absolutely. Because the carbs and the calories are way down, we are cutting the volume and the reps even more. You are about to train with singles, double, and triples!

VA: A common method for getting lean that has been popular with many bodybuilding experts over the years is diet plus high reps, volume, and as much aerobics as your mind can handle. I think this is where your expertise really shines, because your methods are almost totally contradictory. What is the rationale behind your Maximum Muscularity Training Phase?

PT: I know our readers first reaction to our Maximum Muscularity program will be "What the...?! Aren't you supposed to cut up your muscles with ultra-high reps and super 'burn'?" To that I give an emphatic "No, Comrade!" The "burn" you feel from high reps is from lactic acid buildup and does absolutely nothing for toning up your muscles. Pick up a copy of The Guinness Book of World Records, and look up the picture of Captain America, who holds the world record of the most consecutive sit-ups. It's in the ballpark of 25,000! This guy must have "felt the burn" more than anyone else on this planet, and he does not even have a six-pack to show for it, even at his low level of bodyfat. Let me further explain: The reason you feel hard during and after the "burn" is the same reason a corpse is stiff. Your muscle fibers are like mouse traps—they go off by themselves, but need energy to be reset to contract again. A dead body is out of ATP, the energy compound that relaxes the muscles. A "stiff's" muscles are permanently contracted. A high-rep workout exhausts ATP in your muscle and leads to temporary hardness, unlike the rigor mortis! The only way to make such "tone" last is by killing yourself.

VA: Then what is "real" muscle tone and how do you get it?

PT: Real tone is residual tension in a relaxed muscle. The kind of tension that comes from intense muscle contractions, and not energy exhaustion. Strength = tension = tone. It is that simple. Power and definition training is the same thing. Millions of women these days ask "Why am I having trouble getting buns of steel?" The answer is that our glutes have tremendous strength and leverage. When you see a powerlifter squat or deadlift bar-bending weight, their glutes carry the brunt of that multi-hundred pound load! When you do butt squeezes, "fire hydrants," or similar silly moves popular in "muscle sculpting" classes, you do not even come close to tapping the force/tension potential of your body's strongest muscles. You'd better get on a first-name basis with heavy deads if you are after a hard butt!

"Why can't I define my triceps to save my life?" wonder men and women alike. An obscure study done in the early '60s discovered that although the triceps is a "three-headed" muscle, the brunt of the work is performed by its medial head. The other two heads, the long and the lateral, kick in only when the resistance is very high. Research shows that even some powerlifters do not approach the weights needed to recruit the two lazy triceps heads in their training! The most visible part of your triceps is the lateral head on the outside of your arm. It is one of the "bum" pair, and it will remain forever flat and saggy if you keep lifting Ken and Barbie weights! Bottom line: You want to be ripped? Then you need to train heavy!

VA: OK, I know our readers probably want to ask why bodybuilders are more "cut" than powerlifters, and since they look more defined and seem to train with lighter weights than powerlifters, are we missing something?

PT: No. The public stereotype of a weightlifter or powerlifter is that of a 300-lb guy with a beer gut. The lifters in the unlimited class indeed fit this image, because they benefit from the extra weight, even fat. It is much easier to come out of a squat if you have a huge belly and thick calves to bounce off! So these men's rock-hard muscles are buried under slabs of fat. Lighter lifters, on the other hand, tend to be very lean to make the most efficient use of the weight allowed by their class. Check out the anatomy-chart physique of 198-lb Russian Olympic weightlifting legend David Rigert, or the hard body of a petite 123-lb Mary Jeffrey, who bench pressed a whopping world record of 275 lbs! Ironically, these athletes' mind-boggling muscle definition is a side effect, rather than the result, of their training.

Since you are a bodybuilder, and not a lifter, and your appearance is of greater importance than your bench press, you can amplify the muscle-defining effect of heavy-power training by diversifying the limited power arsenal of squats, benches, and deadlifts. Who said that curls or bent-over deltoid raises are not meant to be done for singles? I say question the dogma and succeed.

VA: Well, where do we start?

PT: The standard training protocol in the Maximum Muscularity Training Phase is working up to a heavy, but not impossible, set of one, two, or three reps. For example, a 250-lb bench presser might do 185x3, 205x3, 225x2, 235x1, and 240x1. There is no need to max! Just work up to the heaviest weight you can lift comfortably, without psyching up and doubting the outcome. This is what Eastern European weightlifters call "the training max." Working with training max singles (Tmax singles) is not only safer and more enjoyable than attempting real maxes, but also more effective because it does not burn out your nervous system. Worrying about making a limit attempt spikes your stress hormones, which is a raw deal for the bodybuilder!

To maximize the cut-producing tension, and to limit the drain on the muscle power, we will restrict the volume to 10 to 20 lifts per muscle group per workout. Rest enough between the sets to ensure that the poundage does not suffer. No need for a stopwatch; rest less on lighter sets, and more as you approach the top set. Do not strive to achieve pump; it is does not jibe with a low-carb/low-rep program. And don't forget to stretch between your sets!

VA: Does the rep or volume scheme vary at all during the course of the entire Maximum Muscularity Training Phase?

PT: We take a different approach to small-scale periodization in the Maximum Muscularity Training Phase. We vary the volume by repeating the sequence of working up from a light to a heavy weight or "wave" once, twice, or three times. For the bodybuilder with a 250-lb bench press, three waves may look like this:

Wave 1: 185 lbs x 3 reps, 205 lbs x 3 reps, 225 lbs x 2 reps, 235 lbs x 1 rep, 240 lbs x 1 rep

Wave 2: 205x2, 215x2, 225x2, 235x1, 240x1, 245x1

Wave 3: 205x1, 220x1, 230x1, 235x1

It is OK to stagger your heavy, light, and medium days. For instance, in one workout you could do three waves for your pecs, one for your triceps, and two for your biceps.

On one hand, we need to do a variety of exercises to bring out every striation. On the other hand, we have to work each muscle quite frequently because low volume combined with low reps might lead to a loss of muscle mass. The solution is a powerful three-on and one-off split used by seven-time Mr. Olympia Lee Haney:

Day 1: chest, biceps, triceps
Day 2: legs, calves, abs
Day 3: back, shoulders
Day 4: off

If you do not like a split that does not follow a week, you can do this:

Monday: chest, biceps, triceps
Tuesday: legs, calves, abs
Wednesday: back, shoulders
Thursday: chest, biceps, triceps
Friday: legs, calves, abs
Saturday: back, shoulders
Sunday: off

VA: Is there any special rationale for these body part splits?

PT: Yes. We have picked this championship arrangement over the conventional push/pull split for two reasons. First, it spares your shoulder joints by splitting pec and delt work. Second, you will make greater gains by training your shoulders fresh rather than as a chest chaser. And third, it enables you to blast your biceps, not fatigued by previous lat work, with great intensity.

VA: Posing or constant flexing each body part was a big part of the dieting-down process when I competed. This technique did seem to have a great impact on muscle control and definition. What are your thoughts?

PT: Recall that tension is what makes you ripped! Which is why you should make posing an integral part of your training. Even if you are not a competitive bodybuilder, do it anyway. Constant flexing is the prescription for unreal definition. Cramp and pose at every opportunity! A special Power Breathing technique can also help you achieve the greatest intensity of contraction, especially in your abs.

VA: And what is Power Breathing?

PT: Power Breathing and isometrics actually go hand in hand. Here is an example: Inhale and contract your abs while keeping your glottis closed and your rectal sphincter contracted. Expel your air forcefully in three to five seconds while keeping your tongue pressed against your teeth, and making the "ts" sound. Isometrics or pushing against unmovable objects is another great muscle definer that has been unjustly forgotten. Bruce Lee owed his unbelievable ripples to isometric strength training. Just push or pull while imitating some bodybuilding exercise or making up a new one. Take a normal breath and gradually, over a period of three seconds or so, build up the tension to the max. Stay there for another three seconds and relax. Do not hold your breath. Power breathe or simply breathe shallow. You may incorporate posing and isometrics into your workouts or, better yet, perform them throughout the day whenever you have a private moment.

Perform your lifts also in a nearly isometric "dynamic tension" fashion. Keep all of your muscles, especially your core and your grip, super tight. Squeeze your weights off the starting position, and grind them through to completion. Expect to instantly boost your strength by 30 to 50% while maximizing your training safety.

VA: What about cardio training while on the Maximum Muscularity Diet?

PT: Even though the purpose of the Maximum Muscularity Training Phase is ultimate definition, we advise you to limit your cardio to walking. Interval training and high-intensity aerobics could destroy your muscle mass in this very low-carb/low-calorie phase. Walk! If it is good enough for Dorian Yates, it should be good enough for you.

The Maximum Muscularity Training Phase

- Four weeks long
- Focus on one-to-three-rep power training
- Use a variety of exercises, not just the powerlifts
- Train with low volume, around 10 to 20 reps per exercise
- Work up to a heavy single, double, or triple, but do not max
- Repeat the wave once, twice, and three times in consecutive workouts
- Get enough rest between your sets to keep on lifting heavy poundages
- Don't strive to achieve pump
- Stagger the exercises for different muscle groups to minimize the fatigue
- Lift with dynamic tension, slow and tight
- Keep up your Loaded Passive Stretching (LPS)
- Do plenty of isometrics or/and posing throughout the day
- Employ the Power Breathing technique for your posing and isometrics
- Limit your fat-loss training to walking or similar low-intensity activities

WORKOUT 1: CHEST, BICEPS, TRICEPS

1. Wide-grip bench presses
2. Barbell curls
3. Incline (cambered bar) bench presses
4. One-arm dumbbell hammer curls
5. Close-grip bench press power rack lock-outs
6. EZ bar skull crushers
7. Concentration curls

1. Wide-grip bench presses

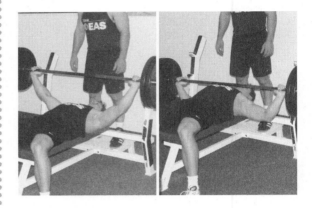

Do not forget to pause for a second on your chest without relaxing. Using the powerlifting style while bench pressing is a lot safer and more effective than the usual bodybuilding habit of bouncing.

2. Barbell curls

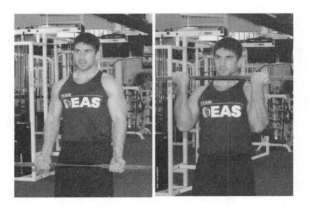

Squeeze the bar and flex your wrists in the beginning of each rep

3. Incline (cambered bar) bench presses

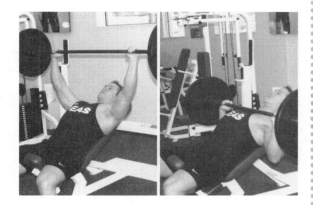

If you have a cambered or McDonald bar that enables you to lower the bar below your chest level, use it. If you don't, don't sweat it.

4. One-arm dumbbell hammer curls

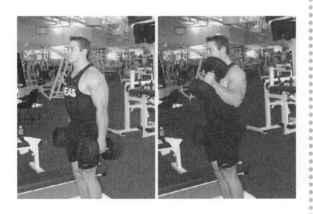

Curl the bell across your body. You are doing it right if you feel tension in your chest.

5. Close-grip bench press power rack lockouts

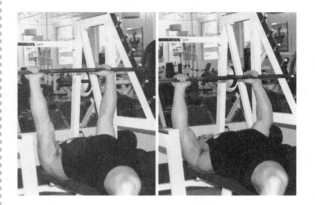

Press the weight two to four inches. Expect to gain horseshoe tris and a mean bench from this exercise.

6. EZ bar skull crushers

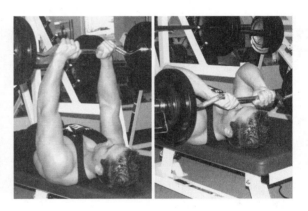

Keep the weight on the meaty parts of your palms below your little fingers. Be sure not to bounce, as it can be rough on your elbows.

7. Concentration curls

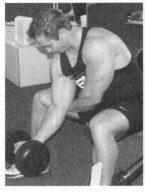

Crush the dumbbell to pulp, and flex your biceps!

WORKOUT 2: LEGS, CALVES, ABS

1. Power squats
2. Hip pull-throughs
3. Hack squats
4. Pause calf raises in the leg-press machine
5. Pause seated calf raises
6. Nautilus crunches
7. Dumbbell side bends

1. Power squats

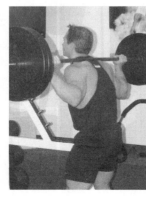

Use a slightly wider stance than usual, and carry the bar low on your back. Squat down

to at least the parallel position, when your thighs are parallel with the floor.

2. Hip pull-throughs

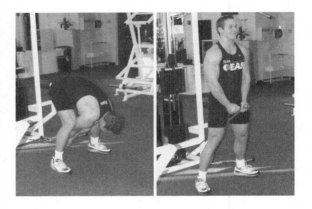

This goodie will annihilate your glutes and hamstrings! Facing away from a cable machine, stick your arms between your legs and grab a triceps pushdown rope attached to the low cable. Keeping your arms straight, take a step forward to load your muscles. Now squeeze your glutes and drive your hips forward while locking out your knees. If your knees stay bent, the drill will not work.

3. Hack squats

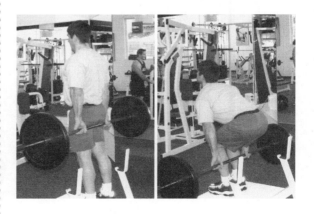

Use a barbell with this exercise. It is safer and more effective than a machine.

4. Pause calf raises in the leg-press machine

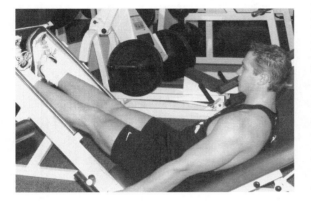

Pause for three seconds in the top position.

5. Pause seated calf raises

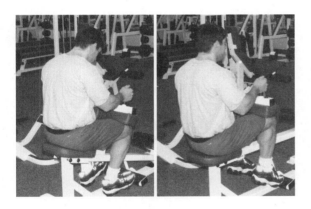

Use a three-second pause, like in the other calf drill.

6. Nautilus crunches

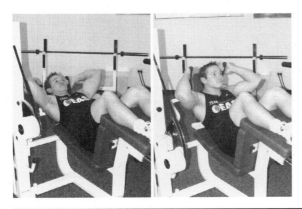

Another machine is fine, just make sure it carries enough plates.

7. Dumbbell side bends

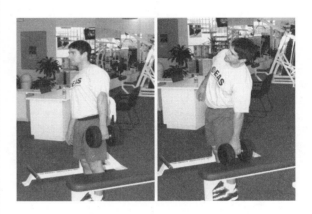

Do not be afraid to overbuild your love handles; low reps will just cut them up. Lift the dumbbell off a bench and do not twist!

WORKOUT 3: BACK, SHOULDERS

1. Deadlift lockouts
2. Wide-grip pull-ups
3. Clean and presses
4. One-arm barbell side presses
5. Cable lateral raises

1. Deadlift lockouts

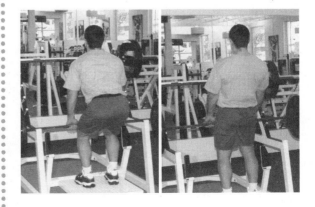

The power rack pull from slightly above the knees is one of the favorite back exercises of the legendary Frank Zane. Use straps or the powerlifting staggered grip, which is one palm facing the other. Keep your triceps flexed to protect your biceps tendons.

2. Wide-grip pull-ups

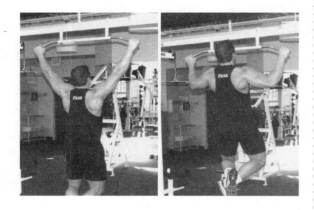

Use the pull-down or Gravitron machine if these are too tough for now.

3. Clean and presses

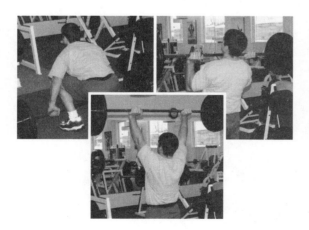

This is a double whammy for the back and shoulders! Keep your abs tight. Curve the bar around your head so you lock out in the press behind your neck in the top position.

4. One-arm barbell side presses

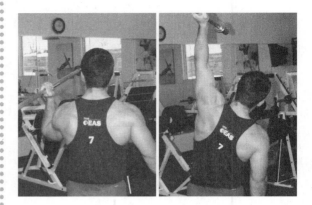

Grab a long bar and press it overhead while leaning to the side opposite the press. The long bar works your muscles with greater intensity than a dumbbell. The sideways lean enables you to use more weight, while discouraging you from leaning back, which is dangerous.

5. Cable lateral raises

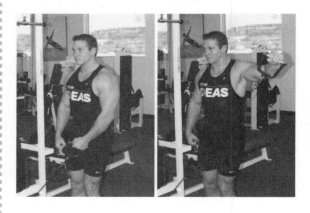

Lift your hand no higher than shoulder level for this exercise.

HARDGAINER TRAINING PHASE

There are many theories regarding not only who is a hardgainer but also how he or she should eat and train. I have my own beliefs regarding this subject, and I am pleased to say that the following training information should be a welcome surprise to the many athletes who feel they are doomed to a skinny body. So let's resume our discussion with Pavel Tsatsouline with respect to training on the Hardgainer Diet.

Vince Andrich: Pavel, many athletes who are on the skinny side seem to get bombarded with the notion that they are overtrained or not training with enough intensity. What is the European view on this subject?

Pavel Tsatsouline: The European view on training for the hardgainer surely bucks the trend! Whereas the consensus for the skinny guy or gal is heavy-duty-style training, or busting your butt with one or two high-rep sets to failure once in a blue moon, we have upped the volume, backed off the failure thing, cut the reps, and upped the weight! Our madness is well-grounded in science, though. A hardgainer's two major problems are weakness and nervousness. Wolff's Law states, "Function precedes the structure." In bodybuilding terms, until you can move some iron, do not expect your coat hanger shoulders to fill out with brawn. Therefore, a powerlifting-style program is the best choice for a hardgainer. Basic exercises, moderate reps, heavy weights, and lots of rest and food. The poundage is cycled and failure is avoided like the plague.

VA: Now we're talking. So how did your theories come about?

PT: Old timers understood that "training on the nerve," or what is known today as training to failure, is a one-way ticket to skinnyhood. Even more so for the already restless hardgainer. Modern endocrinologists know that overstimulating your stress hormones—be it by praying to make that last impossible rep or being chased by a tiger—is highly catabolic. All science aside, if "training to failure and beyond" is so hot, how come your bench has been stuck at 185 lbs since Arnold's first movie? The hardgainer MUST call it quits at least a rep before he or she hits failure! If it is good enough for Ed Coan, it is good enough for you.

VA: What about tempo or rep cadence on the Hardgainer Training Phase?

PT: We have added a wrinkle to the basic powerlifting workout: super slows and pause training. Not only will a different tempo spur new growth; forced slowness will discipline a hardgainer who may be inclined to bounce his or her weights. Steady tension is guaranteed to fire up muscle hypertrophy, especially in an impatient hardgainer whose muscles have not known anything but pump and cheat. A nervous hardgainer needs to overcome the desperate focus on the outcome and learn to enjoy the process of weight training. Exaggeratedly slow lifting will help him or her develop that mind set. It is not a bad idea to take up chi kung or yoga while other bodybuilders are doing their aerobics. Fat loss is not a priority for a hardgainer, but developing a calm demeanor for an optimal anabolic environment is.

VA: What about workout splits on the Hardgainer Training Phase?

PT: A hardgainer should not follow conventional bodybuilding splits. He or she should focus on the three big lifts rather than the body parts, and he or she needs more rest to facilitate the testosterone rebound. Here are my suggestions:

Monday: bench press (heavy), squat (heavy), deadlift (light)

Thursday: deadlift (heavy), bench press (light), squat (light)

What works for a lifter will work for a hardgainer who needs to zero in on strength before worrying about cuts, proportions, and other advanced considerations. You are not going to do any direct biceps, lat, or calf work. Just the big three, plus heavy abs to protect your back. Bear with it; it is worth it.

VA: What are the key points related to the Hardgainer Training Phase?

PT: Here it is—a hardgainer program that actually works!

The Hardgainer Training Phase

- Eight weeks long. A hardgainer does not need to rotate his or her exercises very frequently.
- Never train to failure or max
- Rest for three to five minutes between your sets
- Stick to basics such as squats, deadlifts, bench presses, and heavy ab work.

- Employ a split that focuses on the powerlifts rather than body parts
- Emphasize the four-to-seven-rep range. Try one to three reps if you use super slow or pause techniques
- Train with moderate volume, with 15 to 35 reps per powerlift and its assistance exercises
- Employ super slow reps and/or pause techniques
- Avoid stress, and sleep at least 9.5 hours a night
- Take up chi kung or yoga
- Do not do any cardio

WORKOUT 1: BENCH (HEAVY), SQUAT (HEAVY), DEADLIFT (LIGHT)

1. Bench presses
2. Parallel box squats
3. Spider lifts
   *Follow the 5x5 format for all these exercises

1. Bench presses

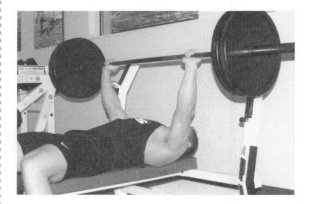

Perform 5x5 in the same manner that was described in the Muscularity Training Phase. Start by doing five crisp reps with a weight you think you could handle for seven repetitions or so. Rest for whole five minutes. Time your rest periods. Do five sets with the same weight. Next week add five to ten pounds and repeat the sequence. Do not get bummed out if you do not get all the fives. Just do as many reps as you can in good form, with no forced reps, and stay with the weight until you make it.

2. Parallel box squats

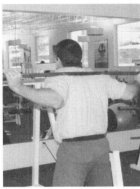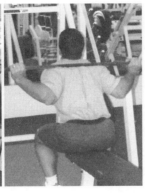

If your back can take it, the box squat is awesome for teaching you textbook technique and increasing your squatting power! Walk out of the squat rack and straddle a bench, which will place your hips at the level parallel to the floor or slightly below once you sit on it. Carefully sit back with a bar on your shoulders. Stick out your butt out as far as possible; you should feel tension in your hamstrings if you do it right. Gently sit on the bench, rock back an inch or so while staying tight, and rock forward to get up. Your knees should not move forward!

3. Spider lifts

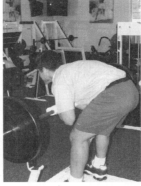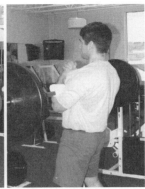

Also known as the Zercher lift, this wicked powerlifting favorite will strengthen your midsection and teach you to stay tight during your squats and pulls. Set a light bar in a power rack slightly above your knee level—you can pull from a deeper level once you get the technique down—and wrap it with a towel.

Bend forward, cross your forearms, and rest the bar in the crooks of your elbows. Inhale, pull up your butt as if you are trying to stop going to the bathroom—and slowly lift the bar until you are standing straight. Keep your abs tight, as if braced for a punch. To your surprise, you should find that you feel hardly anything in your back, but your stomach has to do all the work. This killer move will wean you off lifting belts in no time flat!

WORKOUT 2: DEADLIFT (HEAVY), BENCH PRESS (LIGHT), SQUAT (LIGHT)

1. Graduated deadlifts
2. Superslow bench presses
3. Pause squats
4. Spider squats

1. Graduated deadlifts

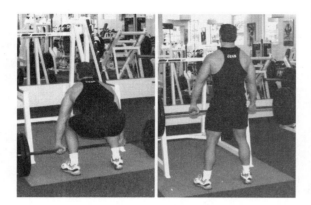

Old-time super deadlifter Bob Peoples used to deadlift a weight heavier than one he could pull from the floor while standing in a pit he had dug out in the back yard. Before every workout, he would add a little dirt in the hole, and before you know it he was pulling a full deadlift with a record weight! This graduated deadlift or "neurological carry-over" technique delivers easy progress, while accustoming you to a heavy weight. It also teaches the important skill of keeping full body tension, the safe and powerful alternative to isolation.

Work up to a set of five that feels reasonably heavy with a bar set in a power rack at your knee level. For example, 95x5, 135x5, 185x5, 225x5, 235x5, and 240x5. At your next workout, do the same, but a notch lower. Keep lowering the barbell until you pull off the floor. Then start from knee level again. If the holes in your power rack are far apart, you may stand on a plate to make smaller jumps. For example, for workout 1, use pin #5; for workout 2, use pin #5 standing on a plate; and for workout 3, use pin #4.

Do not use straps, but employ the stag- gered grip, which is one palm facing the other. Hang on a pull-up bar between sets to decompress your spine.

2. Superslow bench presses

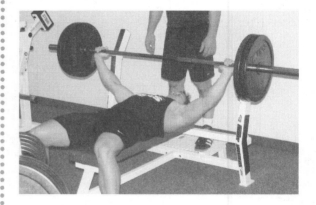

Have a friend with a stopwatch keep you honest by counting out the seconds. Take five seconds to lower the bar to your chest, and ten to lift it! Move very steady, without jerks. Do not hold your breath; breathe shallow. Do sets of one long rep and work up to a heavy single.

3. Pause squats

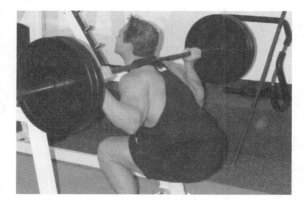

Once you have reached the "hole" or the legal squatting depth (which is just below parallel) stay there for three seconds—make your friend or better yet enemy count them out—before standing up. Work up to a heavy set in triples.

4. Spider squats

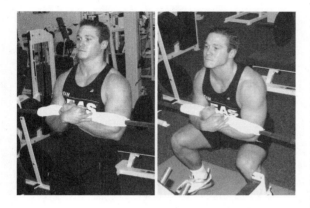

This is almost the same thing as the spider lift except you take a wider stance, sit deeper, and push your knees out as you stand up. Do not let your hips come up first.

"There are only two options regarding commitment. You're either IN or you're OUT. There's no such thing as life in-between."

-Pat Riley

Chapter

17

Miscellaneous Supplements

While the editing team and I were putting together this issue of the *Sports Supplement Review,* we realized there needed to be a place for compounds that can't be categorized as amino acids, herbs, or vitamin and minerals. We decided that a Miscellaneous Supplement Section for all the products that don't fit neatly into a category would be a useful section, since many of these compounds have oftentimes been marketed to bodybuilders and athletes. While these compounds didn't make our "Hot List," many of them can elicit positive effects to your training and exercise programs. And as with any collection of compounds, there is of course some that just do not work for any athletic purpose at all. In this chapter, I'll review some of these "miscellaneous supplements" which will round out your understanding of products that you may have heard of or you think might be of interest to you.

N-Acetyl Cysteine (NAC)

NAC is the acetylated form of cysteine, which provides for better absorption. It is an antioxidant used to increase glutathione content in cells. Glutathione a naturally produced antioxidant in the body, and is responsible for neutralizing many free radicals and toxic chemicals that are present in the environment or due to exercise-induced oxidative stress. Studies indicate its use as an antioxidant and chemopreventative based on its ability to prevent LDL oxidation,[1,2] one of the main causes of atherosclerosis (hardening of the arteries). With respect to athletes, training programs do have specific effects on tissue glutathione metabolism and may in fact impair performance and our ability to maintain lean mass. One study that I am aware of showed that supplemental NAC helped to minimize muscle-protein breakdown associated with intense exercise.[19] Since studies of glutathione-deficient animals unmistakably point toward the importance of having adequate tissue glutathione to protect against exercise-induced oxidative stress,[18] it is probably a good idea to add supplemental NAC to your training regimen if your budget allows it. Athletes usually take from 500 mg up to one gram of NAC during training periods, which require high workloads.

Glucosamine and Chondroitin

Here are two of my personal favorite supplements. If you have been training for several years, you can really appreciate the benefits. Both of these compounds have long been used to help treat mild to moderate cases of osteo arthritis and other joint damage.[3,4] Athletes commonly use these two to alleviate joint pain and to either ward off or assist in the rebuilding process of damaged cartilage. Personally, I take 1,500 mg of glucosamine (either sulfate or HCl) and 1,200 mg of chondroitin daily. Most anecdotal data indicates this stuff starts kicking in around six to eight weeks, so be sure to use it long enough to notice its effects. If you have joint problems or are just a hard-training athlete, I highly recommend this combination especially when combined with a natural anti-inflammatory like boswellia or curcumin.

Phosphatidylserine

Data on this compound indicates its potential as both an anti-cortisol agent and a memory enhancer. The problem with phosphatidylserine is research indicates you need to consume around 800 mg at a time for this compound to lower cortisol levels[5]—which is a little pricey if you add it up. But, if price isn't your primary concern, I highly recommend

you give this product a try, especially as a memory enhancer. Personally, I use phosphatidylserine at a lower dose, on the order of 100-300 mg daily, which seems to work extremely well for cognitive and memory enhancement.

Acetyl-L-Carnitine (ALC)

Anecdotally touted as an anti-catabolic agent, this compound's true benefit is much like phosphatidylserine, which is memory and cognitive enhancement. In a study on 481 human geriatric subjects, the administration of acetyl-L-carnitine produced significant improvement in cognitive function.[6] The authors of the study concluded that acetyl-L-carnitine may be an effective treatment for age-related decline in memory. If you are looking for components of a "brain cocktail," ALC may a good addition. However, I think you'll need about 1,000 mg per day to see any results, which could be cost prohibitive.

Canthaxanthin

Canthaxanthin is one of two major carotenoids in nature, the second being beta carotene. This unique carotenoid has been studied for its effects to combat the deleterious effects of vitiligo, which is a condition, which is defined by white patches of skin resulting from loss of pigment. Any part of the body may be affected and usually many milky-white patches similarly affect both sides of the body.[7] Athletes often use this compound to assist in the tanning process, however caution should be used because this compound is fat soluble. By the way, Dye-O-

Derm™, the skin bronzer used by body-builders to get an instant tan, is also typically used to treat vitiligo.

CLA

Used for many years now, CLA (conjugated linoleic acid) is a great non-essential fatty acid. Often used to help decrease bodyfat and act as a repartioning agent, CLA is a greatly overlooked supplement. CLA is the collective term for the different chemical variations of linoleic acid—one of the omega-6 essential fatty acids that cannot be made by the body but is necessary for thousands of biochemical reactions to take place. In the two decades since its discovery, CLA has been shown in numerous studies to be an anti-carcinogen in several animal models, to reduce the adverse catabolic effects induced by immune stimulation, to enhance growth, and even to improve blood lipid profiles. Of greater interest to exercise enthusiasts, however, is the extent of more recent clinical research studying CLA's effects on metabolism and body composition.

In the latest study conducted at Scandinavian Clinical Research based in Kjeller, Norway, 60 overweight people were randomly administered either a placebo or CLA for 12 weeks to determine the effects of different doses of CLA, from 1.7 grams to 6.8 grams, compared with a placebo. Study participants were given the option to undertake light exercise and moderate their food intake. Results showed that 3.4 grams of CLA daily provided CLA's beneficial effects on lowering bodyfat percentage. Participants who received 6.8 grams daily, the highest dose, compounded the results with a slight increase in lean muscle mass. According to study co-author Jan Wadstein, M.D., Ph.D., associate professor of medicine at Lund University in Sweden, "CLA may be a valuable weight-management supplement to any diet regime. Keeping lean body mass and speeding up fat loss are the keys to a successful weight loss program. We are encouraged by our findings and are involved in further research on CLA's ability to expedite fat loss and preserve muscle mass."

CO-Q 10

A coenzyme for numerous reactions in the body, CO-Q 10 is a powerful antioxidant especially in the cardiovascular system. It does not however appear to have any beneficial effects on lean mass or bodyfat loss. And it may be detrimental to performance.[20]

HCA (Hydroxy Citric Acid)

For years, bodybuilders have used HCA or garcinia cambogia (an herb standardized for HCA) to combat the fat-storing effects of carbohydrates. This compound is reported to have two modes of action. 1) To decrease appetite and 2) To inhibit the conversion of carbohydrates to fat by blocking the enzyme ATP citrate lyase. Unfortunately, several studies have been performed on this compound and have found no significant differences in groups.[8] My advice is that if you've had good luck with HCA in the past, go for it. If not, I would save this one for a rainy day when all else seems to have failed.

ZMA

Briefly touched on in the mineral section, the combination of zinc and magnesium aspartate has become commonplace in the supplement industry. The reason for this is that studies indicate the combination may help to increase levels of testosterone in the body possibly due to a common thread of zinc deficiency in today's diet. Originally developed by SNAC systems, numerous companies offer various formulations and tout this product as a non-hormonal anabolic. Due to today's hectic schedules and not-so-good diets, I highly recommend this combination taken before bed. (It may also help you sleep better.)

Chitosan

Chitosan is a fiber, naturally isolated from shellfish. It has a unique property that allows it to bind with fat. The concept is to take chitosan with your fatty meals, so the chitosan can bind the fat and the body cannot absorb the fat so it gets flushed out. While this works great in a beaker, whether or not this actually happens in the body is another story. The studies I have looked at on this compound indicate that it only helps to increase regularity—not fat loss.[8]

Ipriflavone

This isoflavone otherwise known as 7-ispopropoxy isoflavone has come into the spotlight recently for its beneficial effects on menopausal women and those trying to combat the deleterious effects of osteoporosis. In bodybuilding terms, this compound has been touted by some as an anabolic or anti-catabolic substance to help decrease muscle breakdown and increase protein synthesis. To my knowledge, the only data on this substance available relates to bone, not muscle growth.[9]

Glycerol

Glycerol is what most call the fatty acid backbone. Simply put, it is a three-carbon sugar of which fatty acids attach to form triacylglycerols. Glycerol is often used in bodybuilding to help increase the "cut" look and vascularity before a photo shoot or contest. Of further interest, endurance athletes, to prolong the onset of dehydration, often use glycerol to stay cooler from better hydration. You see, when glycerol is consumed, it drives water into plasma, thus super-hydrating your cells. Keep in mind that this strategy for super-hydration and endurance only works if you take in a specific amount of water with the glycerol. From what I have read, it appears that for every 45 grams of glycerol, an athlete will need to consume at least 36 ounces of water.

Pyruvate

Back in the day, this supplement was touted for its dramatic effects to improve fat loss. Problem was the studies that showed this used outrageous amounts of this compound, on the order of 20-30 grams per day, which simply is not attainable by the consumer. So does pyruvate in smaller doses work? In reviewing the literature the answer seems to be a resounding NO! My recommendation—if you comply with all the warning labels—is to get a good ephedrine and caffeine stack, watch your diet, and train like a madman. However, for individuals sensitive to the aforementioned compounds, products that substitute synephrine for ephedrine are your next best bet. Pyruvate, on the other hand, is probably not worth wasting your time or money on.

MCTs

MCT oils are a purely saturated, medium-length fatty acid. They do, however, posses the unique property that enables them to quickly be converted to energy or ketones in the body. MCT may be beneficial for high-endurance athletes and those on a ketogenic diet. For these purposes a couple of table-spoons daily should do the trick.

Colostrum

This is a subject that seems to be getting a lot of attention these days, but honestly I haven't been keeping a very close eye on the details. Because of this, I recently contacted a colleague of mine who has been spending a good amount of time studying the literature on this compound, Alan Shugarman, M.S., R.D., from Weider Nutrition, and I asked him to give me an update. Here are the highlights of our recent conversation.

Colostrum is the substance that is produced from the breast tissue of mammals immediately following the birth of offspring.

In the case of supplements, we are referring specifically to bovine colostrum.

In order to collect "prime" or "high-quality" colostrum, collection must stop after the first six hours, which usually means only one milking has occurred.

Once past the first six hours, the colostrum has begun to degrade significantly on its way to becoming the stuff we pour on our cereal, milk.

High-quality colostrum contains many interesting and nutritionally relevant compounds. For mammals, this first meal of colostrum provides many benefits to the immune system, gastrointestinal tract, and hormone levels, all of which result in tissue growth and proliferation, causing the offspring to thrive.

Colostrum is made up of both casein and whey proteins, with high concentrations of immunoglobulins (IgG, IgA, IgM, Secretory IgA), antimicrobial agents (lactoferrin and lactoperoxidases) and hormonal factors (IGF I & II), all of which provides a "breakfast of champions" for calves and infants alike.

The nutrition factors found in high-quality colostrum are what make it such a unique food, and they are also what have garnered the interest of scientists looking to improve the human physique and its performance. The question has now been raised as to whether or not a bovine colostrum, with all of its unique growth-promoting factors, has benefits to adult humans such that there will be an improvement in the physique or a measurable athletic parameter.

The bodybuilding claims for colostrum would lead you to believe that improved athletic performance and muscle growth are a forgone conclusion, however if you look closely, the overwhelming amount of research data is focused on immune function and gastrointestinal health. Recently there have been studies performed regarding the muscle-building, performance-enhancing, IGF-1 increasing effects of colostrum, and the literature is neither conclusive nor substantial in support of such claims, however it does indicate it may have some potential in performance athletics.[14] For athletes, it may come down to the simple fact that if you can stay healthier via a stronger immune system, you can train more consistently and recover more effectively. Personally, unless I suffered from repeated training distractions such as colds, flu, or upper respiratory infections, I would wait until more data comes out to spend any limited supplement dollars here.

Gugglesterones

Used for centuries, this compound greatly helps to reduce cholesterol levels. Numerous studies indicate the beneficial effects of this compound on cholesterol, HDL, and LDL levels.[11] Of primary interest to athletes though, this compound reportedly helps to increase thyroid function and output of T4 and thyroxin, which stimulate the metabolism and may provide benefit to those looking to lose fat. Guggulsterones supposedly do a good job of inhibiting the reduction of thyroid hormone when faced with a low-calorie regimen, thus keeping the fat-burning machinery operating at a peak levels. Personally, I haven't heard any rave reviews for gugglesterones and fat loss, but that doesn't mean that they couldn't be of value.

Quercetin

A naturally occurring bioflavonoid, this supplement is reported to act as an antioxidant, anti-allergenic, and many other benefits. Thought most of this data is relatively fresh, it appears that this may be a very effective antioxidant, especially in the cardiovascular system. Many athletes report a synergistic effect when they take about 50 mg of quercetin with caffeine and ephedra, possibly due to increasing intracellular cyclical AMP and a beneficial effect on beta-adrenoceptors.[21] This "synergism" with caffeine and ephedra is, however, purely hypothetical.

Methyl Sulfonyl Methane (MSM)

This supplement is basically a principal source of sulfur. It is reported to act as an antioxidant, mainly dealing with joints. The research I have pulled on this compound indicates very little if no effect on the repair of collaginous tissues.

Fructo Oligosaccharide (FOS)

This soluble fiber also serves as a probiotic, and is associated with increases in immune function and digestion. Other benefits of this compound include cholesterol and blood sugar support. Best of all, this is a great fiber additive to meal replacements, ready-to-drink shakes and protein supplements to naturally increase the sweetness of a product while minimizing sugars and artificial sweeteners.

Phosphates

Numerous products on the market today

utilize phosphates, particularly sodium phosphate, to help increase energy levels and boost metabolism. Phosphates serve as a building block to our body's energy source ATP. I know of many bodybuilders who use phosphate supplementation while on low-energy diets to enhance their resting metabolism. This strategy seems to work at least partly due to an influence of phosphates on peripheral metabolism of thyroid hormones[14]. If you want to give this strategy a try, I suggest using EAS' Myoplex Lite™ meal supplement formulas or Twinlab's Phos Fuel™ capsules.

Melatonin

Melatonin has been used for a number of years now as a sleep aid.[13] Most data indicates that a dose of 1-5 mg will do the trick. However, be sure not to consume melatonin for too long a period of time, as it may shut off the negative feedback loop the body normally relies on to operate its circadian rhythm (natural sleep patterns). Other than this, melatonin may also be an effective antioxidant and help mitigate jet lag, but data is somewhat controversial.[12] Several good companies sell melatonin including Schiff® and Enzymatic Therapy®.

Androstenedione**

The prohormone that really started it all... at least for bodybuilding. This is the most popular of the prohormones, but in reality it appears to be the least effective prohormone from a bodybuilding standpoint. Labeled as just "andro" by the press, the mass media glommed onto this supplement when it became a topic of discussion in Mark McGwire's race for the homerun record.

One metabolic "step" from DHEA, androstenedione is a direct precursor (and metabolite) of testosterone. In fact, androstenedione and testosterone convert back and forth to each other through the enzyme 17-beta hydroxysteroid dehydrogenase.

Since androstenedione is converted (albeit not that efficiently) into testosterone, it was not that much of a scientific stretch to believe that supplementation could increase testosterone production and the androgenic (male characteristic) properties that accompany testosterone.

Here is the biosynthesis pathway (conversion process) in the production of testosterone:

Cholesterol => Pregnenolone => DHEA => Androstenedione => Testosterone

As you can see from a conversion point of view, this compound looks pretty good. Indeed, armed with this biochemical information and studies cited in the original German patent that proclaimed that androstenedione supplementation can elicit an increase in free testosterone levels by as much as 237%, the rush to market "andro," by supplement manufacturers was a forgone conclusion.

But with all the hype, a study funded by EAS clearly showed that androstenedione doesn't increase testosterone at all, but it does increase estrogen levels, which is definitely not good for bodybuilding[16]. This study prompted EAS to stop marketing prohormones such as "andro," since the data did not support the products intended benefits.

CAUTION: Contains prohormones. See warning at end of this section.

4-Androstenediol**

Like androstenedione, 4-androstenediol (4AD) is metabolically converted to testosterone. But unlike androstenedione, this "diol" form converts more efficiently via a different enzyme, 3-beta hydroxysteroid dehydrogenase. This more efficient conversion has been demonstrated through research showing 4-androstenediol converting to testosterone a rate that is threefold to androstenedione. I first heard about this research through Patrick Arnold, whose company LPJ Research funded the study. According to Patrick, Tim Ziegenfuss, Ph.D., supervised the study, which was performed at Eastern Michigan University. What Dr. Ziegenfuss did was give 7 male subjects (average age: 28.1 years) samples of 100 mg androstenedione, 100 mg 4-androstenediol, and 100 mg placebo, all on separate days. The subjects had a portion of blood drawn before and after ingesting the samples. They continued to have blood drawn at intervals of 30, 60, and 90 minutes. Blood samples were then analyzed for total testosterone and free (unbound) testosterone. 4AD caused a 310% greater increase (relative to placebo) in total testosterone compared to androstendione, and a 256% greater increase in free testosterone! Apparently another advantage of 4AD is that because of its chemical structure it **cannot directly** aromatize (aromatization is

the biological process that converts androgens to estrogens) into estrone like androstendione. However, any time you increase testosterone, you run the risk of the additional levels of this hormone converting to estrogens.

In another conversation with Patrick Arnold regarding aromatization and prohormone supplements, he told me that an interesting fact that is becoming apparent is that the route of administration of prohormones makes a big difference on estrogen formation, even for 4-dione. Apparently, blood tests from sublingual and topical prohormones show much less proportional increases in estrogen than when doses are taken orally. This might be due to the fact that the liver is very rich in aromatase, and by avoiding the liver's first pass at these compounds, you may avoid a lot of aromatization. He also stated that it may also be true that adverse blood lipid changes are greatly increased with oral versus extra-oral administration. Although the latter information in particular is very "theoretical," preliminary data for 4AD appears to be the most logical supplemental **prohormone** to boost testosterone.

CAUTION: Contains prohormones. See warning at end of this section.

19-Nor-4-Androstenedione**

19-nor-4-androstenedione (norandrostenedione) is an androstenedione molecule minus the methyl group at the 19th position. Upon conversion by the liver, this subtle structural difference causes the conversion to yield nortestosterone, not testosterone. This conversion uses the 17-beta hydroxysteroid dehydrogenase enzyme—the same enzyme used to convert androstenedione to testosterone.

Nortestosterone has slightly different effects than does testosterone. Nortestosterone tends to be only mildly androgenic, but still possesses anabolic properties.

CAUTION: Contains prohormones. See warning at end of this section.

19-Nor-4-Androstenediol**

Like 4-Androstenediol, 19-nor-4-androstenediol (norandrostenediol) converts more efficiently than its dione counterpart. Still yielding nortestosterone after conversion, norandrostenediol converts through the enzyme 3-beta hydroxysteroid dehydrogenase—the same enzyme involved with androstenediol conversion.

CAUTION: Contains prohormones. See warning at end of this section.

5-Hydroxy-Tryptophan

5-Hydroxy-Tryptophan, a natural metabolite of tryptophan, is used to help regulate brain serotonin levels. Moderated brain serotonin can foster an improved mood, increased sense of well being, and improved sleep patterns.

5-HTP has been studied for its effects on anxiety, panic disorder, sleep abnormalities, and obesity. The obesity research suggests that 5-HTP triggers an increased feeling of satiety and a reduction in carbohydrate cravings. Personally, I just don't have any testimonials from athletes who have tried 5-HTP for weight loss.

7-Keto DHEA

7-Keto DHEA is a non-hormonal cousin to DHEA that has been recently marketed to bodybuilders as a possible fat-loss supplement. In fact, data does exist that supports supplemental 7-Keto DHEA combined with 60 minutes of cross-training (aerobic and anaerobic workouts) exercise can augment your fat-loss efforts.[17] While not nearly as effective as your typical caffeine and ephedra thermogenics, 7-Keto DHEA does not convert to sex hormones such as testosterone or estrogen, and may be a nice addition to a non-ephedra-based fat burner for those who want to avoid ephedra-containing products. Several good companies sell 7-Keto DHEA (which is licensed by Humanetics™ Corporation) such as Twinlab® and Enzymatic Therapy®.

DHEA

DHEA, shorthand for dehydroepiandrosterone (de-hydro-epi-andro-sterone), is often referred to as the "mother hormone." Produced in the adrenal glands and brain, it is metabolized into other hormones including the sex hormones, testosterone, and estrogens. DHEA levels rise during puberty, and reach their peak about the age of 30. After that point, the levels decline drastically in men and women. As people begin to age, their bodies produce less DHEA. These reduced levels have a direct effect on the aging process, including a decline in immune and memory functions. By age 80, people produce about 5% the amount of DHEA that they produced at age 30.

In clinical studies, DHEA has demonstrated

to be a beneficial nutritional substance for its ability to support and restore healthy adrenal function, improve energy, and enhance a sense of well being. On the contrary, it is important to note that these benefits occur only in somebody who is deficient in DHEA or has an imbalance in their DHEA/cortisol ratio. DHEA, a hormonal liaison, is two steps away from converting to testosterone and can be easily converted to estrogen. Personally, most of the anecdotal evidence that DHEA elevates testosterone levels consistently is in woman and older men who are DHEA-deficient. If you feel you are a candidate for DHEA or testosterone deficiency, it would be best to consult your physician before you self medicate. In any event, the availability of 4-androstenediol listed above is probably a better choice over supplemental use of DHEA to support testosterone production.

CAUTION: Contains prohormones. See warning at end of this section.

** **WARNING** Finally, for those athletes who are considering adding prohormones to your supplement program, please do not do so "blindly." These compounds, when designed properly, are very powerful, and can potentially alter your own hormonal environment. This **may not be appropriate** for many athletes, especially women. It appears that the best candidates for prohormones are aging males over 50 or those with hormones such as testosterone that have consistently hovered in the low ranges due to health-related problems or stress. In my view, the best approach to using these compounds is an educated one.

This means that you will need to do a little "homework" on the biological effects of any compound you want to use, and bring this information to your physician. Only after you do this can you have an intelligent conversation with any medical professional concerning your personal needs and if these products are right for you (not your training partner or friends). Your physician should then set up a full blood chemistry exam and analyze your current hormonal status. Once your physician looks at your hormonal status from a medical point of view, he or she can make a proper determination as to what products may benefit you. Remember that this is your endocrine system, and it is very delicate. The endocrine system you have has many built-in "feedback" systems that, if overloaded, may cause untoward health risks. I am sure you can get the most current prohormone data for your physician from the National Library of Medicine at www.nlm.nih.gov. If your physician is unfamiliar with these compounds, you can always ask him or her to seek advice from colleagues. Just remember that the blood chemistry work should be the basis from which your doctor makes how or her recommendations. Prohormones are also on several banned substance lists including the NCAA.

References:

1 Sen CK, Atalay M, Hanninen O. Exercise-induced oxidative stress: glutathione supplementation and deficiency.J Appl Physiol. 1994 Nov;77(5):2177-87.

2 Reid MB, Stokic DS, Koch SM, Khawli FA, Leis AA. N-acetylcysteine inhibits muscle fatigue in humans. J Clin Invest. 1994 Dec;94(6):2468-74.

3 Kreder HJ. Glucosamine and chondroitin were found to improve outcomes in patients with osteoarthritis. J Bone Joint Surg Am. 2000 Sep;82(9):1323. Deal CL, Moskowitz RW.

4 Nutraceuticals as therapeutic agents in osteoarthritis. The role of glucosamine, chondroitin sulfate, and collagen hydrolysate. Rheum Dis Clin North Am. 1999 May;25(2):379-95. Review

5 Monteleone P, Maj M, Beinat L, Natale M, Kemali D. Blunting by chronic phosphatidylserine administration of the stress-induced activation of the hypothalamo-pituitary-adrenal axis in healthy men. Eur J Clin Pharmacol. 1992;42(4):385-8.

6 Salvioli G, Neri M, L-acetylcarnitine treatment of mental decline in the elderly. Drugs Exp Clin Res 1994;20(4):169-76

7 Gupta AK, Haberman HF, Pawlowski D, Shulman G, Menon IA. Canthaxanthin. Int J Dermatol. 1985 Oct;24(8):528-32.

8 Luc JC van Loon, Johannes JM van Rooijen, Bas Niesen, Hans Verhagen, Wim HM Saris and Anton JM Wagenmakers "Effects of acute (-)-hydroxycitrate supplementation on substrate metabolismat rest and during exercise in humans." American Journal of Clinical Nutrition, Vol. 72, No. 6, 1445-1450, December 2000

9 Pittler MH, Abbot NC, Harkness EF, Ernst E Randomized, double-blind trial of chitosan for body weight reduction. Eur J Clin Nutr. 1999 May;53(5):379-81.

10 Arjmandi BH, Birnbaum RS, Juma S, Barengolts E, Kukreja SC. The synthetic phytoestrogen, ipriflavone, and estrogen prevent bone loss by different mechanisms. Calcif Tissue Int. 2000 Jan;66(1):61-5.

11 Singh RB, Niaz MA, Ghosh S. Hypolipidemic and antioxidant effects of Commiphora mukul as an adjunct to dietary therapy in patients with hypercholesterolemia. Cardiovasc Drugs Ther. 1994 Aug;8(4):659-64.

12 Edwards BJ, Atkinson G, Waterhouse J, Reilly T, Godfrey R, Budgett R. Use of melatonin in recovery from jet-lag following an eastward flight across 10 time-zones. Ergonomics. 2000 Oct;43(10):1501-13.

13 Monti JM, Cardinali DP. A critical assessment of the melatonin effect on sleep in humans. Biol Signals Recept. 2000 Nov-Dec;9(6):328-39.

14 Nazar K, et al, Phosphate supplementation prevents a decrease of triiodothyronine and increases resting metabolic rate during low energy diet. J Physiol Pharmacol 1996 Jun 47:2 373-83

15 Mero A, Miikkulainen H, Riski J, Pakkanen R, Aalto J, Takala T. Effects of bovine colostrum supplementation on serum IGF-I, IgG, hormone, and saliva IgA during training. J Appl Physiol. 1997 Oct;83(4):1144-51.

16 King DS, et al, Effect of oral androstenedione on serum testosterone and adaptations to resistance training in young men: a randomized controlled trial, JAMA 1999 Jun 2 281:21 2020-8

17 Colker CM, et. al, Double-Blind, Placebo-Controlled, Randomized Clinical Trial Evaluating the Effects of Exercise Plus 3-Acetyl-7-oxo-dehydroepiandrosterone on Body Composition and the Endocrine System in Overweight Adults, Journal of Exercise Physiology online, ISSN 1097-9751, Volume 2, Number 4, October 1999.

18 Sen CK, Packer L, Thiol homeostasis and supplements in physical exercise. Am J Clin Nutr 2000 Aug;72(2 Suppl):653S-69S

19 Kinscherf R, Hack V, Fischbach T, Friedmann B, Weiss C, Edler L, Bartsch P, Droge W. Low plasma glutamine in combination with high glutamate levels indicate risk for loss of body cell mass in healthy individuals: the effect of N-acetyl-cysteine. J Mol Med 1996 Jul;74(7):393-400

20 Malm C, Svensson M, Ekblom B, Sjodin B Effects of ubiquinone-10 supplementation and high intensity training on physical performance in humans. Acta Physiol Scand 1997 Nov;161(3):379-84

21 Revuelta MP, Hidalgo A, Cantabrana, Involvement of cAMP and beta-adrenoceptors in the relaxing effect elicited by flavonoids on rat uterine smooth muscle. B Auton Pharmacol 1999 Dec;19(6):353-8

"The best inspiration is not to outdo others, but to outdo ourselves."

-Anonymous

Chapter

18

Additional Help

As I mentioned earlier, we, as a society, are smack in the middle of the Information Age. And with that comes access to a plethora of information that is both helpful and confusing. To obtain supplemental information to that found in this book, my colleagues and I have drafted a solid list of reputable information pools. We feel that all of the references and information sources listed throughout this section will provide you with a broader knowledge base on nutrition, training, and supplements.

Governmental Organizations:

Food and Drug Administration (FDA):

As stated in Chapter 2, the FDA is responsible for the policing of the Dietary Supplement Industry. Above and beyond the information that we have already relayed to you on this organization, you can visit their web site for further reference information on dietary supplements. Some of the information they provide on this site is:

- Warning and Safety Information
- Adverse Event Reporting
- Announcements and Meetings
- General Information
- Industry Information and Regulation
- Q&A
- Other Sources for Information

This site also contains two additional sections that address the Latest Announcements and Frequently Requested Information.

The FDA's web site is as follows: www.fda.org

Contact Information:

E-mail: webmail@oc.fda.gov.
Phone: 1-888-INFO-FDA
Food and Drug Administration
HFI-40
Rockville, MD 20857 or
MedWatch Hotline: 1-800-FDA-1088 or www.fda.gov/medwatch/report/hcp.htm
(To report any serious harmful effect or illness from a dietary supplement.)

Federal Trade Commission (FTC):

We have briefly addressed the steps the FTC has implemented to make sure that the advertising efforts of the companies involved in selling dietary supplements are straightforward and not misleading in any way. We urge you to reference their web site if you have any questions or concerns about any of the advertisements that you see in the magazines or other media. Many of you might get lost due to the abundance of information contained on this site, so I will take you through the process of locating the information the FTC provides as guidelines for the supplement industry.

Once you are on the site, click on the "Business Guidance" section, and go to the link for Advertising Policy Statement and Guidance. In this section, you will find the Dietary Supplement section. Under the Dietary Supplement section you can access information on the following:

- Advertising Guide for the Industry
- Dietary Supplement Labels
- Statements concerning Dietary Supplements
- The FTC's website is as follows: www.ftc.gov

Contact Information:

Phone: toll-free 1-877-FTC-HELP (382-4357)
Federal Trade Commission
CRC-240
Washington, DC 20580

National Library of Medicine/PubMed:

PubMed is a search service that provides access to over 11 million citations in MEDLINE, PreMEDLINE, and other related databases, with links to several online journals. You can look up virtually any published study on this web site. It is sometimes difficult, but you should be able to locate most of the references that you see in magazine advertisements on this site. This site can be very technical, so you might not be able to understand all of the medical jargon, but it is a good way for you to investigate those references that often appear in many advertisements.

The web site is as follows: www.ncbi. nlm.nih.gov/PubMed/

Online Information

There is literally a ton of information existing in cyberspace for you to obtain additional knowledge on virtually any topic. The following represents a short list of some reputable and interesting web sites where you can access credible information.

www.eas.com & www.musclemedia.com

These web sites are home to EAS and *Muscle Media* in cyberspace. As you would expect, the EAS web site is full of the latest information regarding performance supplements, nutrition science, and a new section called the EAS Training Zone. The Training Zone is an interactive program that allows you to build sport-specific training routines, nutrition plans, and supplement regimens. This program contains some valuable "tools" that consist of calculators that will help determine your maximum heart rate, your target heart rate, your estimated one-rep max, your VO_2 max, calorie expenditure, and bodyfat percentage. I believe this program is a great tool for athletes who want to specialize in a particular sport or event. Here is how it works:

Log in and complete a form to indicate your gender, sport, playing level, position, and playing season.

Complete the strength test, which consists of three workouts during the course of one week. Keep track of repetitions and the weight used.

After you submit the weight and repetition information, your training program will be generated. Click on the name of the exercise to get a description and a visual example of the exercise and its correct form. The calendar on the right indicates the exercises for particular days. You may track your daily exercise program under "My Progress."

Another great feature is called Muscle Activation and Stretching, which consists of a biomechanically based stretching and exercise program designed specifically to improve each athlete's performance levels. Each exercise is specifically designed for strengthening a movement pattern that is consistent with the movements required for your sport or position. Stretching exercises are also incorporated into your personalized program.

The *Muscle Media* web site contains information on current and back issues for the magazine, plus full text versions of select articles. Additional links on this site contain information on training for "physique conscious" consumers and a full list of answers to frequently asked questions.

www.dragondoor.com

This simple site is home to Dragon Door Publications, and is a great place to get your hands on the videos and training materials of our training expert, Pavel Tsatsouline. Check out these favorites: "Beyond Crunches: Hard Science, Hard Abs" and "Power to the People: Russian Strength Training for Every American." Pavel has a very keen grasp of exercise science that challenges your mind and body.

Eastern philosophies mixed with Russian training techniques are the flavor of this very interesting site. Do yourself a favor and check it out.

www.webmd.com

WebMD is the comprehensive, one-stop source for health-based information. This site gives its users easy access to the latest health news and a vast library of medical articles. Up-to-the-minute medical news, message boards, a physician directory, and a fitness store are just a few of the valuable pieces that reside in this slice of the Internet.

www.charlespoliquin.net

This is the home of Charles Poliquin. Coach Poliquin is a very prolific trainer, writer, and lecturer, and has been involved in the physiology of sport for over 20 years. This site gives readers access to his popular training videos, pamphlets, and books. Point your mouse to this site to see what has made Charles Poliquin a household name in the strength and fitness arena.

www.paulchekseminars.com

The ever-prolific Paul Chek has created this excellent site. This site gives you access to all the Paul Chek goodies. Education materials, articles, videos, products—it's all there. Check out his "Squatology" video, which is probably the best squatting technique video ever produced.

I have met with Paul several times, and it is apparent that he has dedicated his life to the pursuit of excellence in sports sciences, holistic health, and neuromuscular therapy. His unfailing determination and persistent attention to the specific needs of an individual, a group, a team, or an institution invariably results in proof of his innate genius in succeeding where others fear to tread. He has a reputation for solving physiological riddles in a dynamic, medically authentic, and physically empowering way. Visit this site to get your hands on some of Paul Chek's wisdom.

www.musclemonthly.com

Don't let the head wound icon scare you. Muscle Monthly is a free bi-weekly publication that is dedicated to the science of bodybuilding. This online 'zine provides a forum for some of the top minds to discuss subjects like performance enhancement, training techniques, nutrition, dietary modifications, rehab training, and just about anything else you can think of that pertains to the health and fitness world.

www.myodynamics.com

Propelled by strength and conditioning specialist Charles Staley, Myo Dynamics provides a wealth of free information and resources on physical preparation strategies for athletes and fitness enthusiasts. This includes training for strength, flexibility, endurance, fat loss, speed, agility, and power, as well as injury prevention/management, performance nutrition, active recovery, and body composition issues.

www.bodytrends.com

This is an excellent resource for equipment reviews and overviews on all sorts of different training techniques—everything from aerobics to yoga.

www.thinkmuscle.com

Armed with some great up-and-coming writers, ThinkMuscle is bound to be one of the great destination sites of the industry. Their monthly newsletter is filled with interesting and cerebral work covering topics on nutrition and training, dieting, hormone therapies, and the like. Bookmark this one or sign up for their free newsletter.

www.glycemic.com

The Glycemic Research Institute (GRI) is a nonprofit organization based in Washington, DC that conducts ongoing research into foods and supplements and their glycemic responses.

The Glycemic Research Institute has compiled and recorded the Glycemic Index for hundreds of foods and food ingredients (I think the number is over 800). So if you're not quite sure about the glycemic response of a certain food, visit this valuable web site and get solid information that you can trust.

Software

Meticulous, type A, tedious. All these words typically pop into our minds when we think of following a regimented diet and exercise program. Well, you're in luck. Thanks to the never-ending advances in computing, following the zigs and zags of your daily routine are easier than ever to follow.

There are several software packages available to help you track your daily intake, but the most impressive package that I have used is called FitBody 4.0. The folks at Nutrology have been perfecting this software package over the last five years—and their efforts have paid off.

With a familiar, intuitive interface, the FitBody program gives you access to the largest food database, tracks daily intake of supplements, prepares shopping lists, compares food prices, interfaces with your personal trainer, and is accessible from a PDA or any computer via the Internet. And that's not the half of it. The product is around $75 with a $25 yearly membership.

Trainers and dietitians should take note: This software can be used to track all of your clients while providing them with frequent updates and feedback mechanisms. Check out www.nutrology.com for more information on this extremely helpful piece of bits and bytes.

Certifications and Other Industry Information

Whether you want to become a personal trainer, strength and conditioning coach, or just want to gain more knowledge, we have provided a list of the most widely recognized organizations. These entities are literal warehouses of information. Certifications are available on training and nutrition for everyone from the coach and personal trainer to the fitness enthusiast.

American Council on Exercise (ACE)

5820 Oberlin Dr., Suite 102
San Diego, CA 92121-3787
Phone: 858-535-8227 or 800-825-3636
Web site: www.acefitness.org

American College of Sports Medicine (ACSM)

401 W. Michigan St.
Indianapolis, IN 46202-3233
Phone: 317-637-9200
Web site: www.acsm.org

National Strength and Conditioning Association (NSCA)

(CSCS—Certified Strength and Conditioning Coach certification)
1640 L St., Suite G
Lincoln, NE 68508
Phone: 402-476-6669 or 888-746-2378
Web site: www.nsca-cc.org

International Sports Sciences Association (ISSA)

1035 Santa Barbara St.
Santa Barbara, CA 93101
Phone: 800-892-4772
Web site: www.fitnesseducation.com

Books

Some of the web sites that we mentioned above are great resources for some of the hottest and most authoritative books in the business. Here's a quick list of some of the books that you may want to pick up:

Science & Practice of Strength Training, by Vladimir M. Zatsiorsky

Considered a "must" in the library of serious trainers and coaches. This textbook-style work by Dr. Zatsiorsky (a biomechanics expert) delves into the strength-training techniques of the former Soviet Union. This is a science-based book and is not one you'll read while riding the exercise bike.

Power: A Scientific Approach, by Fred Hatfield

An oldie but goodie by Dr. Squat, Fred Hatfield. This is an easy-to-understand overview of how muscles generate and develop power, speed, and strength. This book covers all types of training with solid, well-researched information. This book has been read by some of the greatest in the sports of bodybuilding and powerlifting.

Bodybuilding: A Scientific Approach, by Fred Hatfield

Another Dr. Squat classic. This is the first book that gave me a clear understanding behind the basis of modifying reps, rep speed, and rest between sets, plus all facets of muscle loading. This book is a great place to get acquainted with key bodybuilding principles.

Neuromechanical Basis of Kinesiology, by Roger Enoka

This book is really heavy. If you're a student or graduate of the field of biomechanics, you are probably familiar with Dr. Enoka's work. Like its predecessor, this second edition integrates biomechanics and neurophysiology to provide a unique theoretical framework for the study of human movement. It's also an outstanding reference for sport biomechanists, exercise physiologists, motor behavior specialists, and physical therapists. Like I said, it's heavy.

Strength and Power in Sport, by P. V. Komi (Ed.)

This installment in the IOC and International Federation of Sports Medicine-sponsored series examines all the basic and applied aspects of strength and power in athletic performance. This book will appeal to sports scientists, sports medicine doctors, physical therapists, trainers, coaches, and allied health professionals.

Joint Structure and Function: A Comprehensive Analysis, by Pamela Levangie and Cynthia Norkin

This book is for those who are interested in studying the musculoskeletal system in detail—especially if you are a trainer or physical therapist. The authors present the basic principles needed to understand human kinesiology. This is a heavy textbook and is not for the uninitiated. Check it out in your local science library to glean the relevant nuggets for your particular interests.

The Ketogenic Diet: A Complete Guide for the Dieter and Practitioner, by Lyle McDonald

Lyle has been active in the bodybuilding community for quite some time, and his book is a complete resource for anyone who wants an objective, technical, unbiased look at all aspects of ketogenic/low-carbohydrate diets. Lyle objectively delves into the physiology of these popular diets—including potential negative effects—and gives specific recommendations on how to optimize such a diet.

Two modified ketogenic diets (which involve the insertion of carbohydrates to sustain exercise performance) are also discussed in detail, along with specific guidelines. Exercise is discussed in great detail, including background physiology, the effects of exercise on fat loss, exercise guidelines, and sample workouts. Although technical in its approach, The Ketogenic Diet contains a great deal of basic physiology information so that readers without a technical background will be able

to understand the topics discussed. This is not a magical diet book. The Ketogenic Diet tries to sort out the misconceptions of these diets and is quick to point out the pros and cons of undertaking a ketogenic diet.

Facilitated Stretching, by McAtee

Contains step-by-step information on how to perform 66 facilitated stretches covering all major muscles. This book is a healthy addition to the library of bodybuilders, athletes, coaches, and sports medicine professionals. It includes a section on using facilitated stretching along with soft tissue therapy for reducing pain and restoring range of motion lost due to injury.

The Poliquin Principles, by Charles Poliquin

Like I said in the web site section, Charles Poliquin is a household name when it comes to strength training. The Poliquin Principles has been a source of discussion over the years—both positive and negative. There are people who feel his expertise only resides over the strength training world and that he is "off the back" when it comes to bodybuilding. The nay-sayers and yeah-sayers may have valid points in some regards, but here's what I think: Poliquin knows strength training, and with that knowledge comes an understanding of how to better your weaker parts. I recommend this book because it is an informative and entertaining read that will provide you with immediately usable information. It is easy to understand and should be a welcome addition to both the beginner and advanced bodybuilder's library.

Nutrition Almanac, by Gayla J. Kirschmann

This is a great resource for putting together your meal plans on any of the nutrition phases outlined in this book. This book gives you a handy guide to the amount of proteins, carbohydrates, and fats for just about any food you can imagine. The first three editions of *Nutrition Almanac* sold more than 2.5 million copies. This fourth edition contains a detailed section on nutrients and describes each vitamin and mineral, how it is absorbed and stored, dosage and toxicity, deficiency effects and symptoms, and research findings. It also contains a chapter covering the traditional uses of 70 herbs. And, of course, the book has extensive nutritional information about common foods, showing how they help meet the RDA for each nutrient for both babies and adults.

Life Extension, by Durk Pearson and Sandy Shaw

This book is a classic or should I say THE classic when it comes to advanced supplementation. Although some of the theories have worn thin though the years (the book was written in 1984), this book definitely paved the way for a large number of supplement combinations that are on the market today. This book has had a tremendous impact on people who were looking to improve many aspects of their overall health and extend their life expectancy. Durk and Sandy have established this well-researched opus as one of the most influential works in the industry. If you can find a copy, do yourself a favor and read this groundbreaking, thought-provoking journey into the pursuit of living forever.

The New Encyclopedia of Modern Bodybuilding, by Arnold Schwarzenegger and Bill Dobbins

This follow-up to the highly popular original is a nice stroll down memory lane. This is a great addition to anybody's library. Most exercises are covered in meticulous detail. I will say that you won't discover anything entirely novel, but what you'll get is a great history lesson with some of the best pictures in the business.

Bill Pearl's Keys to the Inner Universe: World's Best Built Man, by Bill Pearl

The sheer number of exercises that are detailed in this book make it perfect for a beginning bodybuilder and a great reference tool. Bill Pearl's approach is a straightforward how-to and when you couple this book with "Getting Stronger," also by Pearl, you get a nice set of bodybuilding texts.

This book is a little older (I think the reprint was in 1992), and as with all books on training, you will rarely find authors that agree on all things.

Joe Weider's Ultimate Bodybuilding: The Master Blaster's Principles of Training and Nutrition, by Joe Weider and Bill Reynolds

Fans of the Weider Principles will undoubtedly love this trip into the past. This 1980's book had an impact—and continues to have an impact—on many beginners, and that's why I have listed it here.

The Strongest Shall Survive, by Bill Starr

This is a football-training book and step-by-step guide for the coach who wants to develop and administer an effective strength program. There are three sections: Weight Training, Nutrition, and a Related Topics section that covers rehab and drug use in athletes.

Serious Strength Training, by Tudor O. Bompa and Lorenzo Cornacchia

The exercise scientist who crafted the concept of periodization, Bompa and Cornacchia present a six-phase training program that maximizes both strength and muscle definition, and is teeming with illustrations. Don't let the name fool you, this is more of a bodybuilder's book than it is a powerlifter's book.

The experienced and knowledgeable Dr. Bompa provides very extensive and detailed programs for achieving bodybuilding goals through periodization. Dr. Bompa also briefly discusses the physiology of strength training—strength, muscle hypertrophy, and fat loss are all covered.

Unleashing the Wild Physique, by Vince Gironda

The Iron Guru Vince Gironda was a true bodybuilding pioneer. From his gym in the San Fernando Valley, Vince has produced some of the world's most aesthetically pleasing physiques, and was certainly way ahead of his time with regard to nutrition and exercise theory. Bodybuilders in the know still rely on many of the concepts that he pioneered in the late '60s and '70s—except now science has begun to understand why they work. Theories such as the cyclical high-protein/low-carbohydrate diet, protein every three hours, and pushing size gains through systematic volume training seemed radical when he introduced them over 30 years ago, and have elevated all of Gironda's work to that of "classics." His book, "Unleashing the Wild Physique" covers many of his early nutrition concepts and delves into specialized exercise selection for attaining "symmetry," which he aptly calls "cosmetic fitness."

Bullet-Proof Abs : 2nd Edition of Beyond Crunches, by Pavel Tsatsouline

Like Pavel's other books, this one is short, easy-to-read, and straight-to-the-point. This former Soviet Special Forces conditioning coach has compiled the most effective exercises for the abdominals, obliques, and other muscles of the torso. He compares crunches to communism and suggests that they should both be put in a pile of historical rubbish. In his own unique style, Pavel further explains why "going for the burn" with endless sets of ineffective crunches is a waste of time, and what works better.

Pavel demonstrates the effectiveness of the Pavelizer, a device that is an effective—but not a necessary—way to do Janda situps, the backbone of his program (see Chapter 16 for more information). Powerfully entertaining, this book will open your eyes to a more effective form of ab training

Writers

The following is a list of authors that you all should keep a lookout for. Whether you're reading a magazine or a book, you should be able to recognize the following names (above and beyond the books and authors I have already listed), as they produce some of the best information this industry has to offer.

Jeff Feliciano—Icon in the Bodybuilding Nutrition Field

Jim Wright, Ph.D.—All facets of Nutrition and Exercise Science

Bill Roberts—Ergogenic Aids

Brian Haycock MS—Performance Nutrition

Patrick Arnold—Nutrition/Prohormone Specialist

Elzi Volk—Performance Nutrition for Women

Jerry Brainum—Performance Nutrition and Exercise

Jeff Everson, Ph.D.—All Facets of Nutrition and Exercise Science

Chad Coy—Strongman Nutrition and Exercise Science

Disclaimers

We do not endorse in any way any of the additional sources of information listed in this chapter. Please verify the veracity of all information on your own before undertaking any reliance. The authors and any content are not under our control, and we are not responsible for the contents of any linked site or any link contained in a linked site, or any changes or updates to such sites. We are providing these links and information sources to you only as a convenience, and the inclusion of any source does not imply endorsement by us.

We hereby expressly disclaim any implied warranties imputed by the laws of any jurisdiction. We consider ourselves and intend to be subject to the jurisdiction only of the courts of the state of Colorado, USA.

If you don't agree with any of our disclaimers above, please do not read the material from any of the sources listed in this chapter.

Winning is not everything.
It's the only thing."

-Vince Lombardi

terms & jargon

Sports Supplement Review, 4th Issue

A number of complicated words and scientific terms and jargon are used in this book. If you refer to this section of the book often, you'll not only expand your functional vocabulary; you'll also be able to derive even more benefits from reading this book. Of course, some of you fitness wizards have already embraced these expressions as your second language, but for others, some of these terms may be new, and an explanation of what they mean will help—a lot!

Additive Effect: This term is often used in scientific jargon when researchers are measuring the effects of two or more substances in a single study. "Additive effect" simply means the combined effect of two or more factors equals the sum of their individual effects in isolation. For example, let's say creatine monohydrate supplementation, by itself, enhances lean body mass by six pounds over a four-week period, and HMB supplementation, by itself, increases lean body mass by two pounds over a four-week period. If their effects are additive, we would expect subjects to gain eight pounds in a four-week period of time when the two products are "stacked."

ADP (Adenosine Diphosphate): This is an important chemical involved in the energy production of a cell. ADP is formed when ATP is broken down within the mitochondria (the cells '"furnaces ") to provide energy for muscular contraction. In order to recreate ATP and replenish cellular energy stores, ADP must combine with creatine phosphate.

Aerobic: This means "requiring oxygen." Aerobic metabolism occurs during low-intensity, long-duration exercises, like jogging.

"All Natural": This is gym jargon for athletes who have not used anabolic steroids for a particular period of time. Usually, natural athletic competitions are open to athletes who have not used steroids or other banned ergogenic aids for a period of no less than 12 months.

Amino Acids: These are a group of nitrogen-containing, carbon-based organic compounds that serve as the building blocks from which protein (and muscle) is made.

Anabolic Steroids: These are synthetic versions of the male hormone testosterone, a hormone that controls many functions and occurs naturally in the body. Among these functions is the promotion of anabolism. Steroids mimic this naturally occurring event, but have the ability to do so at an accelerated rate. Through drastic metabolic changes in the body, anabolic steroids speed up protein synthesis, reduce catabolism, and increase muscle mass and strength in athletes who train with weights. Steroids not only exert their effects on muscles, but unfortunately affect many other parts of the body as well. This is why dramatic gains in muscularity are often accompanied by serious side effects.

Anabolic: This term refers to promoting anabolism, which is the actual building process of tissues, mainly muscle, in the body. This might occur through the body's own natural reactions to muscular work and proper nutrition or through the introduction of drugs. Anabolism occurs by taking substances from the blood that are essential for growth and repair and using them to stimulate reactions which produce tissue synthesis.

Anaerobic: This word means "without oxygen." Anaerobic metabolism in muscle tissue occurs during explosive activities like weightlifting or sprinting.

Anti-Catabolism: This is the halting of cellular breakdown in the body. A number of effective nutritional supplements such as glutamine, AKG, and HMB, as well as anabolic steroids, may help promote anti-catabolism. Slowing down the breakdown of protein tips the scales of protein metabolism in favor of new muscle growth.

Antioxidants: These are little dudes that minimize tissue oxidation and help control free radicals and their nasty effects.

Anti-Proteolysis: This is a specific type of anti-catabolism: namely, the slowing or halting of protein (muscle) breakdown in the body.

Assimilation: This is the process by which foods are absorbed and utilized by the body.

ATP (Adenosine Triphosphate): This is a high-energy molecule stored in muscle and other cells in the body. When a muscle cell needs energy to contract, ATP is broken-down to ADP to provide this energy. ATP can be thought of as the actual fuel that makes muscles move. Oxygen and glucose contribute to the formation of ATP. Many distributors of the supplements alleged to be performance-enhancing or ergogenic aids claim the supplements increase oxygen or glucose delivery to the cells. This would, inturn, increase the usable fuel in the form of ATP, hence increasing the duration of muscular endurance.

Attenuate: This verb means to weaken, diminish, or reduce. This term is often used to describe the diminishing effect of a drug or supplement over time. For example, if you take the herb ephedra every day, its positive effects "attenuate "—they diminish.

Bioavailability: This is the ease at which nutrients can be absorbed. (This differs from potency.)

Biochemical Reaction: This term refers to the broad range of chemical reactions which take place in all living organisms. Examples of biochemical reactions, which occur within the human body, are the conversion of blood sugar into energy, the effects of testosterone on muscle cell growth, and nerve impulse reaction, to name only a few of thousands.

Biological Value (BV): This is a measure of protein quality, assessed by how well a given food or food mixture supports nitrogen retention in humans.

Body Composition: This is the percentage of your body composed of fat versus fat-free mass. Very sensitive methods of body composition measurements, including DEXA, can actually subdivide body composition into more specific categories, such as percentage of bone mineral, body water, hair, etc.

Buffer: This is a substance that minimizes changes in hydrogen-ion concentration (pH). Buffers such as sodium phosphate are used by athletes to help reduce lactic-acid buildup during strenuous exercise.

Carbohydrates: These are organic compounds containing carbon, hydrogen, and oxygen. They're a very effective fuel source for the body. The different types of carbohydrates include starches, sugars, and fibers, and are classified into three groups—monosaccharides, disaccharides, and polysaccharides. Carbohydrates contain four calories per gram. Glucose—blood sugar—is a carbohydrate used by every cell in the body as fuel.

Catabolic: This is the opposite of anabolic. It means the breakdown of tissue. Catabolic states occur with disease, infection, injury, intense training, strict dieting, and immobilization. Catabolic conditions are not conducive to lean muscle mass gains; in fact, they typically cause a loss of lean muscle mass.

Catabolism: This refers to the breakdown or loss of muscle and other bodily tissues.

Chelating Agents: These are soluble organic compounds that can fit certain metallic ions into their molecular structure. These are often used to increase the absorption of minerals within the body. For example, amino acids are very commonly used as chelating agents for iron and other poorly absorbed minerals.

Cholesterol: This is a type of lipid which, although most widely known as a "bad fat" implicated in promoting heart disease and stroke, is a vital component in the production of many steroid hormones in the body. It also plays a vital role in proper cell-membrane structure and functioning. It's a substrate for bile-acid synthesis, as well as sex hormone and Vitamin D synthesis. There are different types of cholesterol: namely, HDL and LDL (HDL being the "good" form and LDL being the "bad" form).

Coenzyme: This is a substance which works with an enzyme to promote the enzyme's activity. Many coenzymes have vitamins as part of their structures.

Complete Proteins: These are proteins that contain all the essential amino acids in the right balance.

Cortisol: This is one of the primary catabolic hormones in the body. However, catabolism, or the breakdown of body tissue, is not the only function of cortisol. It is typically secreted in response to physical trauma or prolonged stress. Its functions include controlling inflammation, increasing muscular catabolism and glycolysis (the energy-yielding conversion of glucose to lactic acid), suppressing immune response, and maintaining normal vascular circulation and renal function, among others. Suppressing cortisol production at key times during the day may help bodybuilders avoid excess muscle breakdown. But, you need some cortisol to survive.

Creatine Phosphate (CP): This is an inorganic phosphate molecule that binds with ADP to form ATP. Supplementing with creatine monohydrate helps increase your muscle's CP reserves, which is good!

Cytokine: This term is used to describe a broad range of molecular protein messenger cells. The cytokine family of proteins includes interleukins (powerful anti-carcinogenic agents), interferons (which can be very effective against viral infection), IGF-1 (insulin-like growth factor-1), etc. Cytokines act directly on cells and are very potent agents which can elicit massive changes in cellular function.

Deficiency: This is a sub-optimal level of one or more nutrients that are essential for good health, most often seen with vitamins. Many natural supplements that are marketed to athletes as ergogenic aids are effective at enhancing performance if an individual is efficient in that nutrient. A deficiency can be caused by poor nutrition, increased bodily demands (especially from intense training), or both.

DEXA: This term stands for "dual-energy x-ray absorptiometry." DEXA is a form of total-body x-ray, which is used to determine body composition. This is probably the most accurate method available for measuring bodyfat, lean body mass, bone mineralization, and body water content. This is a very expensive procedure; however, it's an important part of quality clinical trials.

Dextrose: This is simply another name for glucose—the terms are interchangeable (see glucose).

Dipeptides: These are protein fragments made up of only two amino acids.

Disaccharide: This is a carbohydrate compound made up of two sugars. Examples are sucrose (table sugar), lactose (milk sugar), and maltose.

Diuretic: This term can describe any product that increases the amount of urine excreted by the body. Natural diuretics include black tea, coffee, guarana, and dandelion.

Drug: This is the generic name for any substance (except food) used for the prevention, diagnosis, and/or treatment of a disease, as well as the relief of symptoms. The word medicine is usually preferred to describe therapeutic drugs to distinguish them from the addictive drugs that are used illegally.

DSHEA: This is a term which stands for the "Dietary Supplement Health and Education Act of 1994. " This law was established by Congress and states that "dietary supplements" are defined as: vitamins, minerals, herbs, or other botanicals (except tobacco), amino acids, any "dietary substance for use by man to supplement the diet by increasing the total dietary intake," and "a concentration, metabolite, constituent, extract, or combination of any of the above-listed ingredients."

Efficacious: This means producing the desired effect—that "it works."

Electrolytes: These are substances that, in solution, are capable of conducting electricity. These charged particles are present throughout the body and are involved in many activities such as regulating the distribution of water inside and outside cells in the body. Examples include the bulk minerals, potassium, sodium, and chloride.

Empirical Data: This is information based on observation and experience, not scientific reasoning. Empirical data is often very accurate, although it is not accepted as scientifically sound; however, no area of science is devoid of a real-world/empirical component.

Endogenous: This term refers to things that occur naturally in the body. For example, the testosterone your body produces naturally is "endogenous."

Energy: This is the capacity to do work. The energy in food is chemical energy: It can be converted to mechanical, electrical, or heat energy. Energy is sometimes measured in "calories."

Enzyme: This is a protein molecule that acts as a "helper" in thousands of chemical reactions in the body, including: digestion of food, hormone production, muscle-cell repair—literally thousands and thousands of things.

Ergogenic: This word refers to something that can increase muscular work capacity. Natural supplements that can increase some aspect of athletic performance are said to be ergogenic or performance-enhancing aids.

Essential Fatty Acids (EFAs): These are fats that our bodies can't make, so we must obtain them through our diets. These fats (which include linoleic and linolenic acid) are very important to hormone production, as well as cellular synthesis and integrity. Good sources of these fats are flaxseed oil and safflower oil.

Exogenous: This term refers to things originating outside of the body. For example, if you took a DHEA pill, it would be an "exogenous " source of that hormone.

Fat: This is one of the macronutrients. Fat contains nine calories per gram; it has the most calories of all the macronutrients. Dietary fats may also be referred to as lipids or triglycerides. Fats serve a variety of functions in the body; they act as structural components for all cell membranes, as well as supply necessary chemical substrates for hormone production. There are two types of fat—saturated "bad " fat and unsaturated "good" fat.

Fat-Free Mass (FFM): This refers to all portions of body tissues not containing fat. These tissues include all skeletal bones and muscles, skin, organs, and body water, as well as hair, blood, and lymph. Fat-free mass is a term used frequently in the texts of clinical studies. Often, an increase in fat-free mass equals an increase in skeletal muscle.

Free Radicals: These are troublemakers. They're highly reactive molecules possessing unpaired electrons that are produced during metabolism of food and energy production, and are believed to contribute to the molecular damage and death of vital body cells. Free radicals may be a factor in aging or disease and may ultimately contribute to death. Antioxidants help neutralize free radicals.

Free-Form Amino Acids: These are structurally unlinked, individual amino acids.

Fructose: This is the main type of sugar found in fruit. It's sweeter than sucrose (table sugar) and has a low glycemic index (GI). In other words, eating fructose won't cause nearly as dramatic a release of insulin as glucose (dextrose). Eating a high-fructose diet may increase blood fats. Because of its low glycemic index and because it's metabolized mostly in the liver, fructose is often used as a sugar substitute for diabetics.

Full-Spectrum Amino Acids: These are supplements that contain a combination of all of the essential amino acids.

Glucagon: This is a hormone that is responsible for helping maintain proper blood sugar levels. When blood sugar levels go too low, glucagon activates glucose production in the liver, as well as regulates the release of glycogen from muscle cells. Eventually it may cause the catabolism of muscle cell proteins for glucose. This is considered a catabolic hormone.

Glucose Disposal Agent: A nutrient or complex of nutrients that has the ability to increase insulin sensitivity, thus allowing circulating blood glucose to be readily deposited in to target tissues.

Glucose: This is the simplest sugar molecule. It's also the main sugar found in blood, and is used as a basic fuel for the body. When you eat complex carbs, they're broken down by the body into glucose. Glucose is also found in various fruits, but not in as high concentrations as sucrose and fructose, two other sug-

ars. However, when you eat too much glucose, it's converted to fatty acids and triglycerides by the liver and adipose (fatty) tissue. Due to its quick absorption by the body, it's often used as an invigorating and strengthening agent in many medicinal formulations. It will cause your body to release a rapid and large amount of insulin to counteract the large influx of sugar.

Glycemic Index (GI): This is a measure of the extent to which a food raises the blood sugar (glucose) level as compared with white bread, which has a GI of 100. Glucose (dextrose) scores a 138, brown rice a 81, and fructose (fruit sugar) is all the way down at 31.

Glycemic Response Modifier: A nutrient or complex of nutrients that has the ability to slow down the absorption rate of ingested carbohydrates, thus lowering the glycemic index.

Glycogen: This is the principal storage form of carbohydrate energy (glucose), which is reserved in muscles and in the liver. When your muscles are full of glycogen, they look and feel full/pumped.

Growth Hormone (GH): This is a hormone that is naturally released by the pituitary gland; it is an anabolic hormone. GH promotes muscle growth and the breakdown of bodyfat for energy. GH levels are high in children and in teens, but diminish greatly after age 20. Some sports supplements are supposed to increase the amount of GH that is naturally released in the body, and therefore create an anabolic state and increase fat burning in the athlete. Unfortunately, most have little effect.

HDL: This stands for "high-density lipoprotein." It's one of the subcategories of cholesterol—typically thought of as the "good" cholesterol. HDL cholesterol is the form that is typically used to clear fats from the system, therefore not lending itself to the formation of crud in your arteries that can cause heart attacks. You may be able to raise your HDL cholesterol levels by ingesting quality unsaturated fats like flaxseed oil. Exercise has also been shown to increase HDL levels.

Hormones: These are substances in the body that are very important to bodybuilders. Two important hormone-producing organs are the pituitary gland and the testes. Hormones regulate various biological processes through their ability to activate or deactivate enzymes. Examples of this regulation are the effect of the testosterone hormone on the enzymatic activity relating to protein production of muscle cells. Other hormones, such as insulin and glucagon, control blood sugar levels and energy storage in the body. Hormones can be made of proteins

Hydrolysis: This is a chemical reaction where water reacts with a substance to change it to another substance or substances. For instance,

if you add sodium acetate to water, it hydrolyses into sodium ions and acetate ions.

Hypertrophy: This means to increase in size. Muscular hypertrophy is the increase in size of the muscle cells.

Hypoglycemia: This is low blood sugar/glucose levels, resulting in anxiety, fatigue, perspiration, delirium, and in severe cases, coma. Hypoglycemia occurs most commonly in diabetics, where it is due to either insulin overdose or inadequate intake of carbohydrates. Temporary hypoglycemia is common in athletes and can be overcome with the ingestion of carbohydrates.

Incomplete Proteins: These are proteins that lack or are low in one or more of the essential amino acids.

Insulin Amplifier: A nutrient or complex of nutrients that has the ability to increase the secretion of insulin.

Insulin: This is an anabolic hormone secreted by the pancreas that aids the body in maintaining proper blood sugar levels and promoting glycogen storage. Insulin secretion speeds the movement of nutrients through the bloodstream and into muscle for growth. When chronically elevated, as with a high-carbohydrate diet, insulin can cause you to gain fat. However, short bursts of insulin, caused by consuming high-glycemic carbs, may help enhance the uptake of nutrients like creatine and glutamine by muscle cells.

Jargon: This is specialized language concerned with a particular subject. For example, surfers say "hang ten " which refers to ... well ... I don't know what it refers to, but that's what jargon is—words and catch phrases certain "insiders" know but others don't.

Ketones: These are organic chemical compounds resulting from the breakdown of triglycerides. They are used as an energy source in the body during very-low-carbohydrate diets.

Lactic Acid: This is a molecule produced from glucose during anaerobic metabolism. When oxygen becomes available, lactic acid can be completely broken down to carbon dioxide and water. Lactic-acid buildup is a primary cause of muscle fatigue. Supplements that limit lactic-acid buildup may enhance athletic performance.

LDL: This stands for "low-density lipoprotein" and is a subcategory of cholesterol, typically thought of as the "bad" cholesterol. LDL is the type of cholesterol that circulates throughout the bloodstream and may cause heart disease. Levels of LDL cholesterol can be elevated by ingestion of saturated fats and a lack of exercise.

Lean Body Mass (LBM): This is another term that describes fat-free mass (see fat-free mass).

Limiting Factor: This is an element that prevents a process or reaction from taking place. For example, a lack of protein in the diet can be a "limiting factor" for muscle growth.

Linoleic Acid: This is an essential fatty acid and, more specifically, an omega-6 polyunsaturated fatty acid. Good sources of this fatty acid are safflower oil and soybean oil.

Linolenic Acid: This is an essential fatty acid and, more precisely, an omega-3 polyunsaturated fatty acid. It is found in high concentrations in flaxseed oil.

Lipid: This is simply another name for dietary fats or triglycerides.

Lipogenic: This means making bodyfat (literally translated "fat producing"). This is bad.

Lipolysis: This term refers to the chemical breakdown of bodyfat by enzymes that results in stored bodyfat being used as fuel by the body. This is good.

Lipolytic: This term is usually used to describe something with fat-burning effects. It literally means "to disintegrate fat."

Luteinizing Hormone (LH): This is a powerful hormone that, in men, stimulates the testes to make testosterone. (Yeah!) In gals, LH induces ovulation.

Macronutrients: These are the nutrients that we ingest in large (macro means "big") quantities on a regular basis. These include proteins, carbohydrates, fats, and, I guess, water. All of these macronutrients are necessary to sustain life.

Malabsorption: This big word means bad absorption of nutrients from the digestive tract. This can result in vitamin deficiencies, loss of weight, and poor health. Malabsorption can be caused by intestinal diseases or lack of digestive enzymes.

Meal-Replacement Powders (MRPs): These are a category of supplements which contain protein, carbohydrates, vitamins, minerals, and other key nutrients which are used to replace a regular-food meal for purposes of weight loss, weight gain, or increasing dietary nutrient intake. These supplements may also be referred to as "total-nutrition products," "engineered foods," or "superfoods." (Try finding that definition in Webster's!)

Metabolic Rate: This refers to the rate you convert energy stores into working energy in the body. In other words, it's how fast your "whole system" runs. The metabolic rate is controlled by a number of factors, including: muscle mass (the greater your muscle mass, the greater your metabolic rate), caloric intake, exercise, and use of stimulant or depressant chemicals.

Metabolism: This is a frequently used term that refers to the utilization of nutrients by the body for both anabolic and catabolic processes. It's the process by which substances come into the body and the rate at which they are utilized.

Micronutrients: These are dietary nutrients which we ingest in relatively small (micro means "small") amounts compared to macronutrients. Examples of micronutrients include vitamins and minerals. Many micronutrients are essential dietary nutrients that perform vital functions in the body. Micronutrients are typically ingested in gram quantities or less.

Minerals: These are naturally occurring, inorganic substances that are essential for human life and play a role in many vital metabolic processes.

Monosaccharide: This is a simple carbohydrate made up of one sugar molecule. Examples are glucose and fructose.

Muscle Fatigue: This is the failure of a muscle to continue to perform work, caused by muscle ATP depletion. Lactic-acid buildup also plays a role in muscle fatigue. Some natural supplements marketed to athletes have the ability to postpone muscle fatigue, thus increasing the work potential of the muscle—one of the most potent is creatine, which increases the availability of ATP, which is used for energy.

Myocyte: This means "muscle cell."

Natural: This term is often used to refer to foods or supplements that are not highly refined and which do not contain chemical fertilizers or artificial flavors and colors. The word natural has no legal definition in food supplementation though.

Net Protein Utilization (NPU): This is a method of evaluating protein quality by comparing the amount animals retained to the amount they ingested. Evaluation parameters are digestibility and essential amino acid content. (Don't worry, I don't understand it either.)

Neurotransmitter: This is a substance that is released at the end of one nerve cell when a nerve impulse arrives there. Neurotransmitters diffuse across the gap to the next nerve cell and alter the membrane of that cell in such a way that it becomes less or more likely to fire. Examples include adrenaline and serotonin. Adrenaline is responsible for the "fight-or-flight" response and is an excitatory neurotransmitter; serotonin is the opposite—it makes you sleepy.

Nitrogen Balance: This is when a person's daily intake of nitrogen from proteins equals the daily excretion of nitrogen: a negative nitrogen balance occurs when the excretion of nitrogen exceeds the daily intake and is often seen when muscle is being lost. A positive nitrogen balance is often associated with muscle growth.

Nitrogen: This is an element that distinguishes proteins from other substances and allows them to form various structural units in our bodies, including enzymes and muscle cells.

Nutrients: These are components of food that help nourish the body: that is, they provide energy or serve as "building materials." These nutrients include carbohydrates, fats, proteins, vitamins, minerals, water, etc. Omega-3 is the name of the first spacecraft that landed on the moon. (Nah, I'm just kidding—I was seeing if you were paying attention. This chapter is boring, huh?!) Omega-3 is actually a name for a certain fatty acid. The "3" designates where the first double-bond is located in the fatty acid carbon chain. Linolenic acid is an example of an omega-3 fatty acid. Omega-6 is another name for a fatty acid. Omega-6 refers to the first double-bond on a fatty acid chain which is located at the sixth carbon acid. Linoleic acid is an example of an omega-6 fatty acid.

Optimal Nutrition: This is a term you need to know. It means the best possible nutrition; distinct from merely adequate nutrition that is characterized by no overt deficiency. This term describes people free from marginal deficiencies, imbalances, and toxicities, and who are not at risk for such. All athletes making an effort to increase muscle growth naturally must try to achieve optimal nutrition. In many cases, this requires supplementation of protein, vitamins, and minerals, and possibly other conditionally essential nutrients such as glutamine and creatine.

Over-The-Counter (OTC): This refers to substances that do not require a prescription to be obtained legally.

Oxidation: This is the process of cellular decomposition and breakdown. Oxidation produces free radicals.

Oxygen Debt: What this means to me is "out of breath." It's a deficiency of oxygen in working muscles when performing exercise that is so demanding the cardiovascular system cannot deliver oxygen fast enough to the muscles to support aerobic metabolism. The debt must be repaid by rapid breathing after the activity slows down or stops. Oxygen debt leads to anaerobic metabolism, which leads to

lactic-acid buildup and muscle fatigue.

Peptide: This is a compound made up of two or more amino acids. Protein molecules are broken down into peptides in the gut and absorbed in that form.

Phytochemical: This term means "plant chemical." It's used to refer to a broad spectrum of bioactive plant compounds that are typically used in herbal preparations and a variety of other nutrition supplements.

Pineal Gland: This is an endocrine gland that functions mainly in the secretion of melatonin and a few other peptide hormones.

Placebo: This is a harmless, "inactive" substance which may be given in the place of an effective drug or substance, especially to "control groups" in clinical studies. In many cases, individuals using a placebo will react positively as though they were using an efficacious compound. Some of the positive effects performance athletes experience while using natural supplements are attributed to a "placebo effect." Basically, if you strongly believe a supplement will work, there is a chance that belief alone will produce positive results. It is even theorized that many of the positive effects athletes experience while using anabolic steroids can be attributed to a placebo effect. This is why it's important to do placebo-controlled scientific studies—to separate real effects from "placebo effects."

Polypeptides: These are proteins formed by the union of three or more (usually many) amino acids.

Polysaccharides: These are carbohydrates containing a large number of "sugar groups." Starch, glycogen, dextrin, and cellulose are examples.

Precursors: These are compounds from which another compound is formed. For example, the hormone androstenedione is a direct precursor to testosterone production in the body.

Prohormone: This term refers to a class of chemicals typically found inside various glands in the body, such as the pituitary and adrenal glands. These chemicals are the direct precursors to hormone production: e.g., pro-insulin is the direct precursor to insulin. DHEA and melatonin are also prohormones.

Prostaglandins: These are "hormone-like" chemicals produced in the body. Their structure is much like that of a fatty acid, and they exhibit a wide range of actions on things like blood pressure, water balance, immune system reactions, inflammation, etc. Their synthesis, in almost all tissues in the body, is partially controlled by fatty acid intake.

Protein Efficiency Ratio (PER): This is a measure of protein quality assessed by determining how well a given protein supports weight gain in laboratory animals: namely, rats. The PER is probably not the best rating system because it overestimates methionine needs due to the greater need for methionine in rats for hair production, but whatever.

Proteins: These are highly complex nitrogen-containing compounds found in all animal and vegetable tissues. They are made up of amino acids and are essential for growth and repair in the body. A gram of protein contains four calories. Those from animal sources are high in biological value since they contain the essential amino acids. Those from vegetable sources contain some but not all of the essential amino acids. Proteins are broken up by the body to produce amino acids that are used to build new proteins. Proteins are the building blocks of muscle, enzymes, and some hormones.

Pure: This term is often used to refer to supplements that are unadulterated—that have no other ingredient in them except that which is stated on the label.

Saturated Fats: These are bad fats. They are called "saturated" because they contain no open spots on their "carbon skeletons." Saturated fats include myristic acid, palmitic acid, stearic acid, arachidic acid, and lignoceric acid. These bad fats have been shown to raise cholesterol levels in the body. Sources of these fats include animal foods and hydrogenated vegetable oils, such as margarine. These fats serve no biological function in the body, other than to supply calories.

Stacking: This term refers to taking two or more compounds at once in an attempt to maximize results.

Sublingual: This means "beneath the tongue." Several supplements available to athletes are made to be taken in this manner. This occasionally results in better absorption. Some suggest hormonal preparations be taken sublingually to avoid the harsh environment of the gut.

Sucrose: This is most commonly known as table sugar. Industrially, sucrose is derived from sugar cane or sugar beets. When you eat it, the body breaks sucrose into fructose and glucose. Consequently, it has some of the properties of fructose and some of the properties of glucose. Eating it will elicit a rapid insulin response, but not as high as that caused by glucose.

Supplement: This is a term used to describe a preparation such as a pill, powder, or liquid that contains nutrients. A supplement is to be used as part of a person 's daily food intake to either supply adequate or supraphysiological levels of a nutrient.

Supraphysiological: This big word means amounts greater than normally found in the body. For example, a person consuming ten grams of creatine monohydrate per day will create supraphysiological levels of creatine in muscle cells.

Synergistic: This term refers to an action that is created when things "cooperate" with one another: that is, one supplement could enhance or multiply the effectiveness of another supplement. Many vitamins have been found to be synergistic. Creatine plus carbs is synergistic, as is caffeine plus ephedrine, in the right amounts.

Testes: This term refers to the male reproductive organs. The testes are where many of the hormones that regulate growth, such as testosterone, are produced.

Testosterone: This is the anabolic hormone produced primarily by the testes in men, which makes muscles grow. It literally separates the men from the boys.

Thermogenic: This term means heat producing or fat burning. Taking a thermogenic agent will speed up the metabolism, raise core body temperature, and accelerate calorie expenditure.

Triglyceride: This is the scientific name for a common dietary fat. The backbone of the molecule is a glycerol molecule that is connected to three fatty acid molecules. Triglycerides are also called fats or lipids.

Tripeptides: These are protein fragments that are three amino acids long.

Unsaturated Fats: These are "good" fats. They are called unsaturated because they have one or more open "carbon spots." Unsaturated fats can be divided into two categories: polyunsaturated fats and monounsaturated fats. Unsaturated fats have been shown to help reduce cholesterol and triglyceride levels in the blood. This category of fats includes the essential fatty acids linoleic and linolenic. The main sources of these fats are from plant foods, such as safflower, sunflower, and flaxseed oils.

Up-regulate: This term basically means "increase." For example, creatine monohydrate appears to have the ability to up-regulate or increase the muscle's ability to replenish energy stores.

Vitamins: These are organic compounds which are vital to life, indispensable to bodily function, and needed in minute amounts. They are non-caloric essential nutrients. Many of them function as coenzymes, supporting a multitude of biological functions.

VO$_2$ max: This is the maximum volume of oxygen an individual can consume per minute of work. It is often used to evaluate an athlete's cardiovascular efficiency and, thus, performance capacity.

ZMA Force + is a trademark of Weider Nutrition International

SyntheVol HP is a trademark of EAS

Xenadrine RFA-1 is a trademark of Cytodyne Technologies

Phosphagain 2 is a registered trademark of EAS

Methoxy-Pro is a trademark of Cytodyne Technologies

Diet Fuel is a registered trademark of Twinlab Inc.

Cell-Tech is a trademark of Muscletech Inc.

Ecdysten is a trademark of Thermo-Life International

Myoplex is a trademark of EAS

Promax is a trademark of SportPharma

BetaLean HP is a registered trademark of EAS

CytoPlex is a trademark of Cytodyne Technologies

Speed Stack is a trademark of Weider Nutrition International

Horny Goat Weed is a trademark of Bodyonics Ltd.

3-Andro Extreme** is a trademark of AST Research

BetaStatin-WPI2 is a trademark of BetaStatin

Secretagogue One is a trademark of MHP

Ultimate Orange is a trademark of Next Proteins Inc.

Male Fuel is a trademark of Twinlab Inc.

Methoxy-7 is a trademark of Biotest Laboratories LLC

Super Heavyweight Gainer is a trademark of Champion Nutrition Inc.

Ultra Pure Protein Shake is a trademark of Worldwide Sport Nutrition

Lean Body Bars is a trademark of Labrada Bodybuilding Nutrition

Thermo-Tek is a trademark of Iron-Tek

MX7 is a trademark of GEN

ATP Advantage Serum Creatine is a trademark of Muscle Marketing USA

Muscle Milk is a trademark of CytoSport

index

Sports Supplement Review, 4th Issue

Hard Body, 239
Hardgainer, 7, 23, 33, 61-71, 73, 77, 202, 207, 210, 247-248
Hatfield, 270
Haycock, Brian, 274
HCA, 208, 255
Hip pull-throughs, 244
Histidine, 129, 138-139
HMB, 38, 49-51, 53-57, 59, 68, 72, 83-84, 96, 134-135, 193, 277-278
Horny Goat Weed, 204-205, 207, 291
Hydration, 47, 81, 256
Hypertrophy, 174, 215-217, 229, 247, 273, 284

I

Immunity, 149, 155, 197
Incline alternate dumbbell curls, 222-223
Incline bench presses, 242-243
Indian ginseng, 173
Infection, 135, 159, 170, 279-280
Inflammation, 154, 169, 172, 280, 289
Inositol, 108
Insomnia, 132, 154
Insulin, 12, 18, 29-33, 45, 64-66, 80, 90, 94, 96, 102, 106-114, 120-121, 132, 137-138, 141-143, 148, 152, 159, 162-163, 174, 188, 196-197, 202, 283-284, 289-290
Interferons, 280
Interleukins, 280
International Sports Sciences Association (ISSA), 270
Inzitol, 108
Iodine, 160
Ipriflavone, 199, 256, 263
Iron, 140, 145, 159-163, 191-192, 214, 216-217, 247, 273, 279
Iron-Tek, 208, 291
Isoflavone, 94, 199, 208, 256
Isoleucine, 129, 133-134
Isoquinolone, 170

J

Janda sit-ups, 234-235
Joint, 27, 225, 254, 263, 271

K

Ketones, 45, 48, 257, 285
Kneeling cable crunches, 224-225
Komi, 143, 270

L

Labrada Bodybuilding Nutrition, 208, 291
Lactic acid, 238, 280, 285

Lactose, 89, 281
L-arginine, 32, 113-114, 143, 207
Lat pull-downs, 225-226
Lateral raises, 224-225, 235-236, 245-246
L-carnitine, 140
L-dihydroxyphenylalanine, 120
L-dopa, 120, 205-206
Lean Body Bars, 208, 291
Lean mass stimulator, 198
Leucine, 84, 129, 133-135, 143
Libido, 205
Linoleic acid, 255, 285, 288
Linolenic acid, 282, 285, 287
Lipid, 26, 97, 126, 159, 177, 255, 260, 280, 285
Lipogenic, 285
Lipoic acid, 107, 121, 140
Lipolytic, 82, 285
Liver, 29, 47, 111, 120, 123, 126, 132, 138, 140, 142, 147-148, 150-155, 159-162, 169-170, 172, 177, 260, 283
L-theanine, 118-119, 195
Luteinizing hormone (LH), 286
Lycopene, 155
Lysine, 129, 135, 139, 143

M

Ma Huang, 166, 174, 198, 200, 202, 208
Macronutrient, 24, 31, 41, 45, 64, 77
Magnesium, 18-19, 91, 97, 157-159, 163, 195, 200, 256
Male Fuel, 207, 291
Maltodextrin, 203
Manganese, 121, 161
Max Muscle, 186-187, 200
McAtee, 271
McDonald, Lyle, 48, 236, 243, 271
MCT, 257
Meal-replacement powders (MRPs), 35-37, 50-52, 54-55, 57, 68-71, 75, 77, 79, 81, 97, 133, 182, 193, 286
Medline, 266
Melatonin, 259, 263, 288-289
Menaquinones, 150
Mesomorph, 61
Methionine, 95, 129-131, 137, 139-140, 289
Methoxyisoflavone, 96-97, 104-106
Methoxy-Pro, 199, 208, 291
Methyl sulfoyl methane (MSM), 258
MET-Rx, 2, 183-184, 186-187
MHP, 180, 191, 206, 291
Micronutrient, 155
Military press, 236
Milk protein, 88, 124
Milk thistle, 170
Moderate-grip bench presses, 230-231
Molybdenum, 161

Vitiligo, 254-255
VO2 max, 102, 291

W

Water-soluble vitamins, 150
Weider, 2, 118, 180, 182, 184-185, 257, 273, 291, 300
Weider Nutrition International, 180, 184, 291
Weight gain, 203, 286, 289
Weight Gainer, 198, 207
Weight loss, 15, 44, 61, 82, 84, 109, 148, 151, 204, 255, 261, 286
Weighted crunches, 222, 224
Weightlifting, 80, 217, 239, 278
Whey protein, 78, 87-92, 94-96, 134, 188, 190, 199, 201
White willow bark, 198
Wide-grip bench presses, 225, 230-231, 242
Wide-grip pull-ups, 245-246
Worldwide Sport Nutrition, 183, 186, 207, 291
Wright, Jim, 274

X

X-Ray, 280
Xenadrine, 183, 197-198, 208, 291

Y

Yogurt, 130, 154, 156, 158
Yohimbe, 171-172, 207
Yohimbine, 172

Z

Zatsiorsky, Vladimir, 270
Zinc, 19, 97, 140, 152, 162-163, 195-196, 256
ZMA, 97, 158-159, 195-196, 256, 291
ZMA Force +, 195-196, 291
Zumpano, Michael, 190

"Strive for excellence, exceed yourself, love your friends, speak the truth, practice fidelity and honor your father and mother. These principles will help you master yourself, make you strong, give you hope and put you on the path to greatness."

-Joe Weider

Notes

Notes

Notes

Notes

Notes

Notes

Notes

Notes

Notes

Notes

Notes

Notes

Notes

Notes

Notes

Notes

Notes

Notes

Notes

Notes